Surgery

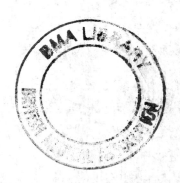

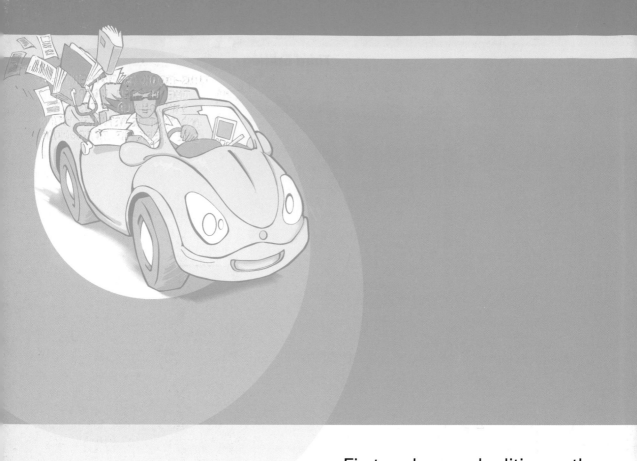

First and second edition authors:

Helen Sweetland

Kevin Conway

James Cook

CRASH COURSE

Third Edition

Surgery

Series editor:

Daniel Horton-Szar
BSc (Hons), MBBS (Hons), MRCGP
Northgate Medical Practice
Canterbury
Kent, UK

Faculty advisor:

Helen Sweetland
MB ChB, MD, FRCS(Ed)
Reader in Surgery
Department of Surgery
School of Medicine
Cardiff University and Honorary
Consultant Surgeon, Cardiff
and Vale NHS Trust, Cardiff, UK

Angeliki Kontoyannis
MB ChB, BSc, MRCS
Specialty Registrar in General Surgery
Queen Mary's Hospital
London, UK

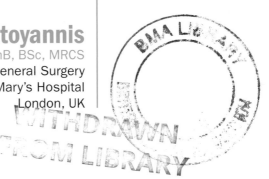

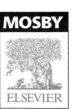

MOSBY

ELSEVIER

Edinburgh • London • New York • Oxford • Philadelphia • St Louis • Sydney • Toronto 2008

MOSBY
ELSEVIER

Commissioning Editor:	Alison Taylor
Development Editor:	Clive Hewat
Project Manager:	Alan Nicholson
Page design:	Sarah Russell
Icon illustrations:	Geo Parkin
Cover design:	Stewart Larking
Illustration management:	Bruce Hogarth

First edition 1999
Second edition 2004
Third edition 2008

ISBN: 978-0-7234-3475-7

British Library Cataloguing in Publication Data
A catalogue record for this book is available from the British Library

Library of Congress Cataloging in Publication Data
A catalog record for this book is available from the Library of Congress

Note
Knowledge and best practice in this field are constantly changing. As new research and experience broaden our knowledge, changes in practice, treatment and drug therapy may become necessary or appropriate. Readers are advised to check the most current information provided (i) on procedures featured or (ii) by the manufacturer of each product to be administered, to verify the recommended dose or formula, the method and duration of administration, and contraindications. It is the responsibility of the practitioner, relying on their own experience and knowledge of the patient, to make diagnoses, to determine dosages and the best treatment for each individual patient, and to take all appropriate safety precautions. To the fullest extent of the law, neither the Publisher nor the Authors assumes any liability for any injury and/or damage to persons or property arising out or related to any use of the material contained in this book.

The Publisher

Patients present to doctors with symptoms rather than diagnoses. Learning how to take a focused history and performing a thorough examination is the first hurdle in coming to a sensible differential diagnosis. An understanding of relevant investigations and the key features to look for can then help narrow the differential or indeed help formulate an accurate diagnosis. The format of the first part of this book follows the above progression, helping the student make sense of what often appears an impossible task. This third edition introduces communication tips. These are pieces of 'wisdom' that the authors have collected from their experience that we hope will help make the transition of diagnosis formation from textbook to reality. Another new addition is the highlighting of surgical emergencies. For a newly qualified doctor a cause for anxiety when assessing a patient is the inability to recognize what condition needs immediate treatment and what can safely wait for more senior review. We hope that this new feature will help junior doctors make confident diagnoses and initiate a treatment plan in often stressful circumstances.

We hope the book helps you make sense of a fascinating subject and helps you get the most out of your surgical attachments.

Angeliki Kontoyannis

Helen Sweetland

More than a decade has now passed since work began on the first editions of the *Crash Course* series, and over four years since the publication of the second editions. Medicine never stands still, and the work of keeping this series relevant for today's students is an ongoing process. These third editions build upon the success of the preceding books and incorporate a great deal of new and revised material, keeping the series up to date with the latest medical research and developments in pharmacology and current best practice.

As always, we listen to feedback from the thousands of students who use *Crash Course* and have made further improvements to the layout and structure of the books. Each chapter now starts with a set of learning objectives, and the self-assessment sections have been enhanced and brought up to date with modern exam formats. We have also worked to integrate material on communication skills and gems of clinical wisdom from practising doctors. This will not only add to the interest of the text but will reinforce the principles being described.

Despite fully revising the books, we hold fast to the principles on which we first developed the series: *Crash Course* will always bring you all the information you need to revise in compact, manageable volumes that integrate pathology and therapeutics with best clinical practice. The books still maintain the balance between clarity and conciseness, and providing sufficient depth for those aiming at distinction. The authors are junior doctors who have recent experience of the exams you are now facing, and the accuracy of the material is checked by senior clinicians and faculty members from across the UK.

I wish you all the best for your future careers!

Dr Dan Horton-Szar
Series Editor

Acknowledgements

For loan of slides for illustration:

From University Hospital of Wales, Cardiff: Mr MCA Purtis for Fig. 8.3 (endoscopic retrograde cholangiopancreatogram); Mr D Webster for Fig. 16.1a (intravenous urogram); Dr C Evans for Fig. 16.1b (intravenous urogram): Mr C Darby for Fig. 32.1 (arteriogram).

From the Royal Glamorgan Hospital: Dr E Hicks for Fig. 23.2 (mesenteric angiogram); Mr M H Lewis for Fig. 29.4 (chest radiograph) and Fig. 32.6 (computed tomogram).

From Kings Mill Centre for Health Care Services: Miss J Patterson for Fig. 21.5 (barium swallow).

Dedication

To all those who have encouraged and supported me in my surgical career.
HS

"The mediocre teacher tells, the good teacher explains, the superior teacher demonstrates, the great teacher inspires." (William Arthur Ward)

To my teachers at the University Hospital of Wales for inspiring me, and to my family for your constant love and support.
AK

Contents

Contents

Abscess   a circumscribed collection of pus appearing in acute or chronic localized infection and associated with tissue destruction and liquefactive necrosis.

Adenoma   a benign neoplasm of epithelial tissue.

Aneurysm   circumscribed dilation of an artery.

Ascites   accumulation of serous fluid in the peritoneal cavity (hydroperitoneum).

Carcinoma   malignant neoplasm derived from epithelial tissue.

Clubbing   a condition affecting the fingers and toes where proliferation of distal tissues, especially the nail beds, results in broadening of the extremities of the digits and makes the nails appear extremely curved and shiny.

Crigler–Najjar syndrome   rare autosomal recessive defect causing a complete absence of the enzyme that conjugates bilirubin. It is characterized by a familial non-haemolytic jaundice and, in its severe form, may cause brain damage and may be fatal.

Dentate line   the line between the simple columnar epithelium of the rectum and the stratified squamous epithelium of the anus. Above the dentate line the area is insensate.

Erythema nodosum   a dermatosis marked by the sudden formation of painful nodes on the extensor surfaces that are self-limiting but may recur. Associated with athralgia and fever.

Embolus   a plug composed of detached thrombus or vegetation or other foreign body occluding a vessel.

Endoscopy   examination of the inside of a hollow viscus by means of a special instrument called an endoscope. For example, oesophagoduodenoscopy, sigmoidoscopy, colonoscopy.

Gilbert syndrome   familial non-haemolytic jaundice caused by reduced activity of the enzyme that conjugates bilirubin. The

hyperbilirubinaemia is brought on at times of stress, exercise, fasting or illness.

Haematocrit   percentage of the volume of a blood sample occupied by cells.

Hernia   protrusion of a viscus or part of a viscus through the tissues normally containing it.

Incarcerated hernia   an irreducible hernia that is neither obstructed nor strangulated.

Intussusception   the infolding of one segment of the intestine into another.

Laparoscopy   examination of the contents of the peritoneum via a specialist instrument (the laparoscope) that is passed through the abdominal wall.

Laparotomy   an abdominal section, usually transabdominal, into the peritoneal cavity.

Liver flap (asterixis)   involuntary jerking movements, particularly in the hands in patients with metabolic encephalopathy. Most commonly seen in patients with impending hepatic coma. Best elicited by asking the patient to extend the arms, dorsiflex the wrists and spread the fingers.

Lymphadenopathy   any disease process that affects the lymph nodes.

Myxoedema   hypothyroidism characterized by a relatively hard oedema of the subcutaneous tissues.

Peritonitis   inflammation of the peritoneum.

Peutz–Neghers syndrome   autosomal dominant condition characterized by multiple hamartomatous polyps of the intestine, more commonly found in the jejunum. Also associated with melanin spots on the lips, buccal mucosa and fingers.

Polyp   a mass of tissue growing upward from the normal surface. They appear spheroidal or hemispheroidal, and can grow from either a relatively broad base or a slender stalk.

Pyoderma gangrenosum   a chronic non-infective eruption of spreading skin ulcers showing central healing and associated with dermal neutrophil infiltration. Seen in patients with ulcerative colitis.

Shifting dullness   a method of eliciting whether there is free fluid in the peritoneum. Fluid is dull to percussion, and if it is free in the peritoneum it will move as the patient shifts. So will the dull percussion note, thereby confirming the presence of ascites.

Spider nevus   a telangiectatic arteriole in the skin with radiating capillary branches. Characteristic of liver disease but also seen in pregnancy, and may also be normal.

Strangulated hernia   a hernia that is constricted so as to prevent the inflow of arterial blood or outflow of venous blood from the mesentery of the bowel.

Thrombosis   formation of a thrombus, clotting within a blood vessel.

Thyrotoxicosis   the state produced by the presence of elevated levels of endogenous or exogenous thyroid hormone.

THE PATIENT PRESENTS WITH

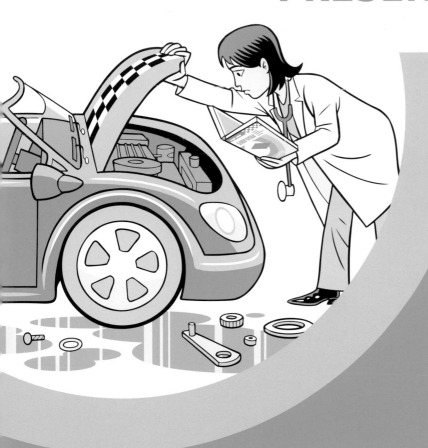

Acute abdominal pain

Learning objectives

You should be able to:

- List the important features relevant to the symptom of abdominal pain.
- Name the nine segments of the abdomen with the organs they contain.
- List a differential diagnosis for pain occuring in each segment.
- Understand the clinical signs of peritonitis.
- Understand the significance of arterial blood gases in the investigation of abdominal pain.
- List features to look for on an abdominal X-ray.

Acute abdominal pain is the most common presenting surgical problem. The main aim of the clinician seeing a patient who has acute abdominal pain is to recognize the serious causes from the not so serious. Many patients are admitted with abdominal pain, but only 20% will need any surgical intervention to speed their recovery. The rest may need investigations to find out the cause of the pain, but there is a group of patients who are labelled as having 'non-specific abdominal pain (NSAP)'.

DIFFERENTIAL DIAGNOSIS OF ACUTE ABDOMINAL PAIN

The differential diagnosis of acute abdominal pain is given in Fig. 1.1.

Medical conditions mimicking an acute abdomen include:

- Lower lobe pneumonia.
- Inferior myocardial infarction. MI
- Hypercalcaemia.
- Hyperglycaemia. DKA

HISTORY TO FOCUS ON THE DIFFERENTIAL DIAGNOSIS OF ACUTE ABDOMINAL PAIN

A full and thorough history of abdominal pain will be the most useful guide to establishing a likely cause.

Site

Many abdominal pains change site as the disease progresses (Fig. 1.2). For example, in acute appendicitis, the pain is initially in the central abdomen and then moves to the right iliac fossa. The abdominal viscera have no somatic sensation, so the pain is often felt initially in the dermatome (usually in the midline) that is related to the embryological development of the gut. It may be:

- Epigastric—indicating foregut pathology.
- Central—indicating midgut pathology.
- Suprapubic—indicating hindgut pathology.

This is often an important start to finding the cause.

As inflammation progresses the parietal peritoneum overlying the organ becomes inflamed and this causes a localized pain in that area.

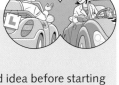

A patient may find annoyance in repeating his symptoms to more than one staff member, particularly if in pain. It is a good idea before starting to take the history to ensure analgesia has been given and to comment that you have read the notes of the nurse or the doctor that came before you but that it is useful to also hear the history from the patient directly.

3

Fig. 1.1 Differential diagnosis of acute abdominal pain

System involved (by location)	Pathology
right upper quadrant	gallbladder disease
epigastrium	peptic ulcer, peptic perforation and pancreatitis
left upper quadrant and umbilical	small bowel obstruction, early appendicitis, mesenteric ischaemia and gastroenteritis
right or left flank	ureteric colic, pyelonephritis and leaking abdominal aortic aneurysm
suprapubic	cystitis, acute urinary retention and pelvic appendicitis
right iliac fossa	appendicitis, carcinoma of caecum, mesenteric adenitis, Crohn's of the terminal ileum, ovarian cyst, salpingitis and ectopic pregnancy
left iliac fossa	diverticulitis, carcinoma of sigmoid colon, ulcerative colitis, constipation, ovarian cyst, salpingitis, ectopic pregnancy
groin	irreducible hernia

Onset

Is the pain sudden in onset or more insidious?

- An inflammatory condition tends to produce a gradual onset of pain that increases as the inflammatory reaction progresses.
- A ruptured viscus typically causes a sudden onset of pain.

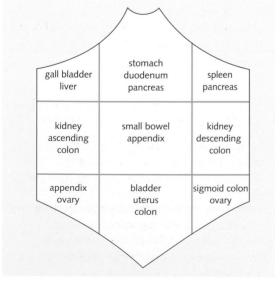

Fig. 1.2 Organs causing pain in the different abdominal regions.

- Smooth muscle colic, as in bowel obstruction or ureteric colic, has a rapid onset.
- Hormonally induced smooth muscle colic, such as biliary colic, has a slow onset because the hormone (in this case cholecystokinin) only gradually increases in concentration.

Severity

Ask the patient to grade the pain on a scale of 1 to 10.

Ureteric colic is said to be one of the worst pains. Many women say that it is worse than childbirth.

Nature

The pain may be described in many terms by the patient. The more common include:

- Aching—a dull pain that is often poorly localized.
- Burning—this may be used to describe symptoms of a peptic ulcer (see Chapter 2).
- Stabbing—a short sharp sudden pain, as may be felt with ureteric colic. (Note, however, that the pain associated with a stabbing is often described as burning in nature.)
- Gripping—often associated with smooth muscle spasm as seen in bowel obstruction. The patient will often describe it with a wringing motion of their hands (as if wringing out a cloth).

Progression

How has the pain changed over time?

- It may be constant—seen in peptic ulcer.
- It may be colicky—each sharp pain may last seconds (bowel), minutes (ureteric) or tens of minutes (gallbladder).
- It may change character completely. Appendicitis starts as a colicky central abdominal pain that then localizes to the right iliac fossa as a sharp pain that is worse on movement.

Radiation

The pain may seem to 'go through' to another part of the body. Often this can be quite revealing as to the cause of the pain. Good examples of radiation and causative organs are:

- Back—pancreas and other retroperitoneal structures.
- Shoulder tip—referred diaphragmatic pain (C4 dermatome—phrenic nerve).
- Scapula—gallbladder.
- Sacroiliac region—ovary.
- Loin to groin—typical description of ureteric colic.

Cessation

Does the pain go away slowly or quickly?

- Colicky pains, such as ureteric colic or bowel colic, usually have an abrupt ending.
- Inflammatory pain resolves slowly.
- Biliary colic also resolves slowly.

Exacerbating and relieving factors

Abdominal pathology causing inflammation of the peritoneum causes pain on movement so the patient lies still.

Ureteric colic is neither exacerbated nor relieved with movement and patients roll around trying to get comfortable.

Food may relieve or exacerbate the pain (see Chapter 2).

Associated symptoms

These may include:

- Nausea and vomiting (see Chapter 3).
- Constipation—there is a sudden onset of constipation, especially absolute constipation (where neither feces nor flatus is passed) associated with vomiting faeculent fluid and colicky abdominal pain in bowel obstruction. These same features in the absence of colicky pain may be seen in ileus.
- Anorexia—a sudden onset of loss of appetite can be associated with any intra-abdominal pathology and should always be investigated further.
- Rectal bleeding (see Chapter 6).
- Fever and malaise—associated with inflammatory and infective conditions.
- Menstrual irregularity—a gynaecological history should be obtained from all women who have abdominal pain as menstrual irregularity may indicate ectopic pregnancy or chronic salpingitis.

EXAMINATION OF PATIENTS WHO HAVE ACUTE ABDOMINAL PAIN

General appearance

The patient's general appearance can give clues to the underlying pathology:

- Sweating—may be associated with a pyrexia and is also seen in hypotension due to intra-abdominal bleeding or sequestration of fluid (as seen in peritonitis or pancreatitis).
- Pallor—the patient may be anaemic due to bleeding, but may also be 'peripherally shut down' in hypotensive states.
- Peritonitic facies—pale sweaty face with sunken eyes and a grey complexion.

Attitude in bed

The clinician's first impression of the patient in bed may suggest the diagnosis. The patient may be:

- Restless—typically seen in colic (either of the gastrointestinal tract or ureteric colic).
- Still—with movement exacerbating pain (as in peritonitis).
- Drawing up their knees—this position is often associated with severe peritonitis.
- Sitting forward—this lifts retroperitoneal structures away from the spine so may be a feature of the patient who has pancreatitis.

Temperature

The patient's temperature may be:

- Low—in states of shock such as severe peritonitis or pancreatitis.
- Increased—if the patient has infective pathology, especially pyelonephritis.

Vital signs

Check the following:

- Blood pressure—may be low in cases of haemorrhage or more frequently in peritonitis, where large volumes of fluid can be 'lost' in the gut and there is no intake of fluid.
- Pulse—a rapid pulse also reflects hypovolaemia (usually before a drop in blood pressure) and the pulse may be increased in infective conditions.
- Respiration—shallow, rapid breaths are associated with generalized peritonitis.

Abdominal examination

Inspection

The abdomen should be carefully inspected for:

- Scars—there may be adhesions inside the abdomen from previous surgery, causing obstruction. The previous operation may have been for malignant disease, making a diagnosis of recurrent tumour high on the list of differential diagnoses.
- Masses—large masses may be visible.
- Movement—the patient who has peritonitis breathes shallowly and minimizes abdominal movement.
- Pulsatility—epigastric pulsation can be seen in the normal resting abdomen, but very prominent pulsations may be associated with an aortic aneurysm.
- Hernias—check the hernial orifices because irreducible hernias can cause small bowel obstruction.

In an anxious patient reluctant to allow palpation due to perceived pain, it is sometimes helpful to start by auscultation and slowly increase the pressure applied. Convinced you have not hurt them, it is more likely they will allow you to proceed with the rest of the examination.

Palpation

Gentle palpation is very important for gaining useful information. Starting with deep palpation will cause the patient to voluntarily tense their abdominal muscles to avoid further discomfort. Examination may demonstrate masses and tenderness. Signs of peritoneal inflammation include:

- Rigid abdomen—the abdominal muscles are contracted involuntarily. This is a sign of generalized peritonitis.
- Guarding—a localized area of involuntary muscle spasm indicating underlying peritoneal irritation.
- Rebound tenderness—the release of pressure on the peritoneum causes irritation as the peritoneum rubs against the inflamed organ. This should not be done routinely as it causes unnecessary discomfort to the patient.

Percussion

Solid or fluid-filled masses and gas-filled structures can be distinguished by percussion. Percussion is also probably the best test for rebound tenderness and is far more gentle than pressing the hand into the abdomen and pulling away sharply.

Auscultation

Bowel sounds are absent in ileus due to peritonitis. Loud high-pitched bowel sounds are heard in bowel obstruction.

Rectal and vaginal examination

These form an essential part of the abdominal examination. Rectal examination may reveal:

- Tenderness associated with a pelvic appendicitis.
- Boggy swelling of a pelvic abscess.
- A large prostate gland causing urinary retention.
- Rectal carcinoma.

Vaginal examination may reveal:

- Vaginal discharge in salpingitis.
- Cervical tenderness or excitation in salpingitis or ectopic pregnancy.
- Retained tampon causing toxic shock.
- Pelvic mass such as ovarian cyst, pelvic abscess or fibroid uterus.

INVESTIGATION OF PATIENTS WHO HAVE ACUTE ABDOMINAL PAIN

An algorithm for the investigation and diagnosis of acute abdominal pain is given in Fig. 1.3.

Blood tests

Full blood count

Findings may include:

- Low haemoglobin in cases of gastrointestinal haemorrhage or chronic blood loss.
- High haemoglobin in patients who are severely dehydrated and have peritonitis or pancreatitis.
- Increased white cell count in infective conditions.

Urea and electrolytes

These are measured to assess renal function and reveal dehydration. The potassium level is important if anaesthesia is required for a surgical operation.

Liver function tests

Liver function may be deranged as a result of diseases of the gallbladder, biliary tree and liver (see Chapter 8).

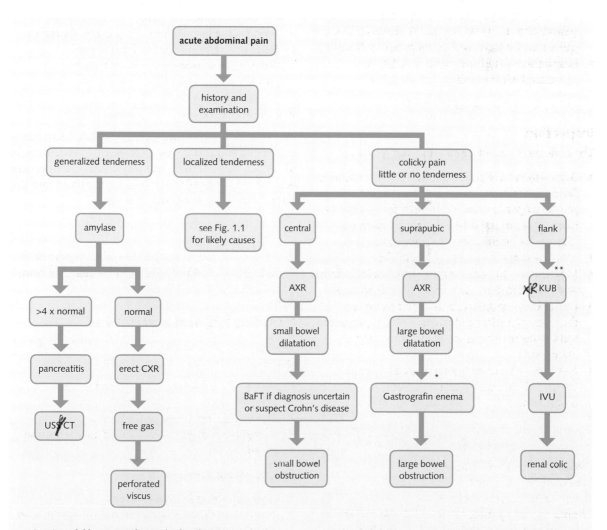

* water-soluble contrast if any risk of perforation
** plain AXR does not always include the bladder

Fig. 1.3 Investigation and diagnosis of acute abdominal pain. (AXR, abdominal radiography; BaFT, barium follow-through; CT, computed tomography; CXR, chest radiography; KUB, kidneys, ureter and bladder radiography; IVU, intravenous urography; USS, ultrasound scan.)

Amylase

This is primarily measured to diagnose pancreatitis. Typically, the amylase level will be increased more than four times the upper limit of normal (normal ranges vary between hospitals). Other conditions such as a perforated duodenal ulcer or ischaemic bowel may also give rise to a high amylase level, so the test should not be used alone to diagnose pancreatitis.

Arterial blood gases ABG.

Acidosis may be a sign of severe sepsis or ischaemic bowel.

Group and save

Blood should be sent for a group and save pending the full blood count and if there is any possibility that the patient will be having an operation.

Urine

Urine should be tested with a dipstick for the presence of:

- Red cells—seen in ureteric colic and infection.
- White cells—seen in infection.
- Nitrites—a breakdown product of urea seen in infection.

If any of these are present in the urine then urine should be sent for urgent microscopy and culture.

All premenopausal women who could be pregnant should have a pregnancy test.

Radiography

Chest radiography

An erect chest radiograph may show:

- Subphrenic free gas—indicating a perforation of a hollow viscus.
- Subphrenic bubbles—may be seen in cases of a subphrenic abscess.
- Lower lobe pneumonia—may cause hypochondrial pain.

Approximately 30% of acute perforations are not evident on an erect chest radiograph.

Abdominal radiography

Plain abdominal radiography may show:

- Dilated loops of bowel associated with an obstruction—large bowel obstruction with a competent ileocaecal valve is a closed loop obstruction and without backflow of colonic contents into the small bowel the caecum is at risk of perforation. Right iliac fossa pain and X-ray findings of a dilated caecum (>10 cm) with no small bowel dilatation is a ⚡SURGICAL EMERGENCY⚡ Dilated large and small bowel loops are seen in large bowel obstruction with an incompetent ileocaecal valve. In small bowel obstruction only small bowel loops are visible in the classic ladder pattern.
- Free gas—may be seen outside the lumen of the bowel.
- Thick-walled inflamed bowel—is suggested by the presence of a widened space between adjacent loops of bowel.
- Stones may be seen—over 90% of kidney stones and less than 10% of gallstones are visible on a plain film.
- Gas in the biliary tree—is seen following the passage of a gallstone into the bowel lumen, as in gallstone ileus or in cholangitis.

Ultrasonography

This may demonstrate:

- Gallstones, dilated common bile duct, thick-walled gallbladder.
- Inflamed pancreas or pseudocyst.
- Liver metastases or cysts.
- Aortic aneurysm.
- Large bladder.
- Dilated pelvicalyceal system in ureteric obstruction.
- Ovarian cysts.
- Hydro- or pyosalpinx.
- Abdominal or pelvic collections.
- Masses.

Computed tomography

Computed tomography (CT) is better for demonstrating retroperitoneal structures such as the pancreas. It also gives better definition of masses.

Both CT and ultrasound can be used in the urgent assessment of a sick patient where an abdominal pathology is thought to be the cause.

Limited barium or Gastrografin enema

If the plain abdominal film shows dilated large bowel and an empty rectum an unprepared single contrast barium enema can reveal any mechanical obstruction. If there is any possibility of perforation, a water-soluble contrast should be used. A CT scan can also be used in these situations.

Beware of a silent perforation in the elderly and patients on corticosteroids.

Laparotomy

Sometimes, despite investigations, the diagnosis is not clear. A sick patient showing signs of peritonism should undergo a laparotomy to treat the underlying cause, if they are fit enough for general anaesthesia. Occasionally, a diagnosis of pancreatitis is made at laparotomy, but this is preferable to missing a perforated duodenal ulcer or colon.

Laparoscopy

This is used increasingly to diagnose the cause of lower abdominal pain in women.

Learning objectives

You should be able to:

- Define the symptom of dyspepsia.
- List a differential diagnosis for dyspepsia.
- Understand how duodenal ulcers can be distinguished from gastric ulcers based on the effect of food.
- Understand the significance of the finding of Virchow's node on clinical examination.
- List the ways in which *Helicobacter pylori* is detected.

Dyspepsia describes an epigastric discomfort felt in many conditions. It is generally a symptom of upper gastrointestinal disease, but other conditions can produce similar symptoms. Patients may describe the symptoms of 'heartburn' (a retrosternal discomfort) or 'waterbrash' (the feeling of acid coming up into the throat).

DIFFERENTIAL DIAGNOSIS OF DYSPEPSIA

The differential diagnoses of dyspepsia are given in Fig. 2.1.

Site of pain

Dyspepsia is concerned with the upper gastrointestinal tract and therefore tends to produce epigastric pain, but there may be pain elsewhere:

- Retrosternal pain is suggestive of gastro-oesophageal reflux and oesophagitis.
- Gallbladder pain is typically referred to the tip of the right scapula (note that pain at the tip of the shoulder is usually diaphragmatic pain, i.e. C4).

Characteristics of pain

Most dyspepsia is described as a 'burning pain', but variations in the character of pain are typical of different conditions:

- The pain of oesophagitis may be described as a tightness or crushing pain and can be confused with myocardial pain of ischaemia.
- Biliary colic is a severe pain that usually starts after eating fatty food and slowly builds up to constant pain lasting over 20 minutes with slow relief of pain

Oesophageal pain may mimic angina. Both may be relieved by glyceryl trinitrate. Electrocardiogram and cardiac enzymes need to be checked. Aortic dissection and leaking thoracic aneurysm are rare differentials but ones not to be missed in the presence of sudden-onset retrosternal pain. Check for a widened mediastinum on chest X-ray and have a low threshold for requesting a contrast CT.

Exacerbating and relieving factors

Food can either exacerbate or relieve dyspepsia depending upon the condition:

- Gastric ulcer pain is typically made worse by food.
- Duodenal ulcer pain is relieved by food and exacerbated by starvation, so the patient may complain of pain at night.

Certain types of food may exacerbate the pain:

Fig. 2.1 Differential diagnosis of dyspepsia

System involved	Pathology
duodenum	duodenal ulcer
stomach	gastric ulcer and gastritis
stomach cancer	gastric cancer
oesophagus	hiatus hernia, oesophagitis and gastro-oesophageal reflux disease GORD
gallbladder	gallbladder disease
intestinal	irritable bowel syndrome

- Fatty food typically produces biliary colic.
- Hot and spicy foods exacerbate the pain of gastric and duodenal ulcers.
- Milky foods help relieve the symptoms of peptic ulcer, but their fat content can worsen the pain of biliary colic.

Gastro-oesophageal reflux and oesophagitis are made worse when the patient lies down or bends over. Obesity exacerbates the problem.

Associated symptoms

Symptoms associated with dyspepsia include:

- Vomiting and nausea.
- Jaundice.
- Bloating.
- Weight loss.

Nausea is common with most causes of dyspepsia. Vomiting may be associated with a gastric outflow obstruction associated with duodenal ulcer or gastric malignancy (see Chapter 3). Jaundice is associated with biliary disease (see Chapter 8). Marked weight loss is usually associated with gastric malignancy. Irritable bowel syndrome often presents with the triad of colicky pain, abdominal bloating and alternating bowel habit. It is a diagnosis of exclusion, but a triad of such symptoms may alert the clinician to the possibility of this diagnosis at an early stage.

Drugs

A careful drug history (including alcohol and cigarettes) should be obtained:

alcohol, smoking, NSAIDs, bisphos.

- Non-steroidal anti-inflammatory drugs and corticosteroids are well-known causes of peptic ulceration.
- Cigarette smoking is associated with an increased incidence of peptic ulcer.
- Excessive alcohol intake is a risk factor for peptic ulcer and can, in acute ingestion, cause severe gastritis.

EXAMINATION OF PATIENTS WHO HAVE DYSPEPSIA

General examination

General examination of the patient should look for:

- Signs of recent weight loss suggestive of malignancy.
- Anaemia in the absence of any overt blood loss—may indicate an occult source of blood loss such as a chronic ulcer or malignancy.
- Jaundice.
- Lymphadenopathy, especially in the left supraclavicular fossa (Virchow's node)—may indicate upper gastrointestinal malignancy.

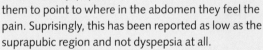

Before assuming that a patient's report of 'pain in the stomach' is dyspepsia, ask them to point to where in the abdomen they feel the pain. Suprisingly, this has been reported as low as the suprapubic region and not dyspepsia at all.

Unexplained anaemia requires examination of the upper gastrointestinal tract and colon with endoscopy or contrast studies.

Abdominal examination

The abdomen should be examined carefully, noting areas of tenderness and any palpable masses (see Chapter 1).

INVESTIGATION OF PATIENTS WHO HAVE DYSPEPSIA

An algorithm for the investigation and diagnosis of dyspepsia is given in Fig. 2.2.

Weight

The patient should be weighed and his or her weight compared with any previous recorded weight or the patient's estimate of his or her weight.

Blood tests

These may include:

- A full blood count—to check for anaemia (especially chronic iron deficiency).
- Urea and electrolytes—if there is a history of vomiting (see Chapter 3).
- Liver function tests—may show derangement in the presence of gallstone disease (see Chapter 8).

Barium meal

Contrast studies of the stomach can reveal many pathologies, including:

- Hiatus hernia.
- Reflux—can be demonstrated with fluoroscopic screening.
- Large gastric ulcers and tumours.
- Scarring of the duodenum.

Endoscopy

This is a better investigation for dyspepsia. With the exception of active reflux, all of the above may be seen at endoscopy and it is possible to visualize and biopsy the mucosal abnormalities to look for:

- Barrett's oesophagus.
- Malignant change in gastric ulcers.
- *Helicobacter pylori.*

Ultrasonography

This is primarily used for assessing the biliary tree, to look for gallstones, any dilatation of the biliary tree, and gallbladder wall thickness, indicating the presence or not of inflammation.

Manometry and pH monitoring

These are used to assess acid reflux. A probe is passed via the nose into the oesophagus and records pH. Regular falls in pH are associated with acid reflux.

achalasia .

Helicobacter pylori testing

Helicobacter pylori is an important factor in the pathogenesis of peptic ulcer and should be tested

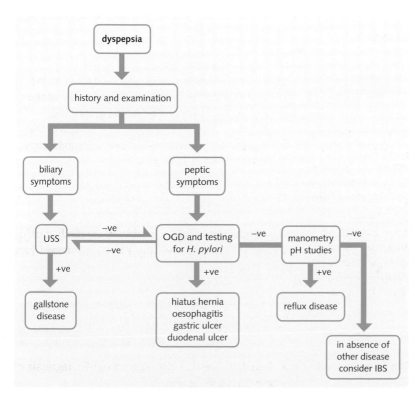

Fig. 2.2 Investigation and diagnosis of dyspepsia. (IBS, irritable bowel syndrome; OGD, oesophagogastroduodenoscopy; USS, ultrasound scan.)

for in cases of dyspepsia, especially if the patient has peptic ulcers. Testing can be by:

- Histology.
- Urease testing of biopsies—*Campylobacter*-like organism (CLO) test. Biopsies are placed in a small amount of medium containing urea. *Helicobacter* splits urea to form ammonia, which turns a pH indicator in the medium bright pink.

- Presence of antibodies in the blood (enzyme-linked immunosorbent assay).
- Breath ($[^{13}C]$urea) test—urea containing ^{13}C is fed to the patient and *Helicobacter* splits it, creating $^{13}CO_2$, which is detected in exhaled breath (overtaken now by the use of the CLO test).

Vomiting, haematemesis and melaena

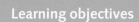

Learning objectives

You should be able to:

- Define the symptom of melaena.
- List a differential diagnosis for vomiting.
- Understand how the timing and nature of the vomitus indicates the site of the problem.
- Understand the significance of the succussion splash.
- List the features that distinguish small from large bowel obstruction on abdominal X-ray.

Vomiting is a common consequence of many non-specific illnesses. If the vomitus contains blood the vomiting is termed 'haematemesis'. The blood may be either bright red blood or partly digested blood, which often has the appearance of 'coffee grounds'.

Melaena is the passage of altered blood rectally and is characterized by offensive-smelling, black, tarry stool.

Both haematemesis and melaena represent bleeding from the upper gastrointestinal tract. Bleeding from the lower gastrointestinal tract is dealt with in Chapter 6.

DIFFERENTIAL DIAGNOSIS OF VOMITING, HAEMATEMESIS AND MELAENA

The differential diagnoses of vomiting, haematemesis and melaena are given in Fig. 3.1 and Fig. 3.2.

Pain

Pain often precedes the vomiting and its location can help to diagnose the primary cause (see Chapter 1). Colicky abdominal pain is associated with obstruction of a viscus. Dyspepsia is associated with several causes of haematemesis (see above and Chapter 2).

A patient's embarrassment about discussing the colour, odour, texture of vomitus or stool can be avoided if it is explained beforehand how important these details are to the establishment of the level of the problem along the gastrointestinal tract.

Timing of vomiting relative to food

Generally speaking, the higher the obstruction, the sooner the vomiting occurs after eating or drinking (Fig. 3.3):

- Oesophageal obstruction—immediate vomiting.
- Gastric outlet obstruction—within 30 minutes.
- Small bowel obstruction—after several hours.
- Large bowel obstruction—vomiting may not occur until very late in the disease process.

Content of the vomitus

The content of the vomitus gives some indication (in the case of obstruction) of the level involved:

- Food and acid—suggests gastric outflow obstruction due to pyloric ulcer, duodenal ulcer or carcinoma of the stomach.
- Bile—suggests obstruction distal to the sphincter of Oddi. It may also be seen with a gastritic-type

Fig. 3.1 Differential diagnosis for vomiting

System involved	Pathology
oesophagus, stomach, small and large bowel	mechanical obstruction
appendix, biliary ducts, fallopian tube and ureter	obstruction of other small muscle tubes
irritation of nerves of peritoneum or mesentry	gastritis, perforation of viscus, intra-abdominal sepsis and torted ovarian cyst
chemically induced central nervous systems disorders	drugs and alcohol vestibulitis and motion sickness

Fig. 3.2 Differential diagnosis for haematemesis and melaena

System involved	Pathology
duodenum	duodenal ulceration
stomach	gastric ulceration, gastritis, gastric cancer
oesophagus	oesophagitis, Mallory–Weiss tear, oesophageal malignancy and oesophageal varices

Fig. 3.3 Features of vomiting

Nature	Timing after eating	Associated symptoms	Site of problem
undigested food	immediately	dysphagia	oesophagus, gastric cardia
partially digested food	soon	epigastric pain	stomach, duodenum
bilious, partially digested food	few hours	abdominal distension, abdominal pain	small bowel
bilious, no food	any	dizziness	neurogenic, vestibular
haematemesis	any	–	oesophagus, stomach, duodenum

picture when there is some reflux of bile into the stomach.
- Faeculent—indicates distal small bowel obstruction. The liquid is contaminated with bacterial flora, hence the faeculent nature.
- Fresh blood—indicates a recent fairly brisk bleed.
- 'Coffee grounds' altered blood indicates a less recent or 'not so severe' bleed.

Symptoms of intestinal obstruction are:
- Colicky abdominal pain.
- Abdominal distension.
- Vomiting.
- Absolute constipation.

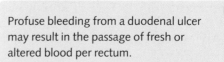
Profuse bleeding from a duodenal ulcer may result in the passage of fresh or altered blood per rectum.

Nausea and loss of appetite

An acute loss of appetite is always important and should be investigated further.

Drug history

Many drugs have side effects of nausea and vomiting. This may be due to a central action or a direct irritant action on the stomach mucosa.

Some drugs are associated with upper gastro-intestinal haemorrhage, for example:

- Non-steroidal anti-inflammatory drugs. *NSAID*
- Corticosteroids.   *warfarin   aspirin plavix*

Chronic cigarette smoking and alcohol intake predispose to peptic ulceration, which is the commonest cause of haematemesis.

EXAMINATION OF PATIENTS WHO HAVE VOMITING, HAEMATEMESIS AND MELAENA

General examination

Weight loss may indicate malignancy.

Long-standing gastric outflow problems due to benign disease can also lead to nutritional deficits.

Persistent vomiting results in dehydration, which may manifest as decreased skin turgor, tachycardia, hypotension and low urine output.

Marked blood loss from haematemesis and melaena cause anaemia and cardiovascular collapse.

Abdominal examination

For the most part, this is the same as for an acute abdomen (see Chapters 1 and 40), but several specific features may be associated with vomiting:

- Scars from previous abdominal operations.
- Large palpable gastric tumours.
- In neonates, the mass of a pyloric stenosis may be palpable as a small mass in the epigastrium on test feeding.
- An irreducible tender hernia may be the cause of intestinal obstruction.

Succussion splash

This is due to chronic gastric outflow obstruction and is produced because the distended stomach contains fluid and gas.

An algorithm for the investigation and diagnosis of vomiting, haematemesis and melaena is given in Fig. 3.4.

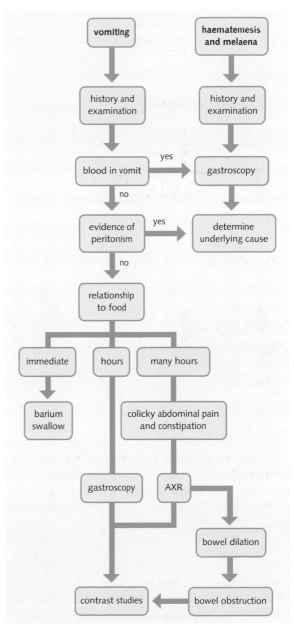

Fig. 3.4 Investigation and diagnosis of vomiting, haematemesis and melaena. (AXR, abdominal radiography.)

INVESTIGATION OF PATIENTS WHO HAVE VOMITING, HAEMATEMESIS AND MELAENA

Blood tests

Full blood count

This may show:

- Anaemia—associated with haematemesis or melaena or due to chronic blood loss.
- Increased white cell count—in infection.
- Increased haematocrit—in dehydration due to persistent vomiting.

Urea and electrolytes

Measurement of urea and electrolytes, including chloride, may show:

- Increased urea and creatinine levels—seen in dehydration.
- Increased urea but normal creatinine—seen in upper gastrointestinal haemorrhage.
- Low chloride—in gastric outflow obstruction due to loss of hydrochloric acid in the vomitus.

Increased serum urea (>10 times normal) but normal creatinine suggests an upper gastrointestinal bleed.

Blood gases

Loss of hydrochloric acid in gastric outflow obstruction leads to an alkalosis. This in turn can lead to a hypokalaemia as the kidneys try to preserve hydrogen ions (H^+) at the expense of potassium ions (K^+).

Using a urine dipstick to test vomit for blood is a waste of time. Vomitus invariably contains sufficient traces of haemoglobin to cause a positive reaction.

Radiography

Abdominal radiography

Dilated small or large bowel may be seen on plain abdominal radiography and the level of obstruction can be estimated. Some distinguishing features include:

- Small bowel is arranged more centrally and has bands that traverse its entire diameter (the plicae circulares or valvulae conniventes) (see Fig. 42.2).
- Large bowel lies more peripherally and has bands (haustra) that do not extend across its diameter.
- Both large and small bowel may be distended if there is large bowel obstruction with an incompetent ileocaecal valve.
- It is helpful to start at the rectum and try to follow the course of the bowel proximally. No air in the rectum is a sign of a proximal obstruction. *white*

Other features may also show up on a plain abdominal radiograph, such as:

- Ureteric stone—over 90% are visible on plain film.
- Gallstone—less than 10% are visible on plain film.

Chest radiography

An erect chest radiograph can show free gas under the diaphragm indicating a perforated viscus that may be causing peritonitis.

Contrast studies

Barium swallow can be used to investigate vomiting due to oesophageal or gastric pathology. In suspected small bowel obstruction, a barium follow-through can be performed to assess the level of obstruction. An unprepared barium enema can show obstructing lesions in the colon.

Oesophagogastroduodenoscopy (OGD)

This is used to diagnose causes of haematemesis and melaena, including:

- Oesophagitis.
- Gastritis.
- Gastric ulcer.
- Duodenal ulcer.
- Gastric and oesophageal cancer.

Change in bowel habit

4

Learning objectives

You should be able to:

- Define the symptom of tenesmus.
- List a differential diagnosis for altered bowel habit.
- List extra-abdominal signs of inflammatory diesease.
- Understand the importance of carcinoembryonic antigen.

Normal bowel habit is a very variable phenomenon. It can range from three to four times a day to just once a week. The frequency and consistency of stool is not the most important finding, but the change in habit is.

DIFFERENTIAL DIAGNOSIS OF A CHANGE IN BOWEL HABIT

The differential diagnoses of a change in bowel habit are given in Fig. 4.1.

HISTORY TO FOCUS ON THE DIFFERENTIAL DIAGNOSIS OF A CHANGE IN BOWEL HABIT

Constipation or diarrhoea

what is normal for you?

Ask the patient how the bowel habit has changed. Worsening diarrhoea may be associated with inflammatory bowel disease, infective colitis, villous adenoma or colonic carcinoma.

The patient may complain of increasing difficulty in opening the bowels, suggestive of:

- Stenosing carcinoma of the colon.
- Diverticular stricture.
- Obstructing lesions of the rectum or anal canal.
- Hypothyroidism.

Left-sided colonic tumours can cause constipation or diarrhoea.

Associated symptoms

Rectal blood or mucus

Blood may be passed in the stool with or without mucus (see Chapter 6):

- Fresh blood—usually due to anorectal disease, either a carcinoma, a polyp or perianal disease.
- Dark blood (partly altered blood)—usually from the sigmoid colon or above.
- Mixed with stool—usually above the sigmoid colon (stool is softer and has time to mix with the blood).
- Blood and mucus—inflammatory bowel disease or colorectal carcinoma.
- Mucus but no blood—typically seen in irritable bowel syndrome.

Villous adenomas cause diarrhoea as a result of excess mucus production and may cause hypokalaemia.

Pain

The patient may complain of abdominal pain associated with the change in bowel habit. This may be:

- Colicky central abdominal pain (small bowel colic). If associated with diarrhoea, the cause may be infective diarrhoea or Crohn's disease, but may be a feature of small bowel obstruction due to a caecal cancer.

Fig. 4.1 Differential diagnosis of a change in bowel habit

System involved	Pathology
colon	colonic carcinoma, ulcerative colitis, diverticular disease, benign colonic polyps
small and large bowel	Crohn's disease
anus	anal carcinoma
endocrine system	endocrine disorders

- Colicky lower abdominal pain is usually associated with colonic pathology. If associated with absolute constipation it can be a sign of complete bowel obstruction. Localized sharp pain in the left iliac fossa may be due to diverticulitis.

Weight loss

Weight loss may be seen with:

- Inflammatory bowel disease, especially Crohn's disease.
- Carcinoma of the colon.

Tenesmus

This describes the sensation of incomplete emptying of the rectum. It is usually associated with a rectal mass lesion, either carcinoma or a large polyp, but may also be seen in inflammatory bowel disease affecting the rectum.

Abdominal distension | bloating

This may be due to either obstruction of the bowel or ascites (see Chapter 5). Patients who have irritable bowel also describe bloating of the abdomen, usually following meals, which may be associated with colicky abdominal pain.

Family history

Certain conditions may be hereditary, for example:

- Familial polyposis coli—autosomal-dominant inheritance.
- Carcinoma of the bowel—increased risk if a relative under 50 years of age has carcinoma of the bowel.

- Inflammatory bowel disease—associated with certain major histocompatibility antigens (e.g. HLA-B27).

Social history

Foreign travel is common these days and acquired infective causes should be sought. Common infections include:

- Giardiasis.
- Shigellosis.
- Salmonellosis.
- *Campylobacter* infection.

Less common infections are:

- Amoebic dysentery.
- Typhoid.
- Cholera.

Drug history

Many drugs can cause constipation, including:

- Opioid analgesics.
- Anticholinergics.
- Antidiarrhoeal medication.

Others drugs cause diarrhoea, including:

- Laxatives.
- Antibiotics.

Antibiotics can also destroy the natural flora of the gut and so lead to pseudomembranous colitis.

EXAMINATION OF PATIENTS WHO HAVE A CHANGE IN BOWEL HABIT

General examination

Look for signs of:

- Anaemia—due to blood loss from the gastro-intestinal tract from a polyp or malignancy. Anaemia may also result from malabsorption of vitamin B_{12} due to terminal ileal disease in Crohn's disease.
- Weight loss.
- Jaundice—due to metastases from carcinoma of the bowel.
- Lymphadenopathy—especially Virchow's node in the left supraclavicular fossa associated with intra-abdominal malignancy.

- Clubbing—may be seen in inflammatory bowel disease.
- Skin changes—both pyoderma gangrenosum and erythema nodosum are associated with inflammatory bowel disease.

Mouth

Inspection of the mouth may reveal:

- Pigmentation of buccal mucosa—associated with Peutz–Jeghers syndrome.
- Aphthous ulcers—seen in Crohn's disease.

Abdominal examination

This is carried out as for the acute abdomen (see Chapters 1 and 4) paying particular attention to the presence of:

- Masses—associated with colonic carcinoma, diverticular disease or Crohn's disease.
- Tenderness—diverticulitis (see Chapter 1).

Rectal examination

This is essential for the patient who has a change of bowel habit. An algorithm for the investigation and diagnosis of patients who have a change in bowel habit is given in Fig. 4.2.

For intimate examinations such as the rectal examination, insist on the presence of a chaperone. Not only is this a requirement for medicolegal reasons, but also an assistant helps place the patient in the correct position, often a difficult task with elderly patients. A chaperone can also talk the patient through the examination while you are not able to talk face to face.

Fig. 4.2 Investigation and diagnosis of a change in bowel habit. (IBS, irritable bowel syndrome; TFTs, thyroid function tests.)

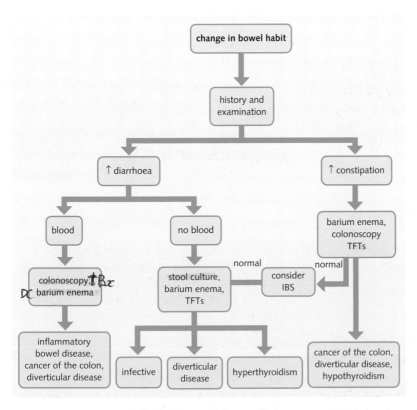

INVESTIGATION OF PATIENTS WHO HAVE A CHANGE IN BOWEL HABIT

Blood tests

Full blood count

A hypochromic microcytic anaemia is associated with a chronic blood loss (e.g. due to carcinoma of the bowel). A macrocytic picture may be associated with malabsorption due to terminal ileal Crohn's disease.

White cell count

This can be increased in infective diarrhoea, but may also be increased in active inflammatory bowel disease.

Thyroid function tests

The thyrotoxic patient may have diarrhoea, whereas the myxoedematous patient may be constipated.

C-reactive protein and erythrocyte sedimentation rate

These markers of acute inflammation are fairly non-specific, but are markedly increased in inflammatory bowel disease.

Carcinoembryonic antigen CEA

This tumour marker may be increased in carcinoma of the colon.

Stool culture and microscopy

Cultures should be sent to diagnose bacterial causes of diarrhoea.

Microscopy should be performed for parasitic infections.

Tests for *Clostridium difficile* toxin should be performed if pseudomembranous colitis is suspected.

Endoscopy

Rigid sigmoidoscopy

Sigmoidoscopy allows visualization of the rectum and lower sigmoid. Any neoplastic lesions or inflammatory changes in this area can be seen and biopsied.

Flexible sigmoidoscopy and colonoscopy

Flexible sigmoidoscopy allows visualization of the colon to the splenic flexure and colonoscopy can give views to the caccum. Biopsies can be taken or polyps removed.

Radiography

Double-contrast barium enema

This gives good imaging of the colonic mucosa. It may be useful for visualizing colon:

- Proximal to a stricture through which a colonoscope cannot pass.
- If colonoscopy is not possible because the colon is tortuous or there is severe diverticulosis.

A barium enema does not visualize the rectum well and therefore a rigid sigmoidoscopy must also be performed.

Abdominal mass and distension

5

Learning objectives

You should be able to:

- Give a differential of an abdominal mass.
- Recognize the symptoms and signs suggesting the presence of an abdominal aortic aneurysm.
- Understand the significance of shifting dullness.
- Understand the difference between an exudate and a transudate.

It is rare for a patient to present with an abdominal mass as a primary symptom. Usually, it is a discovery made after presentation with other symptoms. Abdominal swelling, however, is often noticed by the patient when clothes no longer fit.

DIFFERENTIAL DIAGNOSIS OF ABDOMINAL MASS OR DISTENSION

The differential diagnoses of an abdominal mass or distension are given in Fig. 5.1.

The classic causes of abdominal distension are the five Fs:

- Fat.
- Flatus.
- Feces. *Fuck - CA*
- Fluid. *ascites - liver disease, malig .*
- Fetus.

To these must be added the more specific diagnoses:

- Tumour.
- Inflammatory mass.
- Aneurysm. *AAA*
- Hernia.
- Organomegaly (including bladder).

fibroids, cysts .

HISTORY TO FOCUS ON THE DIFFERENTIAL DIAGNOSIS OF AN ABDOMINAL MASS OR DISTENSION

Timing

Take a careful history of how the swelling has developed:

- A rapid onset of generalized swelling is associated with a bowel obstruction.
- A rapid onset of painful lower abdominal swelling can occur if there is acute retention of urine.
- Other causes of swelling usually take much longer to increase in size or for the patient to become aware of it.

Associated symptoms

The clinician should be alerted to the possibility of bowel obstruction when a patient presents with the following symptoms, especially in the presence of colicky abdominal pain:

- Nausea.
- Vomiting.
- Absolute constipation (passing neither feces nor flatus).

Fig. 5.1 Differential diagnosis of abdominal mass or distension

System involved (by location)	Pathology
right upper quadrant pain	cancer of the hepatic flexure of the colon, distended gallbladder and hepatomegaly
epigastrium	gastric tumour, transverse colon tumour, hepatomegaly, pancreatic tumour, and pancreatic pseudocyst
left upper quadrant	cancers of the descending colon, splenomegaly and pancreatic pseudocyst
right or left flank	renal tumour and polycystic kidney
suprapubic	uterus (fibroids, uterine cancer, pregnancy), ovarian mass and distended bladder
right iliac fossa	distended caecum, caecal tumour, appendix mass, Crohn's disease and ovarian mass
left iliac fossa	sigmoid colon tumour, diverticular abscess or mass, ovarian mass and constipation

The classic history of ascites is a long history of increasing abdominal distension without much pain, but associated with swelling of the legs and shortness of breath. The shortness of breath is due to splinting of the diaphragm with increasing intra-abdominal pressure, but may also be associated with a pleural effusion, which is seen in about 60% of patients who have ascites.

Pain

If pain is associated with the swelling, its character and site can give some clue about the nature of the swelling:

- Back pain is associated with retroperitoneal structures such as the pancreas and aorta. Pancreatic malignancy can present as an unrelenting back pain due to direct invasion by the tumour.
- Aortic aneurysms can present with different types of pain. Dull pain in the back is associated with direct pressure of the aneurysm. The pain may become more intense as the aorta stretches rapidly, and there is severe pain when it dissects or ruptures.
- Hernias rarely cause severe pain except when they become strangulated. They may also present with obstruction.
- Symptoms of rapidly expanding organs such as the liver and spleen can cause abdominal pain due to distension of their relatively inelastic capsules.

Patients with a ruptured abdominal aortic aneurysm may complain of flank or groin pain, which may be mistaken for ureteric colic.

Identify symptoms of malignancy

Any of the following symptoms may be due to underlying malignancy:

- Unexplained weight loss.
- Anorexia.
- Change in bowel habit.
- Night sweats.

Careful direct questioning about these symptoms is required.

- Malignancy may be the underlying cause of many of the differential diagnoses, including:
  - Ascites—due to peritoneal spread of tumour.
  - Hernia—due to straining to pass a stool by a patient who has carcinoma of the colon.
  - Hepatomegaly—due to metastatic disease.
  - Bowel obstruction—due to direct mechanical obstruction by tumour.

Drug history

Some drug therapies can cause abdominal swelling:

- Opioid analgesics can cause severe constipation.
- Many psychotropic drugs can cause bowel inactivity leading to pseudo-obstruction of the bowel.
- α-Blockers (α-adrenoceptor antagonists) can cause urinary retention leading to an enlarged bladder.
- Corticosteroid therapy results in deposition of body fat in a central distribution and can lead to increased abdominal fat layers.

EXAMINATION OF PATIENTS WHO HAVE AN ABDOMINAL MASS OR DISTENSION

General examination

The clinician should observe general signs such as anaemia, weight loss and lymphadenopathy, which may indicate underlying malignancy. Signs of liver failure suggesting that the swelling is due to ascites include:

- Palmar erythema.
- Jaundice.
- Spider naevi (more than five on the body).
- Liver flap.

Cardiovascular examination

Absent peripheral pulses and poor circulation indicate atherosclerotic disease and an increased risk of aneurysmal disease. Peripheral oedema may be associated with ascites of any cause, but also may be a sign of congestive cardiac failure with hepatomegaly, and ascites.

Respiratory examination

Watching the patient breathe may reveal some signs of diaphragmatic splinting, and auscultation may reveal small effusions associated with ascites.

Abdominal examination

Inspection will indicate whether abdominal swelling is generalized, such as ascites, or just a localized swelling. Redness or oedema of skin over the swelling can indicate local inflammation. Distended abdominal wall veins are seen in patients who have liver disease and ascites.

If abdominal distension is suspected, it is useful to ask the patient directly if this is the normal size of his or her abdomen and whether they have noticed a change. Patients come in a variety of sizes.

Palpation

The position of any mass and a knowledge of abdominal anatomy is crucial to aiding differential diagnosis (Fig. 5.1) Asking the patient to straight leg raise both legs will contract the abdominal wall muscles and accentuate any abdominal wall masses and hernias. Deep masses will be impalpable with the abdominal muscles contracted.

Percussion

Distended bowel associated with obstruction is hyperresonant. Shifting dullness is pathognomonic of ascites.

Auscultation

High-pitched tinkling bowel sounds are associated with bowel obstruction. Absent bowel sounds can indicate an ileus or pseudo-obstruction.

INVESTIGATION OF PATIENTS WHO HAVE AN ABDOMINAL MASS OR DISTENSION

An algorithm for the investigation and diagnosis of abdominal swelling is given in Fig. 5.2.

Blood tests

Full blood count

An increased white cell count may be associated with bowel obstruction as well as inflammatory masses.

Liver function tests

These may show liver dysfunction. A low albumin is a marker of poor liver synthetic function and may also cause ascites.

Tumour markers

These include:

- Carcinoembryonic antigen (CEA)—a marker for colonic carcinoma.
- CA125—a marker for ovarian carcinoma.
- β-Human chorionic gonadotrophin (BHCG)—a marker for teratoma.
- α-Fetoprotein (AFP)—a marker for primary hepatoma and teratoma.

Fig. 5.2 Investigation and diagnosis of an abdominal swelling. (AXR, abdominal radiography; USS, ultrasound scan.)

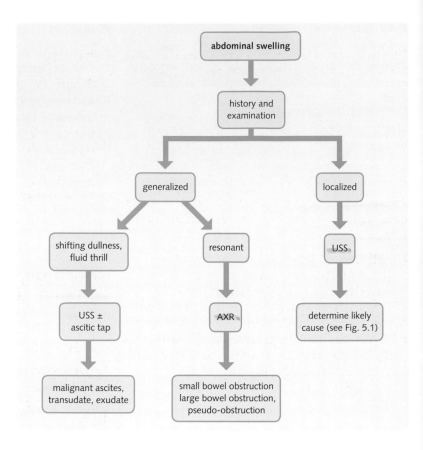

Radiography

Abdominal radiography

Distended loops of bowel filled with gas or fluid are indicative of obstruction or pseudo-obstruction. Distended loops of small bowel indicate small bowel obstruction, whereas colonic or pseudo-obstruction is indicated if there is colonic dilatation with or without small bowel dilatation. A 'ground-glass' appearance suggests the presence of ascites. Certain masses may have calcification in their structure (e.g. aortic aneurysms).

Intravenous urogram

An intravenous urogram (IVU) is performed when a mass is thought to be of renal origin, to assess the anatomy and function of the kidney.

Contrast studies

Double-contrast barium enema

Double-contrast barium enema is indicated when a mass is thought to arise from the large bowel. This method is more successful for imaging caecal masses, as the colonoscope frequently fails to intubate the caecum.

A single-contrast enema is used to differentiate large bowel obstruction from pseudo-obstruction.

Barium meal and small bowel follow-through

Barium meal and small bowel follow-through can be used to investigate masses thought to arise in the small bowel.

Ultrasonography

This can reveal:

- Ascites.
- Abnormally enlarged organs.
- Malignant masses.
- Large cysts in ovaries or kidneys.
- Abscesses.
- Inflammatory masses.

Computed tomography

This may show the same pathology as ultrasonography, but is more useful in showing retroperitoneal structures.

Magnetic resonance

Magnetic resonance (MR) scanning is increasingly being used to assess pelvic masses and liver lesions.

Radioisotope imaging

Radioisotope imaging is used when other methods have failed to identify an abdominal mass accurately.

- Iodine labelled meta-iodobenzylguanidine ([^{131}I]MIBG) scans are used to identify phaeochromocytomas (see Chapter 29).
- Indium-III-labelled leukocyte scans are used in the identification of abdominal masses.
- Technetium dimercaptosuccinic acid (^{99}mTc DMSA) scans are used when the mass is thought to be renal in origin to assess the degree of function in the kidney.

Special investigations

Ascitic tap

This is used to:

- Assess the protein content of the ascites to determine its aetiology (i.e. whether it is a transudate or an exudate). Causes of an exudate include renal, hepatic or cardiac failure. A transudate should raise the suspicion of malignancy.
- Look for the presence of malignant cells.

Ascitic tap: An exudate has a protein content of >25 g/litre and a transudate has a protein content of <25 g/litre.

Biopsy

A fine-needle aspiration cytology, core biopsy or ultrasound-guided biopsy of a mass or palpable lymphadenopathy can provide a histological diagnosis.

Learning objectives

You should be able to:

- Understand how the relationship of blood with the stool indicates the level of the bleeding in the bowel.
- List the important associated symptoms that are suggestive of malignancy.
- Know the common features to look for and exclude when performing a digital rectal examination.
- Understand the significance of the dentate line, particularly when treating haemorrhoids.
- List the types of scope available for direct visualization of the anorectum and large bowel.

This chapter is concerned with the causes of fresh rectal bleeding. Rectal bleeding can be a source of great embarrassment for patients and they may suffer with the problem for a long time before presenting to a clinician. Sudden onset of a large volume of rectal bleeding may be a reason for an acute surgical admission.

DIFFERENTIAL DIAGNOSIS OF RECTAL BLEEDING

The differential diagnosis of rectal bleeding is given in Fig. 6.1; the causes of rectal bleeding are given in Fig. 6.2.

Patients who have a colonic carcinoma may also have haemorrhoids. Do not assume rectal bleeding is due to the presence of haemorrhoids.

HISTORY TO FOCUS ON THE DIFFERENTIAL DIAGNOSIS OF RECTAL BLEEDING

Age

Haemorrhoids and fissure in ano are prevalent at every age. Diverticular disease and cancer are rare in people under 40 years of age.

Character of the bleeding

Bright red blood is usually indicative of anorectal pathology. Dark altered blood is associated with colonic pathology and, occasionally, it is due to a brisk bleed from an upper gastrointestinal source.

Upper gastrointestinal bleeding is usually darker in nature (i.e. melaena; see Chapter 3).

Relationship of bleeding to stool

Mixed with stool

Blood mixed with the stool is indicative of a bleeding source high up in the colon. The softer stool and the time taken to evacuate stool from here means that the blood and stool can mix. It is unusual for this to happen as a result of bleeding from a site below the descending colon.

On surface of the stool

Blood on the surface of the stool is usually from the sigmoid colon or rectum. Isolated streaks of blood on the stool and associated with severe pain on defecation are associated with a fissure-in-ano.

Blood separate from stool

Blood that is separate from stool is usually produced after defecation and is associated with anorectal conditions such as haemorrhoids. The patient will often describe dripping of blood into the toilet after defecation.

Fig. 6.1 Differential diagnosis of rectal bleeding

System involved	Pathology
anus	haemorrhoids, fissure-in-ano, carcinoma
colon and rectum	inflammatory bowel disease, rectal polyp or adenoma, carcinoma and angiodysplasia

diverticulitis & enteritis

Blood on the toilet paper

This is usually associated with anorectal conditions such as haemorrhoids and fissures where the bleeding is not as brisk and a small bloody residue is left on the anal skin.

Mucus

A discharge of mucus may accompany the bleeding if it is due to ulcerative colitis, Crohn's disease of the rectum or an adenoma.

Associated symptoms

Pain

Anorectal pain is not usually a major feature of haemorrhoids or carcinoma of the colon (see Chapter 7).

Severe pain on defecation may be associated with an anal fissure.

Colicky abdominal pain is a feature of an impending obstruction from a carcinoma of the colon (see Chapter 1).

Angiodysplasia of the colon or diverticular disease may cause sudden brisk painless bleeding with clots.

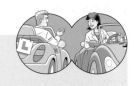

Bleeding is frightening for patients, and especially a large-volume diverticular bleed. Mentioning that most diverticular bleeds are self-limiting is reassuring. Treatment initially will be conservative, but it is important to monitor how much blood volume is lost to monitor progress and assess the need for transfusion. Informing the patient of this makes it more likely that they report any further rectal bleed to nursing staff, allowing for more accurate monitoring.

Change in bowel habit

Change in bowel habit is discussed in Chapter 4.

Tenesmus

Tenesmus is a feeling of incomplete evacuation. It is usually caused by a space-occupying lesion of

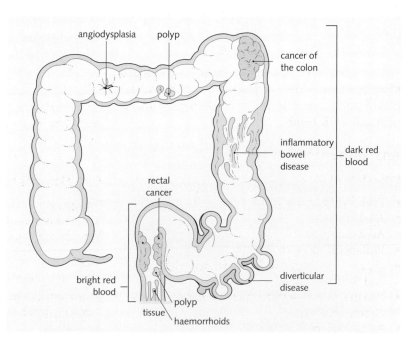

Fig. 6.2 Causes of rectal bleeding.

the rectum, but may also be associated with acute inflammatory conditions of the rectum.

Weight loss

In the elderly this suggests malignancy, but in the younger patient, inflammatory bowel disease such as Crohn's disease or ulcerative colitis is more likely.

Family history

Some patients have several first-degree relatives who have had carcinoma of the bowel and their risk of developing bowel cancer may be as high as 1 in 2 based on 'cancer family' genetic screening.

Familial polyposis coli, in which patients have more than 100 polyps in the colon, is an autosomal-dominant condition and is associated with an almost 100% risk of developing bowel cancer.

EXAMINATION OF PATIENTS WHO HAVE RECTAL BLEEDING

General examination

A general examination of the patient is carried out, looking in particular for clinical signs of anaemia associated with chronic blood loss. If the patient has been admitted as an acute admission to hospital and has marked rectal bleeding, their pulse, blood pressure and urine output must be monitored.

Abdominal examination

This is often normal, but there may be a palpable mass due to a colonic tumour or an inflammatory mass due to Crohn's disease, or tenderness associated with ischaemic colitis.

Anal inspection

Inspection of the anus may reveal:

- Prolapsed haemorrhoids.
- Anal fissure.
- Anal tumours.
- Prolapsing low rectal tumour.
- Skin tags—which may be associated with fissures and fistulae.
- Perianal sepsis—which may be associated with Crohn's disease.
- Rectal prolapse.

Digital rectal examination

Insertion of a finger into the rectum can reveal many conditions:

- The sphincter tone is usually high in patients who have a fissure, and this condition is also very painful. A complete examination may not be possible acutely.
- Presence of blood or mucus on the gloved finger indicates the need for further investigation.

Low rectal tumours are palpable up to 7 cm.

Proctoscopy and sigmoidoscopy

The proctoscope is used to look for anorectal problems and can be particularly useful for visualizing haemorrhoids, which are impalpable.

The sigmoidoscope is used to provide a view of the rectum and the lower sigmoid colon. Lesions can be directly inspected and biopsied.

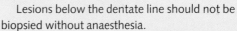

Symptomatic haemorrhoids can be treated at the time of protoscopy with injection sclerotherapy or by the application of rubber bands.

Lesions below the dentate line should not be biopsied without anaesthesia.

INVESTIGATION OF PATIENTS WHO HAVE RECTAL BLEEDING

An algorithm for the investigation and diagnosis of rectal bleeding is given in Fig. 6.3.

Blood tests

Full blood count

This provides an assessment of the degree of blood loss. Chronic blood loss will be reflected as a hypochromic microcytic anaemia.

Haemorrhoids do not bleed sufficiently to cause anaemia.

Fig. 6.3 Investigation and diagnosis of rectal bleeding. (GI, gastrointestinal; OGD, oesophagogastroduodenoscopy; RBC, red blood cell.)

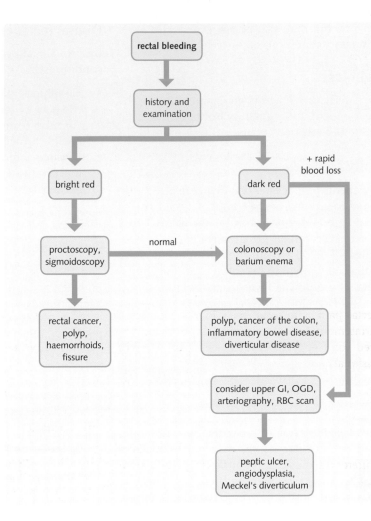

Carcinoembryonic antigen

This tumour marker can be increased in colonic carcinoma (see Chapter 5).

Barium enema and colonoscopy

A flexible colonoscopic investigation has advantages over barium enema because it is the only method for visualizing areas of angiodysplasia and small polyps.

Further investigations

Gastroscopy

This is not usually a first-line investigation for rectal bleeding but, if there has been marked loss of dark blood, a bleeding peptic ulcer may be the cause.

Labelled red cell scan

This is mainly used for diagnosing bleeding from a Meckel's diverticulum or if other tests are normal.

Angiography

This is a specialized investigation to identify the bleeding source if there is rapid bleeding and surgical intervention may be required. A radio-opaque contrast is selectively injected into each mesenteric artery in turn and screening is used to show the site of blood loss into the gut. The patient has to be bleeding at 1–1.5 mL/min for the test to be helpful. Computed tomography angiography is also now being used. The images provide greater anatomical detail, there is no catheter, and the contrast is injected into an arm vein, rather than a large groin vein, and the procedure is therefore quicker and less uncomfortable for the patient.

The usual causes of rapid blood loss from the colon are bleeding from a diverticulum or angiodysplasia.

Anorectal pain, like rectal bleeding, is a cause of embarrassment for many patients and it may be suffered for some time before the patient seeks professional help.

DIFFERENTIAL DIAGNOSIS OF ANORECTAL PAIN

The differential diagnosis of anorectal pain is given in Fig. 7.1.

HISTORY TO FOCUS ON THE DIFFERENTIAL DIAGNOSIS OF ANORECTAL PAIN

Pain

A history of the nature of the pain should be taken, as with all painful complaints, but particular attention should be paid to the timing of the anal pain (i.e. in relation to defecation).

- Severe anal pain at the time of defecation that eases afterwards is often associated with an anal fissure.
- Sudden onset of pain and swelling after passing a bulky stool may indicate a perianal haematoma or prolapsed haemorrhoids.

Abscesses usually present with a gradual onset of throbbing pain that increases in intensity, but may be suddenly relieved if the contents discharge (see below).

The patient may indicate that the site of the pain is external and describe the pain as 'soreness'. This is usually associated with local skin irritation.

Carcinoma of the rectum or anus does not usually present with anal pain but, if there is pain, this often indicates invasion by the tumour of the anal sphincter. The pain is usually severe and persistent without any respite and no exacerbating factors.

A history of a fall onto the base of the spine followed by pain on opening the bowels may suggest a coccygeal injury.

The patient may describe a sharp shooting pain of sudden onset that is deep inside the anal canal and often occurs at night. There appears to be no relation to bowel habit and the pain disappears quickly. This is the typical presentation of proctalgia fugax (flitting anal pain).

Bleeding

Causes of rectal bleeding are dealt with in Chapter 6 and the history should be taken in the manner described.

Discharge

A history of any discharge or 'wetness' should be obtained. Patients often do not describe a discharge but, on direct questioning, may describe staining of underwear. Nearly all of the diagnoses mentioned in this chapter can lead to some form of excess moisture

Fig. 7.1 Differential diagnosis of anorectal pain

System involved	Pathology
anus	fissure-in-ano, perianal haematoma, thrombosed haemorrhoids, fistula-in-ano, perianal abscess, pruritis ani (local irritation), carcinoma, pilonidal abscess, coccydynia, proctalgia fugax
rectum	rectal carcinoma, inflammatory bowel disease and rectal prolapse

in the perianal region and may also cause local irritation of the skin. Fecal soiling of the underwear raises the possibility of a fistula or incontinence.

Fecal soiling of the underwear raises the possibility of a fistula.

EXAMINATION OF PATIENTS WHO HAVE ANORECTAL PAIN

General examination

General examination of the patient should of course be carried out in all cases. Attention should be paid to:

- Signs of weight loss—should alert the clinician to malignancy or Crohn's disease.
- Anaemia—due to severe rectal bleeding.
- Pyrexia and tachycardia—indicate a source of sepsis.

Inspection

Close inspection of the external anal skin may reveal excoriated inflamed skin.

Skin tags may be associated with fissure in ano and multiple skin tags can be associated with Crohn's disease.

Suspect an anal fissure if a patient complains of severe pain on defecation and there is an anal skin tag on examination.

An abscess may be visible as a swelling in the perianal region, with reddened, indurated overlying skin.

There may be a small perianal opening discharging pus or fecal material. The position of the opening should be noted because it will guide the clinician in looking for the internal communication of a fistula. Fistulae with anterior external openings open directly into the anal canal or rectum, whereas fistulae with external openings posterior to the midline usually open in the midline of the anal canal or rectum (Goodsall's rule, Fig. 7.2).

Thrombosed piles and perianal haematomas may be confused, but several differences will distinguish one from the other:

- Thrombosed piles are recognized as dark blue swellings protruding from the anal canal covered in oedematous dusky mucosa.
- Perianal haematomas are subcutaneous swellings on the anal verge and are covered in skin.
- Thrombosed piles are exquisitely tender to touch.
- Perianal haematomas, although causing quite marked pain to the patient, are usually not tender to the touch.

If the piles have been prolapsed and thrombosed for some time they may be excoriated and ulcerated and may be confused with a protruding anorectal carcinoma.

Pilonidal abscesses *(sinus)* usually lie at the top of the natal cleft and there may be associated midline pits. In all cases of pilonidal abscess there is association with excess hair in the natal cleft.

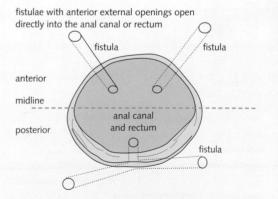

fistulae with anterior external openings open directly into the anal canal or rectum

fistula — fistula

anterior

midline

anal canal and rectum

posterior

fistula

fistulae with external openings posterior to the midline usually open in the midline of the anal canal or rectum

Fig. 7.2 Goodsall's rule.

Digital rectal examination

Once inspection of the external anus has been completed a gloved finger should be inserted. Digital rectal examination may not be possible in patients with acute anal problems because of severe pain and in this case no further investigation should be performed without anaesthetic.

Features to look for include:

- Sphincter tone—is usually high in patients who have anal fissure.
- Any irregularity in the anal canal—anal fissures are often palpable as small indurated or even 'sharp' lesions on the anal verge. The patient will tell you that touching this area is extremely painful.
- Any palpable masses—both size and position (related to clockface) should be recorded.
- Prostatic features in the male (see Chapter 17).

- Coccygeal pain—the coccyx is palpable posteriorly and backward pressure over this causes severe pain in coccydynia.

INVESTIGATION OF PATIENTS WHO HAVE ANORECTAL PAIN

An algorithm for the investigation and diagnosis of anorectal pain is given in Fig. 7.3.

Proctoscopy and sigmoidoscopy

The anal canal and rectum should be inspected directly and attention paid to any mucosal abnormality. An internal opening to a fistula may be seen if there is discharge of pus into the rectum. Any lesions above the dentate line (the limit of somatic sensation in the anal canal) may be biopsied.

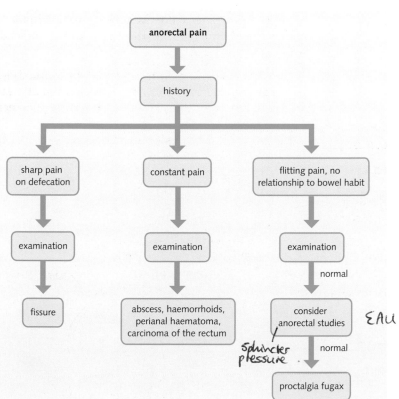

Fig. 7.3 Investigation and diagnosis of anorectal pain.

Even inspection of the anus may not be possible as simple parting of the glutei can aggrevate the pain. The patient may refuse the examination altogether. It is helpful to reassure the patient and give oral analgesia and topical treatment such as ice and lignocaine gel 30 minutes before returning to perform the examination. If still not tolerated then an examination under anaesthetic will be necessary (EUA).

Special investigations

Endoanal ultrasonography

A modified ultrasound probe is inserted into the rectum and is used in the investigation of anal pain, sepsis, fecal incontinence and malignancy.

Anorectal physiology

Assessment of sphincter pressure and coordination can be made with anorectal manometry. This may detect high pressures associated with anal fissures or painful spasms due to sphincter instability.

Learning objectives

You should be able to:

- Define jaundice and give a differential diagnosis for prehepatic, hepatic, and posthepatic jaundice.
- List features of the social history that are important when assessing a jaundiced patient.
- Define Murphy's sign and Courvoisier's law and understand their significance.
- Understand how liver function tests can help distinguish between hepatocellular and obstructive jaundice.
- Define ERCP, what it involves, and its role as an investigative and therapeutic procedure.

Jaundice describes the yellow discoloration of the skin associated with the deposition of bile pigments in the skin and sclera. It is clinically visible when serum bilirubin rises above 30 mmol/litre.

Causes of jaundice can be split into prehepatic, hepatic and posthepatic causes.

DIFFERENTIAL DIAGNOSIS OF JAUNDICE

The differential diagnosis of jaundice is given in Fig. 8.1.

HISTORY TO FOCUS ON THE DIFFERENTIAL DIAGNOSIS OF JAUNDICE

Presentation of jaundice

- Jaundice associated with a common bile duct stone has a rapid onset and is usually painful.
- A past history of self-limiting transient episodes of jaundice suggests the passage of smaller stones.
- Infectious hepatitis is usually preceded by a flu-like illness. The jaundice is usually gradual in onset and progressive.
- Carcinoma of the pancreas has an insidious onset of jaundice, but is progressive.

Urine and stool change

The change of urine colour to dark brown and of the stool to a pale clay colour is classically associated with obstructive jaundice, but may not represent true posthepatic jaundice because 'medical' causes can cause compression of the intrahepatic bile ducts.

Pain

Any pain associated with the jaundice should be explored and noted:

- Intermittent severe pain is associated with biliary colic and common bile duct stones.
- A dull ache in the right upper quadrant can be associated with viral hepatitis and cholestatic jaundice of any cause that gives rise to oedema and swelling of the liver, stretching the liver capsule.
- Carcinoma of the pancreas can present painlessly or, if there is local invasion by the tumour, it may cause severe relentless back pain.
- Haemolytic jaundice is painless.

Social history   ABCDEF of jaun

The social history can give many clues when trying to establish 'non-surgical' causes of jaundice:

- History of contact with known hepatitis carriers, blood transfusion, history of intravenous drug abuse and sexual liaisons with new partners

co-amoxiclav
contraceptives
Chlorpromazine
flucloxacillin, dapsone, steroids

A broad
Bld transf
Contacts
Drugs.

Ethanol
F tbc
Gallstones.

37

Fig. 8.1 Differential diagnosis of jaundice

System involved	Pathology
prehepatic	haemolytic disorders, congenital hyperbilirubinaemia
hepatic	viral hepatitis, alcoholic liver disease, drug-induced metastatic disease
posthepatic	common bile duct stones, carcinoma of the head of the pancreas, ampulla or bile duct, biliary stricture (benign or malignant), external biliary compression (Mirizzi's syndrome, i.e. gallstone impacted in the neck of the gallbladder, but compressing the bile duct), enlarged nodes in the porta hepatis \gastric CA

(especially homosexual males) are all risk factors for viral hepatitis B and C.

- Foreign travel to the Far East and Asia may warn of contact with hepatitis A.
- Alcohol ingestion should also be noted to establish the risk of alcoholic liver disease.

Alcoholism in the elderly is underreported. It is usually secondary to depression relating in turn to either bereavement, loneliness or caring for an ill and elderly spouse. This age group is less likely to talk about these issues directly. Awareness may help you pick up silent body language. It is more useful to ask questions regarding their social circumstances rather than about their addiction behaviour directly. Psychiatrists for the elderly may be able to give specialist advice regarding medical treatment but also provide options for social support such as home help or day centre visits.

Drug history

Recent medications should be recorded. Many drugs can cause cholestatic jaundice even after one dose (e.g. chlorpromazine).

Associated symptoms

Lethargy and general malaise along with an influenza-like illness may be associated with hepatitis.

Haemolytic disorders also produce malaise and lethargy but, because of the associated anaemia, also cause breathlessness and often weight loss.

The presence of rigors and high fevers should alert the clinician to the possibility of cholangitis.

Cholangitis produces 'Charcot's triad' of fever, rigors and jaundice. The patient is seriously ill and requires prompt treatment to prevent septicaemia.

Pruritus due to bile salts is a feature of posthepatic jaundice.

EXAMINATION OF PATIENTS WHO HAVE JAUNDICE

General examination

The clinician should look for evidence of recent weight loss. A careful search should also be made for stigmata of chronic liver disease (see Chapter 26, Fig. 26.2). Other physical signs are pyrexia, lymphadenopathy and anaemia.

Abdominal examination

Inspection of the abdomen may reveal further evidence of liver disease:

- A caput medusae (distended veins around the umbilicus)—indicative of portal hypertension associated with chronic liver disease.
- Distension—due to gross ascites.

The size and texture of the liver should be noted:

- A large tender smooth liver is a feature of hepatitis.
- An enlarged irregular liver may indicate the presence of multiple metastases.

Other masses associated with jaundice may be:

- The presence of a palpable gallbladder is usually indicative that the jaundice is not due to stone disease and in many cases points towards biliary or pancreatic malignancy (Courvoisier's law, see Chapter 26, Fig. 26.10).

- Large pancreatic tumours.
- Gastric malignancies, which can cause lymphadenopathy around the porta hepatis giving rise to bile duct compression.
- Other abdominal primary malignancies leading to liver metastases.

Courvoisier's law—if in the presence of jaundice the gallbladder is palpable then the jaundice is not usually due to gallstones.

Murphy's sign—pressure in the right hypochondrium below the costal margin causes the patient to stop inspiration as the inflamed gallbladder impinges on the examiner's fingers. This is only positive in the absence of this sign in the left hypochondrium. It is a sign of acute cholecystitis.

Ascites may be present due to hypoproteinaemia associated with liver disease or an intra-abdominal malignancy, including malignancy of the pancreas, stomach, colon or ovary.

Abdominal examination should include a rectal examination. Pale stool may be seen, or there may be a palpable rectal tumour that has given rise to liver metastases.

INVESTIGATION OF PATIENTS WHO HAVE JAUNDICE

An algorithm for the investigation and diagnosis of jaundice is given in Fig. 8.2.

Blood tests

Full blood count

This may show:

- Anaemia associated with haemolysis—if haemolysis is suspected a reticulocyte count should also be performed.
- An increased white cell count associated with sepsis.

Liver function tests

These can give some indication to the cause of jaundice as well as some idea of the severity of disease:

- Alkaline phosphatase [ALP] is a ductal enzyme and is increased in obstructive causes of jaundice.
- Alanine transaminase (ALT) and aspartate transaminase (AST) are hepatocellular enzymes, which are increased in hepatocellular dysfunction.

The results of liver function tests should never be interpreted in isolation because severe obstructive jaundice can cause hepatocellular failure.

Amylase

Serum amylase may be normal in exacerbations of chronic pancreatitis and in acute pancreatitis that presents late. Acute pancreatitis may be a sequel to obstructive jaundice due to a stone at the lower end of the common bile duct, but chronic pancreatitis may also be the cause of bile duct obstruction.

Other blood tests

Reliable hepatitis serology is available for hepatitis A, B and C. Autoantibodies (antimitochondrial, antinuclear and anti-smooth muscle) should be checked in suspected autoimmune chronic active hepatitis and primary biliary cirrhosis.

Tumour markers

The marker CA19-9 is not specific and rises in both pancreatitis and pancreatic carcinoma. If liver metastases are suspected, measurement of other tumour markers, such as CEA for colon cancer, may be useful if the primary is unknown.

Urinalysis

The presence of bilirubin in the urine can be tested with a simple ward dipstick test. The presence of bilirubin in the urine demonstrates the presence of conjugated bilirubin, which is water soluble. This indicates cholestasis or inability to excrete bilirubin due to: post-hepatic.

- Hepatocellular dysfunction (intrahepatic cholestasis).
- Duct obstruction (extrahepatic cholestasis).

Jaundice without bilirubin in the urine is seen with:

- Haemolytic jaundice.
- The more common hyperbilirubinaemias such as Gilbert syndrome and Crigler–Najjar syndrome.

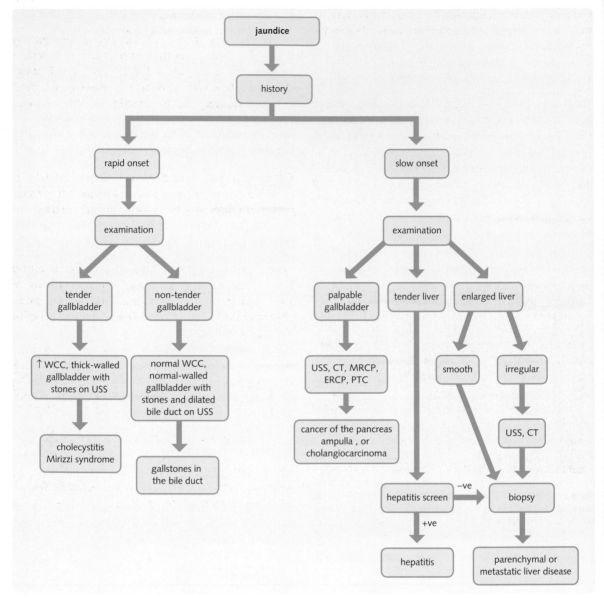

Fig. 8.2 Investigation and diagnosis of jaundice. (CT, computed tomography; MRCP, magnetic resonance cholangiopancreatography; ERCP, endoscopic retrograde cholangiopancreatography; PTC, percutaneous transhepatic cholangiography; USS, ultrasound scan; WCC, white cell count.)

Ultrasonography

This is a very useful tool in the investigation of jaundice. It can demonstrate:

- Dilated biliary ducts (intra- and extrahepatic) associated with biliary obstruction.
- Common bile duct stones.
- Architectural disturbance of the liver itself in association with liver parenchymal disease.

- Metastases.
- Pancreatic swelling or masses.

Computed tomography

Plain or contrast-enhanced computed tomography (CT) may be performed. Computed tomography is better than ultrasound for imaging the pancreas, and contrast-enhanced CT can provide good visualization of metastases. Computed tomography may also demonstrate other intra-abdominal malignancies.

Cholangiography

This can be performed either by endoscopy (endoscopic retrograde cholangiopancreatography—ERCP) or by direct puncture of the intrahepatic ducts (percutaneous transhepatic cholangiography). Either of these methods can be used to demonstrate the presence of stones or tumour. In the case of ERCP a sphincterotomy can also be performed to remove stones, or a stent can be inserted (Fig. 8.3) if there is a tumour.

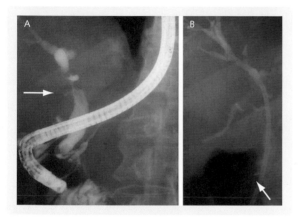

Fig. 8.3 (A) Endoscopic retrograde pancreatogram showing a stricture in the common bile duct (arrow). (B) Subsequent placement of a stent (arrow) across the stricture.

Magnetic resonance

Magnetic resonance cholangiopancreatography (MRCP) is becoming increasingly available and is replacing pure diagnostic ERCP. MRCP can identify stones or tumours causing bile duct obstruction and does not require the injection of contrast or an endoscopy.

Endoscopic ultrasonography

Endoscopic ultrasound (EUS) is performed via an endoscope and is used to evaluate benign and malignant disease of the pancreaticobiliary tree.

Liver biopsy

When no extrahepatic cause for jaundice is found (i.e. there is no duct dilatation and no evidence of haemolysis) a liver biopsy may indicate the cause of liver dysfunction or provide histological proof of metastatic disease.

Hepatobiliary pathology is often difficult for patients to understand but essential, particularly when they give their consent for some of the invasive investigations. A simple anatomical drawing of the biliary tree with annotations when explaining their condition often aids understanding and reduces anxiety (see Fig. 26.3)

Learning objectives

You should be able to:

- Define dysphagia and grade its severity.
- List causes of dysphagia arising from the oesophagus and as a result of systemic diseases.
- Identify signs in the hands related to diseases that can cause dysphagia.
- Recognize on barium swallow characteristic appearances of conditions that can present with dysphagia.
- Understand the role of oesophageal manometry and pH monitoring.

Dysphagia is defined as difficulty in swallowing and may be associated with odynophagia, which is painful swallowing.

DIFFERENTIAL DIAGNOSIS OF DYSPHAGIA

The differential diagnosis of dysphagia is given in Fig. 9.1.

Patients with acute-onset dysphagia due to bolus obstruction are often distressed as they percieve they cannot breathe. Try reassuring them. Explain to them that the dull ache they are feeling in their chest is the blockage but that this is not in their windpipe. They are not choking. Ask them to concentrate on their breathing. This often calms them down.

HISTORY TO FOCUS ON THE DIFFERENTIAL DIAGNOSIS OF DYSPHAGIA

Degree of dysphagia

The patient may have dysphagia only to solid foods such as meat and potatoes, or may only be able to

swallow liquids. Inability to swallow any fluid, including saliva, is a medical emergency and the patient requires immediate admission to hospital and investigation.

To ascertain the severity of dysphagia, ask about the ease of swallowing the following foods—dysphagia is progressively worse as you move down the list:

- Meat.
- Fish.
- Mashed potatoes or vegetables.
- Minced meat.
- Liquids only.

Onset

The onset and progression of dysphagia varies with the diagnosis:

- A sudden onset of dysphagia at the time of eating is suggestive of a bolus obstruction.
- A progressive dysphagia is commonly associated with malignancy.

Associated symptoms

Any associated symptoms should be elicited by direct questioning if necessary and may include:

Fig. 9.1 Differential diagnosis of dysphagia

System involved	Pathology
oesophagus:	
in the lumen	foreign body _GORD_
in the wall	inflammatory stricture, caustic stricture, achalasia, tumour of oesophagus or gastric cardia, pharyngeal pouch, Plummer–Vinson syndrome, diffuse oesophageal spasm, scleroderma and oesophageal web
outside the wall	retrosternal goitre, enlarged left atrium and bronchial carcinoma
general	bulbar palsy, myasthenia gravis and hysteria

- Dyspepsia—a long history of dyspepsia, reflux and progressive dysphagia is suggestive of benign stricture due to oesophageal reflux.
- Weight loss—may be associated with malignancy, but may just reflect the inability of the patient to ingest enough calories to maintain their normal weight due to the severity of the dysphagia.
- Nocturnal cough—aspiration of the contents of a pharyngeal pouch or a dilated oesophagus may trickle down the trachea on lying flat at night, causing a coughing reflex.
- Haematemesis—this may arise from either a bleeding lesion in the oesophagus or may be related to a peptic ulcer (which may be associated with hyperacidity that also causes a stricture of the oesophagus).
- Fatigue—may be due to anaemia, which may be secondary to upper gastrointestinal haemorrhage or chronic blood loss. Anaemia is also classically associated with Plummer–Vinson syndrome, where it is linked to the presence of an oesophageal web.
- Breathlessness—this may be due to anaemia, but may also be associated with a bronchial carcinoma causing dysphagia or recurrent aspiration pneumonia.
- Other neurological symptoms—diseases such as polio, myasthenia gravis, bulbar palsy and syringomyelia may lead to oesophageal motility problems, and so questions about altered sensation and power (especially in the upper limbs) may be relevant.

EXAMINATION OF PATIENTS WHO HAVE DYSPHAGIA

Anaemia is very non-specific, but it is usually due to chronic blood loss from oesophageal carcinoma or gastric carcinoma or reflux oesophagitis.

Examination of the hands may reveal:

- Clubbing of the fingers—associated with a bronchial carcinoma.
- Waxy and tight fingers consistent with scleroderma or Raynaud's phenomenon—as part of CREST syndrome (Calcinosis, Raynaud's, [O]Esophageal motility disorders, Scleroderma, Telangiectasia).

Palpation of the neck may reveal lymphadenopathy in the supraclavicular fossa (Virchow's node) associated with a gastric or intrathoracic malignancy.

The thyroid can also be palpated to assess goitre (but enlargement of the thyroid causing dysphagia is usually retrosternal).

Respiratory examination including auscultation may reveal an underlying bronchial carcinoma or chest infection. A monophonic wheeze or pulmonary collapse may be diagnosed clinically.

INVESTIGATION OF PATIENTS WHO HAVE DYSPHAGIA

An algorithm for the investigation and diagnosis of dysphagia is given in Fig. 9.2.

Radiography

Chest radiography

This is a simple non-invasive investigation that may reveal:

- Primary lung carcinoma.
- Mediastinal mass.
- A large retrosternal goitre.
- An air–fluid level in the mediastinal shadow, which is often diagnostic of the dilated oesophagus associated with achalasia.
- Aspiration pneumonia.

Barium swallow

This is the 'gold standard' primary investigation for dysphagia. It will direct the clinician to the level of the problem. In motility disorders it is often more

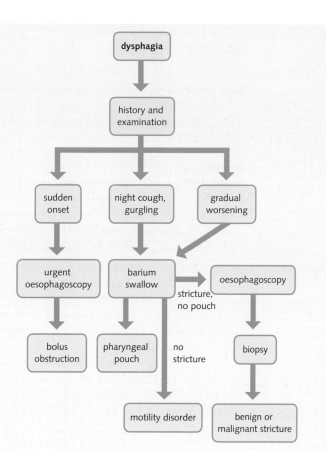

Fig. 9.2 Investigation and diagnosis of dysphagia.

informative than endoscopy, although oesophageal manometry may be required to confirm the diagnosis.

- Pharyngeal pouches and oesophageal webs in the upper oesophagus can be visualized.
- Achalasia appears as a dilated oesophagus above a 'rat-tail' narrowing at the cardia.
- Oesophageal motility disorders can give rise to many appearances on the barium swallow, but fluoroscopic surveillance during the swallow shows muscular incoordination. Diffuse motility problems can give rise to the dramatic appearances of 'corkscrew oesophagus'.
- The appearances of a benign stricture associated with reflux or a carcinoma may be similar and endoscopy is often needed for tissue diagnosis, but the contrast study will show the clinician the length of the stricture.

Achalasia produces a characteristic 'rat's tail' or 'bird's beak' as the dilated oesophagus tapers in the lower oesophagus.

Endoscopy OGD ± Bx.

Oesophagoscopy can be used to visualize directly the cause of dysphagia and biopsies of the lesion can be taken for tissue diagnosis. However, endoscopy can be complicated by perforation, especially in the case of pharyngeal pouch, and for this reason barium studies should be the first-line investigation. Endoscopy is of little diagnostic value in motility disorders.

Bronchoscopy

This may be performed if a primary carcinoma of the bronchus is suspected as a cause of the dysphagia, especially if chest radiography is abnormal.

Computed tomography

This is not a primary diagnostic tool, but can be useful for assessing the stage of oesophageal carcinoma (i.e. the involvement of other structures).

Endoscopic ultrasonography

This is used to assess and stage malignancy in the upper gastrointestinal tract. It is able to assess submucosal disease that may not be visible on endoscopy. Staging is more accurate using this technique than with computed tomography or magnetic resonance imaging.

Transoesophageal ultrasonography

This is used to evaluate bronchial carcinomas and perform guided biopsies of enlarged lymph nodes.

Oesophageal manometry and pH monitoring

Manometry is used to assess coordination and strength of peristaltic movement in the oesophagus and also the sphincter pressures. It can be useful if other modalities have failed to show a cause for dysphagia. pH monitoring may reveal the underlying cause for a benign stricture of the oesophagus.

Breast lump

Learning objectives

You should be able to:

- List a differential diagnosis for a benign breast lump.
- Understand the importance of the menstrual and reproductive history in relation to a breast lump.
- Recognize the distinguishing features of a breast cyst and a fibroadenoma.
- List the features that would raise the suspicion that a breast lump is cancer.
- Understand the principle of triple assessment when investigating and diagnosing a breast lump.

Breast cancer is a well-publicized diagnosis and most women who present with a breast lump are concerned that it is a cancer. It is important for the clinician to evaluate the lump carefully and reassure the patient without giving false hope to those who actually have a malignant tumour.

It is helpful to comment on how common breast lumps are. This is in itself ressuring as the patient feels they are not alone in facing this. Do not fall into the trap of proclaiming that a benign-feeling lump will prove benign. Be empathetic by saying that waiting for results is a difficult time and compliment the patient for doing the right thing and getting the lump checked.

DIFFERENTIAL DIAGNOSIS OF BREAST LUMP

The differential diagnosis of breast lump is given in Fig. 10.1.

HISTORY TO FOCUS ON THE DIFFERENTIAL DIAGNOSIS OF BREAST LUMP

Presentation

How did the patient first become aware of the lump?

- Many lumps are incidental findings discovered while in the shower or washing, and may have been present for a long time before discovery. Women who regularly examine their breasts will be more accurate in their assessment of the duration of the lump than the casual examiner.
- Some women notice asymmetry of their breasts when in front of the mirror; often they notice skin changes or dimpling, and this is suggestive of a carcinoma.
- A history of trauma preceding the discovery may alert one to the possibility of fat necrosis, but may just have been the incident that caused the discovery of a pre-existing lump.
- A lump presenting suddenly in a breast-feeding mother is likely to be a galactocoele or abscess.

Changes

How has the lump changed since its discovery?

- A lump that alters in size during the menstrual cycle is more likely to be a hormone-related benign breast change than a carcinoma.
- A lump that slowly grows in size is more likely to be a solid lump (benign or malignant), but one that doubles in size over a few days is more likely to be cystic. ↑in size ↑ over what time period.

Associated symptoms

Pain

Breast abscesses are acutely painful and tender. A rapidly enlarging breast cyst may also cause pain. Carcinomas of the breast are rarely painful.

47

Fig. 10.1 Differential diagnosis of a breast lump

System involved	Pathology
breast cancer	breast carcinoma
benign breast lumps	fibroadenoma, cystosarcoma phyllodes, benign cyst, fat necrosis, breast abscess, galactocoele, duct ectasia and duct papilloma

Discharge

Ask about any discharge:

- A bloody discharge from a single duct of the nipple can be a sign of malignancy, but may also be associated with benign papillomas of the duct and may also be caused by trauma during breast-feeding.
- A creamy or greenish discharge from multiple ducts is associated with duct ectasia.
- A profuse discharge of milky fluid from multiple ducts is occasionally associated with a prolactinoma.

Fever

This is usually associated with an abscess.

Previous history

A woman who has developed a cyst or fibroadenoma is more likely to develop further cysts or fibroadenomas (but is no less likely to develop breast cancer). Similarly, a past history of carcinoma should raise one's suspicions regarding any further breast lumps.

Family history

Overall one in 10 women will develop breast cancer in their lifetime. Certain genes increase a woman's risk, and therefore a careful history about any first- or second-degree relatives who have had breast or ovarian cancer (particularly at an early age) should be obtained.

Drug history

Increased exposure to oestrogen is associated with an increased risk of breast cancer, so a history of prolonged use of the oral contraceptive and hormone replacement treatment may be relevant.

Menstrual and reproductive history

Early menarche and late menopause are associated with an increased oestrogen exposure and risk of breast cancer. Breast-feeding children for more than 3 months seems to have some protective effects against breast cancer.

A full breast history should include details on:
- Menarche.
- Menopause.
- Pregnancies.
- The pill.
- Lactation.
- Family history.
- Previous breast problems.

EXAMINATION OF PATIENTS WHO HAVE A BREAST LUMP

Inspection

The patient's breasts should be inspected in the seated position and any asymmetry noted. In particular, certain signs are suggestive of underlying malignancy:

- Skin dimpling.
- Unilateral nipple inversion or indrawing.
- Destruction or ulceration of the nipple.
- Peau d'orange.

Ask the patient to identify the lump first. It may save fumbling around normal breast tissue and being unable to identify any abnormality.

Palpation

The whole of both breasts should be examined, remembering that the breast tissue extends into the axilla and paying attention to any irregularity in the breast tissue. The characteristics of any lump (i.e. size, shape, position, texture, mobility and any associated inflammation or discharge) should be carefully noted.

Texture

Hard irregular masses are characteristic of carcinoma. Benign lumps tend to be well defined and smooth.

Cysts do not exhibit signs of fluctuance unless they are very large and lax; most cysts feel firm and may be slightly tender. They can be difficult to distinguish from solid benign lesions.

Areas of tender nodularity, especially in the upper outer quadrants, are characteristic of benign breast change.

Mobility

Benign lumps are relatively mobile, especially a fibroadenoma, which is commonly referred to as a 'breast mouse' because of the way it tends to dart away from under the examiner's fingers.

Any lump that is fixed to the skin or underlying muscle is malignant until proved otherwise.

Discharge

During palpation of the breast it may be possible to express some discharge from the breast. Attention should be paid to whether the discharge is coming from single or multiple ducts. The quadrant of the breast from where the discharge appears to be coming should be palpated carefully. A small duct papilloma may be palpable in the subareolar region.

Other examination findings

Lymphadenopathy

Breast cancers spread via lymphatics draining to the axilla, supraclavicular fossa and internal mammary chain. Axillary and supraclavicular areas should be carefully examined and the character of any palpable lymph nodes recorded.

- Malignant lymph nodes generally feel hard and craggy and may be fixed to each other or adjacent structures.
- Benign reactive lymph nodes feel soft and smooth and may be associated with inflammatory breast disease.

- With advanced malignant nodes there may be lymphoedema of the upper limb.

Hepatomegaly

Advanced carcinoma of the breast may present with liver metastases, so the size and texture of any liver edge should be noted.

INVESTIGATION OF PATIENTS WHO HAVE A BREAST LUMP

An algorithm for the investigation and diagnosis of a breast lump is given in Fig. 10.2.

Assessment of any breast lump is usually made in three ways:

- Clinical examination.
- Radiological investigation.
- Histological examination.

This approach leads to a confident diagnosis.

Radiography

Mammography

Mammography is the investigation of choice for breast lumps in women over 35 years of age:

- Classically, breast cancer appears as a spiculated dense lesion.
- Fibroadenomas and cysts tend to appear as well-defined dense lesions; long-established fibroadenomas can appear calcified.

The pattern of calcification can also give a clue about the nature of the lump:

- Well-defined coarse calcification tends to be benign.
- Malignant calcification appears powdery and is very variable in size and shape.

Ultrasonography

Breast tissue is much denser in younger women, so mammography is of limited value and ultrasound is used more frequently.

- Cysts appear as echo-poor well-rounded lesions.
- Fibroadenomas are well circumscribed and have internal echoes.
- Carcinomas are less well defined with irregular echoes and have characteristic acoustic shadowing behind the lesion.

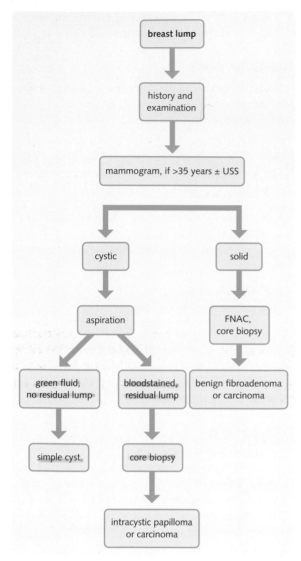

Fig. 10.2 Investigation and diagnosis of a breast lump. (FNAC, fine-needle aspiration cytology; USS, ultrasound scan.)

Tissue sample

Fine-needle aspiration cytology

Cells from the lump can be withdrawn using a 21-gauge needle and a 10-mL syringe. The cells can be examined by the cytology department and assessed for malignancy.

Needle aspiration can also be therapeutic in the case of cysts. Benign breast cyst fluid is yellow-green in colour, but if there is any bloodstaining, further assessment is required.

> It is important even when results prove a lump to be benign to encourage further self-examination and re-presentation if further lumps are found. Reassure the patient that this is not a waste of time nor a waste of resources.

Wide-bore needle biopsy

A wide-bore/core biopsy is taken using local anaesthetic and can be taken under clinical or ultrasound guidance. It allows the pathologist to make a precise diagnosis of benign and malignant pathology.

Excision biopsy

Sometimes the diagnosis can only be truly established by diagnostic excision of the lesion but, in most cases, the diagnosis is established using the biopsy techniques described above.

Most neck pathology presents as a neck swelling. To understand neck swellings, it is important to understand the basic anatomy of the neck and structures within each area (Fig. 11.1).

DIFFERENTIAL DIAGNOSIS OF A NECK LUMP

The differential diagnosis of a neck lump is given in Fig. 11.2.

HISTORY TO FOCUS ON THE DIFFERENTIAL DIAGNOSIS OF A NECK LUMP

General questions relating to lumps are covered in Chapter 39.

Specific questions should cover the following.

Head and neck symptoms

Ask about pain in the mouth, nose and sinuses.

Hoarseness

This may be due to laryngeal pathology or recurrent laryngeal nerve palsy. Interference with the recurrent laryngeal nerve by a neck lump is due to direct compression and suggests a malignant infiltration, usually by thyroid cancer (due to its close relationship to this gland).

Shortness of breath

This may be due to the lump pressing on the trachea (e.g. by a large retrosternal goitre), or the neck swelling may be due to lymphadenopathy associated with a laryngeal or bronchial malignancy as the primary cause of shortness of breath.

Dysphagia

This is discussed in Chapter 9.

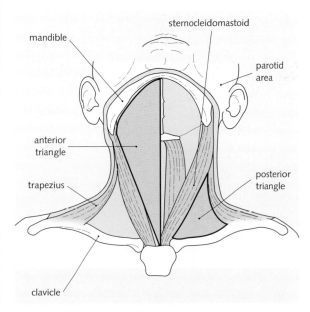

Fig. 11.1 Surface anatomy of the anterior neck.

Fig. 11.2 Differential diagnosis of a neck lump

System involved	Pathology
midline	thyroid goitre, thyroglossal cyst, thyroid carcinoma
anterior triangle of the neck	lymph node, submandibular gland tumour, branchial cyst, carotid artery aneurysm, carotid body tumour, laryngocoele and pharyngeal pouch
posterior triangle	lymph node, cystic hygroma, cervical rib and subclavian artery aneurysm
parotid region	parotid gland tumour, parotid calculus, parotitis

Haemoptysis

A history of coughing up fresh blood may be associated with bronchial carcinoma or carcinoma of the larynx.

Weight loss

This may be associated with any malignant process of the upper gastrointestinal tract, which in turn can lead to cervical lymphadenopathy.

If a neck lump is thought to be malignant, it is necessary to obtain an ear, nose and throat (ENT) assessment early.

Weakness of movements of the face

This indicates involvement of the facial nerve in the underlying process. It is unusual for this to be solely due to the effect of pressure and usually indicates malignant infiltration of the nerve.

Features of hypo- and hyperthyroidism

Features of hyperthyroidism include nervousness or tremor, palpitations, weight loss despite increased appetite, diarrhoea, preference for cold weather, sweating and amenorrhoea.

Features of hypothyroidism include an increase in weight, deposition of fat on the shoulders and neck, lethargy and general slowness, intolerance of cold weather, hair thinning and loss (especially outer third of the eyebrows), muscle fatigue and constipation.

Head and neck cancers usually present with local symptoms or lymph node metastases and not generalized weight loss and malaise.

Exacerbating factors

Some lumps will only appear at certain times:

- A lump appearing behind the sternocleidomastoid on swallowing liquids may be a pharyngeal pouch.
- A laryngocoele is a small mucous outpouching that becomes prominent in the anterior triangle on coughing and sneezing.

EXAMINATION OF PATIENTS WHO HAVE A NECK LUMP

Number

Multiple neck lumps are nearly always lymph nodes.

Thorough examination of head, neck, chest, abdomen and oral cavity

Lymphadenopathy can be associated with disorders in any of these regions and they should therefore be inspected for signs of the primary condition, whether inflammatory or malignant.

Seventh cranial (facial) nerve

Full examination of the facial nerve (i.e. all major divisions) should be made if there is swelling in the parotid area to assess any invasion of the nerve by a malignant process.

Does the lump move?

Thyroid swellings typically move on swallowing. Thyroglossal cysts move on protruding the tongue.

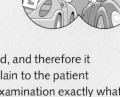

When assessing thyroid swellings, offer the patient a glass of water. It can be very difficult to swallow nothing repeatedly. Explain clearly that they are to take a gulp and keep it in their mouth until you tell them to swallow.

Pulsation

Is the lump pulsatile or expansile:

- Carotid aneurysms should be expansile.
- Carotid body tumours are pulsatile, but not expansile.

The neck is a sensitive area and some neck lumps can be tender. Neck examination is best performed from behind, and therefore it is especially important to explain to the patient beforehand and during the examination exactly what it is you are going to do. Wait until you are facing the patient again to explain any findings.

Eye signs

There may be ocular signs of thyroid disease, including:

- Retraction—the upper lid is higher than normal, but the lower lid is in the normal position.
- Lid lag—the upper lid does not move at the same rate as the eye on downward gaze.

- Exophthalmos—protrusion of eyes, difficulty in convergent gaze and loss of forehead wrinkling on upward gaze.
- Ophthalmoplegia—most commonly this affects the inferior oblique (i.e. affects looking upward and outward).
- Chemosis—oedema of the conjunctivae due to obstruction of venous and lymphatic drainage associated with increased retrobulbar pressure.

Transillumination

Cystic hygromas are found in the base of the posterior triangle and are brilliantly transilluminable. Thyroglossal cysts may also be transilluminated.

INVESTIGATION OF PATIENTS WHO HAVE A NECK LUMP

An algorithm for the investigation and diagnosis of a neck lump is given in Fig. 11.3.

Special investigations

These depend upon the location of the lump and initial clinical impression.

Suspected lymphadenopathy

A series of blood tests should be performed as a routine lymphadenopathy screen, including:

- Full blood count—anaemia may be associated with lymphoma.
- Cytomegalovirus serology—infection by this virus is associated with lymphadenopathy.
- Toxoplasma serology.
- Paul–Bunnell test—for infectious mononucleosis (glandular fever due to Epstein–Barr virus infection).

Testing for human immunodeficiency virus (HIV) may also be considered, but only after appropriate counselling and for high-risk patients.

Thyroid swelling

Thyroid function tests are carried out to assess over- or underactivity of the gland

An ultrasound scan of the thyroid will establish the nature of the lump (i.e. whether it is solid or cystic).

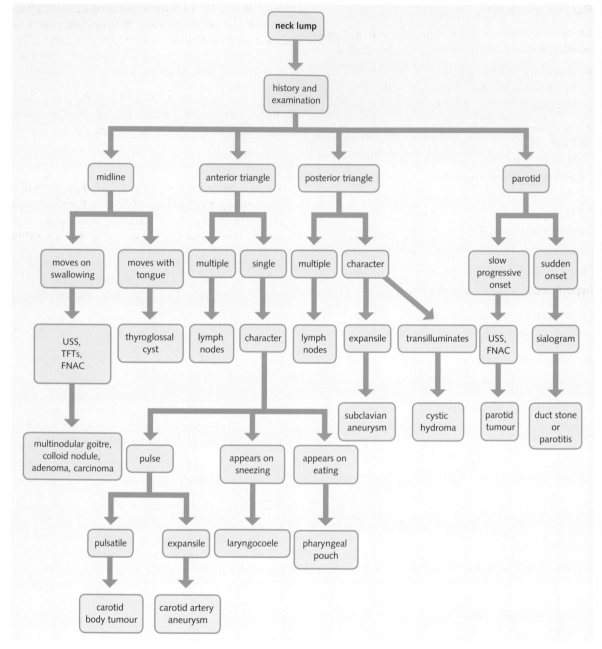

Fig. 11.3 Investigation and diagnosis of a neck lump. (FNAC, fine-needle aspiration cytology; TFTs, thyroid function tests; USS, ultrasound scan.)

In the past, isotope scanning was performed on solitary thyroid nodules in euthyroid patients. However, fine-needle aspiration cytology (FNAC) has now replaced isotope scanning. Isotope scanning is used in thyrotoxic patients with a solitary nodule to ascertain whether the nodule is functioning (hot) or non-functioning (cold). Twenty per cent of cold nodules are malignant.

Malignant thyroid nodules do not usually take up radiolabelled isotopes and are therefore referred to as cold nodules.

Parotid swelling

An ultrasound scan of the parotid will establish whether the swelling:

- Is cystic or solid.
- Extends deep to the facial nerve—this is important in planning surgery.

A sialogram is a contrast study of the salivary duct and will demonstrate an obstructing stone.

Mumps is a viral parotitis caused by paramyxovirus. It is bilateral in 90% of cases.

Mirror examination and fibreoptic endoscopy of larynx and hypopharynx

This is essential to look for laryngeal and hypopharyngeal primary tumours. It can also be used to look at vocal cord function to assess the recurrent laryngeal nerve in the case of hoarseness, or as a preoperative assessment before thyroid surgery.

Computed tomography

This is useful to assess the size and extent of neck tumours and may help to confirm the likely anatomical source of indeterminate swellings.

Barium swallow and endoscopy

These may be performed to assess a pharyngeal pouch or upper oesophageal tumours. Supraclavicular fossa lymphadenopathy is classically associated with stomach carcinoma, so endoscopy may be useful to look for this condition.

Ischaemic limb

Learning objectives

You should be able to:

- Define ischaemia and claudication.
- List the presenting symptoms and signs of acute ischaemia.
- Understand the term acute on chronic ischamia.
- Distinguish between embolus and thrombus and which type of ischaemia is likely to occur as a result of each.
- Define Buerger's angle and Buerger's sign.

Ischaemia is defined as an inadequate blood supply to an organ or limb to enable normal function. Ischaemia of a limb is often described as acute, chronic, or acute on chronic. Management and investigation depends on the speed of onset of the symptoms.

DIFFERENTIAL DIAGNOSIS OF AN ISCHAEMIC LIMB

The differential diagnosis of an ischaemic limb is given in Fig. 12.1.

HISTORY TO FOCUS ON THE DIFFERENTIAL DIAGNOSIS OF AN ISCHAEMIC LIMB

Onset and progression

The most important part of the history is how the disease presents and progresses:

- A sudden onset of severe pain, paraesthesia and paralysis in a previously asymptomatic patient suggests an acute embolic event.
- A long history of reduced walking distance (see below) is suggestive of atherosclerotic disease (chronic ischaemia).
- A sudden worsening of symptoms in a patient who has a long history of claudication may suggest thrombosis of a critically stenosed vessel (acute on chronic ischaemia).

- The onset of pain on activity in a patient under 30 years of age is unlikely to be due to atherosclerotic disease and more likely to be due to a compression or entrapment syndrome.

Claudication

Claudication is the cramping pain associated with anaerobic exercise of a muscle due to ischaemia. The pain is alleviated by rest. The severity is related to the distance walked before the onset of pain. The site at which the pain occurs gives the level of the vessel disease:

- Calf—femoropopliteal.
- Thigh—iliofemoral.
- Buttock—aortoiliac.

Rest pain

Pain at rest implies severe disease leading to ischaemia in the non-active muscle. The pain is often felt in the foot or toes. Patients will describe pain coming on at night (when the leg is elevated in bed) and relieved by hanging the limb out of bed.

Previous medical history

The following conditions are associated with thromboembolic disease:

- Cerebral embolus.
- Transient ischaemic attacks.
- Amaurosis fugax.

Fig. 12.1 Differential diagnosis of an ischaemic limb

System involved	Pathology
acute	embolus, thrombosis and trauma
chronic	peripheral vascular disease, Buerger's disease, external compression (popliteal artery entrapment or thoracic outlet syndrome) and arteritis (i.e. systemic lupus erythematous, Takayasu's aortitis)

Patients are more likely to present with thrombosis of a chronically ischaemic limb than to present with acute limb ischaemia due to an embolus.

Conditions that increase the likelihood of occlusive disease are:

• Diabetes mellitus.
• Hypertension.
• Hyperlipidaemia.

Other cardiovascular events that may be associated with an increased risk of emboli include:

• Recent myocardial infarction.
• Atrial fibrillation.

Family history

Family history of the above conditions and vascular disease is associated with an increased risk.

Social history

Smoking is a major risk factor in peripheral vascular disease. The risk is partly dose related, but any history of smoking is an important factor.

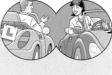

Patients often continue to smoke despite living with the consequences of atherosclerotic disease. Stressing the importance of smoking cessation is not enough. There is specialist help available. Offer the patient an appointment with a specialist vascular nurse in a risk modification clinic.

EXAMINATION OF PATIENTS WHO HAVE AN ISCHAEMIC LIMB

Inspection

General inspection

Chronic ischaemia of a limb can lead to:

• Hair loss.
• Ulceration.
• Blistering of the skin.

Colour

The ischaemic limb will look pale in comparison to a normal limb. Other discoloration may be seen:

• Dusky purple—deoxygenation of the tissues may give a cyanosed appearance when the limb is dependent.
• Black—necrotic patches may be seen, especially on the toes.

Other conditions, although not truly ischaemic, may also cause colour change.

• Blue—in deep venous thrombosis the superficial veins become engorged and a deep blue swollen limb occurs (phlegmasia cerulea dolens).
• White—a milky white limb occurs with severe oedema associated with a deep venous thrombosis (phlegmasia alba dolens) of the iliofemoral veins.

Buerger's angle

The normal limb can be raised to 90° without loss of colour, but an ischaemic limb will blanch on raising the limb above horizontal. The angle at which this occurs is called Buerger's angle. A Buerger's angle of less than 20° indicates severe ischaemia.

After the limb has been raised, the time for the colour to return can also give an indication of perfusion. In severe disease, this may be over 20 seconds.

If the ischaemic limb is then suspended over the edge of the examination couch, it will turn from white to pink and then a dusky red-purple. This is called Buerger's sign.

Venous filling

In the normal limb, the veins appear full when the limb is horizontal. Ischaemic limbs may have underfilled veins, which leave grooves in the skin:

so-called 'guttering' of veins. Where the veins have some filling, the angle at which they become guttered can give some idea of the degree of ischaemia.

Palpation

Temperature

The ischaemic limb will feel cool in comparison to the normal limb.

Use the back of your fingers to assess temperature. The palmar surfaces are often warm and moist and may give a false impression of temperature.

Capillary refilling

Pressure on the toe blanches the skin and the time for normal colour to return is noted. An abnormal result is more than 2 seconds.

Pulses

Peripheral pulses (femoral, popliteal, dorsalis pedis and posterior tibial) must be carefully palpated, noting their presence and quality (i.e. strong, weak, or absent; see Chapter 40).

Pulses may be palpable in the small-vessel disease seen in diabetes and also in Raynaud's disease.

Aneurysm of aorta or popliteal artery

Palpate for the presence of an abdominal aortic aneurysm. Note that, in thin people and those who have excessive lordosis, a normal aorta may be easily palpable, but bimanual palpation of the aorta will indicate whether or not the aorta is dilated.

An easily palpable popliteal artery is usually indicative of an aneurysm. Most popliteal aneurysms are bilateral, and the presence of one aneurysmal popliteal artery and absence of the other popliteal pulse should alert one to the possibility of a thrombosis of the aneurysmal vessel.

Auscultation

Bruits

Listen over the femoral pulses and also in both iliac fossae for bruits, which indicate turbulent flow through a narrowed section of artery.

An objective assessment of the patient's disability using a corridor-walking test or a treadmill is helpful as a baseline.

INVESTIGATION OF PATIENTS WHO HAVE AN ISCHAEMIC LIMB

An algorithm for the investigation and diagnosis of an ischaemic limb is given in Fig. 12.2.

Blood tests

These may include:

- Full blood count—to exclude polycythaemia as a cause of slow perfusion and thrombosis.
- Urea and electrolytes—long-standing ischaemia may lead to muscle necrosis, myoglobinaemia and renal failure.
- Erythrocyte sedimentation rate—a marker of inflammatory vasculitic processes. ESR
- Clotting screen—abnormalities of clotting may lead to thrombosis of venous or arterial vessels.
- Glucose—diabetic arteriopathy may be the first major complication of undiagnosed diabetes mellitus.
- Lipoproteins, triglyceride and cholesterol—increased levels of these are associated with an increased risk of atherosclerosis.
- A thrombophilia screen should be performed if an underlying thrombotic cause is thought to be the reason for ischaemia.

Electrocardiogram

An electrocardiogram (ECG) should be performed in any patient over 55 years of age. Some patients may require more detailed cardiac assessment, depending on their symptoms.

Radiography

Chest radiography

Occlusive vessel disease is a global disease of the body and patients who have peripheral vascular disease are more likely to have coronary artery disease and cardiomyopathy.

Doppler ankle pressures

This uses a Doppler probe to measure the occlusive pressure required to stop blood flow to the ankle

Fig. 12.2 Investigation and diagnosis of an ischaemic limb. (AF, atrial fibrillation; MI, myocardial infarction; USS, ultrasound scan.)

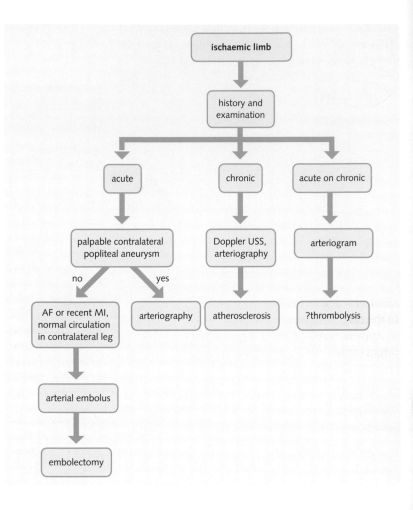

ABPI

vessels. It is often expressed as a ratio to the brachial artery pressure. It may be normal in patients who have intermittent claudication, and a treadmill test may then be performed. Patients are exercised on a treadmill and have Doppler ankle pressures measured at regular intervals—a drop in pressure during the exercise is abnormal and indicates some occlusive disease.

Critical limb ischaemia is defined as rest pain for more than 2 weeks, ulceration and an ankle systolic pressure <50mmHg. Revascularization is essential to avoid limb loss.

Ultrasonography

An ultrasound scan of the abdomen should be performed to exclude an asymptomatic abdominal aortic aneurysm.

Duplex Doppler sonography

This can be used to show blood flow through vessels and can indicate the site and severity of stenoses.

Arteriography

This will demonstrate the anatomy of the vessels, any sites of stenosis and any collateral circulation.

Magnetic resonance angiography

Magnetic resonance angiography (MRA) is performed when angiography is not possible because the femoral artery is not palpable to cannulate. MRA demonstrates the aorta and pelvic vessels well, but the limb vessels are less well demonstrated.

13

An ulcer is defined as a breach in an epithelial surface. In the case of leg ulcers, this is the skin.

Approximately 95% of leg ulcers are vascular in origin (either arterial or venous).

DIFFERENTIAL DIAGNOSIS OF A LEG ULCER

The differential diagnosis of a leg ulcer is given in Fig. 13.1.

HISTORY TO FOCUS ON THE DIFFERENTIAL DIAGNOSIS OF A LEG ULCER

Chronicity and progression of the ulcer should be noted and specific questions should be asked about the following.

Pain

Pain occurs in arterial, infective and sickle cell ulcers.

Neuropathic and venous ulcers are usually painless.

Venous insufficiency

A past history of deep venous thrombosis or varicose veins may be relevant.

Arterial history

A detailed history of ischaemic symptoms, such as claudication and rest pain, should be obtained (see Chapter 12).

Trauma history

There may be a history of recent trauma to the limb. The trauma itself may have been minor, but may lead to an ulcer that is slow to heal due to underlying vascular disease that has been otherwise asymptomatic.

Bowel history

A history of altered bowel habit, suggestive of ulcerative colitis, may be fairly specific to pyoderma gangrenosum.

Previous medical history

This should include any history of:

- Diabetes mellitus.
- Neurological disease.
- Spinal injury.
- Coagulopathy.
- Periods of immobilization.

Social history

A detailed history should be obtained for:

- Smoking—this is associated with atherosclerotic disease.

Fig. 13.1 Differential diagnosis of a leg ulcer

System involved	Pathology
venous	varicose veins and deep vein thrombosis
arterial	ischaemic ulcers
neuropathic	diabetes mellitus, chronic alcohol abuse and other neurological disease
traumatic	bedsores, accidental injury and self-inflicted injury
neoplastic	squamous cell carcinoma, basal cell carcinoma and Marjolin's ulcer
infectious	syphilis
other	sickle cell anaemia, pyoderma gangrenosum

- Alcohol intake—may lead to vitamin deficiencies and peripheral neuropathy.
- Untreated venereal disease—tertiary syphilis can lead to the development of skin ulcers and neuropathies.

EXAMINATION OF PATIENTS WHO HAVE A LEG ULCER

Ask the patient to stand for several minutes before assessing varicosities.

When examining long-standing ulcers, it is often useful to ask the patient for the most recent comments of their community nurse or of their podiatrist. This often yields important information the patient may otherwise omit telling you.

Site of the ulcer

The site may give some clues to aetiology:

- Venous ulcers occur in the lower leg, especially over the medial malleolus.

- Pressure sores and neuropathic ulcers occur over bony prominences such as the heel and malleoli.
- Arterial ulcers occur on the anterior aspect of the shin or dorsum of the foot.

Shape of the ulcer

Careful examination of the edges of the ulcer may help in diagnosis (see Chapter 18, Fig. 18.1).

Neuropathies in diabetic patients result in an incorrect pattern of weight bearing and ischaemic necrosis over pressure points of the foot, causing ulceration.

Other skin changes in the limb

Arterial disease can lead to hair loss and discoloration.

Venous disease may be accompanied by varicosities, varicose eczema, haemosiderin deposits in the skin and a unilateral swollen limb.

Inguinal lymphadenopathy may be secondary to infection or a malignant ulcer.

Arterial examination

The arteries of the lower limb should be examined (see Chapters 12 and 40).

INVESTIGATION OF PATIENTS WHO HAVE A LEG ULCER

An algorithm for the investigation and diagnosis of a leg ulcer is given in Fig. 13.1.

Blood tests

The following blood investigations may be of use:

- Full blood count—to check for anaemia and polycythaemia.
- Sickle cell test—in Afro-Caribbean patients to exclude sickle cell disease or trait.
- Glucose—to exclude undiagnosed diabetes mellitus.
- Erythrocyte sedimentation rate—to check for vasculitis.

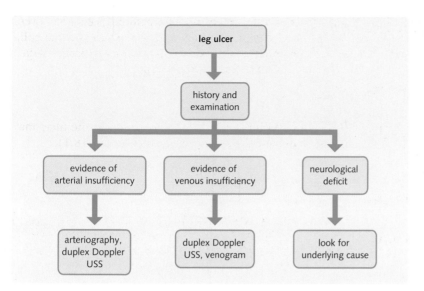

- Antibody screen—to exclude vasculitis.
- Venereal disease research laboratory (VDRL) test—for suspected syphilis.

Culture swab

The organism responsible for an infective ulcer may be cultured in the microbiology laboratory. Most ulcers are colonized by bacteria and so the results must be interpreted with due consideration.

Arterial investigations

If arterial disease is suspected, investigations (as detailed in Chapters 12 and 40) should be carried out.

Venography and duplex ultrasonography

These may be performed to assess the patency of the deep venous system as well as to demonstrate the

existence of incompetent valves at the saphenofemoral and short saphenopopliteal junctions, which leads to varicose veins. Duplex ultrasonography can accurately identify incompetent perforator veins, which can also produce varicose veins.

Biopsy of ulcer

Suspected malignancy should be investigated by biopsy of the lesion. Long-standing venous ulcers can undergo malignant change (Marjolin's ulcer), and so the edges of these should be biopsied too.

Any suspicious ulcers should be biopsied to exclude malignancy.

Swelling in the groin is one of the most common presenting complaints in the general surgical outpatient clinic, and to a lesser degree on the acute surgical intake.

DIFFERENTIAL DIAGNOSIS OF A GROIN SWELLING

The differential diagnosis of a groin swelling is given in Fig. 14.1.

HISTORY TO FOCUS ON THE DIFFERENTIAL DIAGNOSIS OF A GROIN SWELLING

The patient usually presents to the general practitioner because he or she has discovered a lump but, occasionally, a hernia is an incidental finding. In either scenario, several important questions about the lump should be asked during the routine history.

How did the lump first appear?

A history of sudden appearance of the lump following lifting or straining is usually a good indication that the lump may be a hernia, although the event in question may have just brought the lump to the patient's attention.

Is the lump present all the time?

Uncomplicated hernias and a saphena varix may disappear on lying down. Incarcerated or irreducible hernias are present all the time, as are other swellings in the differential diagnosis list (Fig. 14.1).

An irreducible femoral hernia may appear suddenly with no past history of a hernia.

Any associated symptoms?

If the lump is a lymphadenopathy it may be associated with general malaise, an influenza-like illness or recent skin infection.

Is the lump painful?

Characteristic pain patterns include the following:

- Sudden onset of a tender irreducible hernia suggests that the hernia is strangulated.
- Colicky abdominal pain with vomiting and distension may indicate intestinal obstruction.
- Sudden severe pain and generalized abdominal pain may indicate peritonitis resulting from a strangulated hernia.
- Lymphadenopathy can be very tender, but does not usually cause pain at rest.
- Pain on hip extension may be associated with a psoas abscess, but may be due to direct pressure of enlarged lymph nodes.

Direct questioning

Underlying causes of hernias include any cause of increased abdominal pressure, such as:

Fig. 14.1 Differential diagnosis of a groin swelling

System involved	Pathology
groin swelling	inguinal hernia, femoral hernia, lymphadenopathy, saphena varix, hydrocele of the cord, femoral artery aneurysm, lipoma or other adnexal mass, psoas bursa or abscess, undescended or retractile testis

- Straining to pass urine.
- Constipation.
- Chronic cough.
- Heavy manual labour.

There may be a history of lower limb trauma, producing ascending infection and lymphadenopathy.

EXAMINATION OF PATIENTS WHO HAVE A GROIN SWELLING

General examination

Examination should include the whole of the abdomen, looking for abdominal masses and ascites. Remember to examine the perineum and rectum. Anal tumours may give rise to lymphadenopathy in the groins, and prostatic enlargement may be the underlying cause for hernias.

Examination of the lump

The groins should be examined when the patient is standing and lying down. The characteristics of the different lumps in the differential diagnosis are as follows.

When trying to establish whether a hernia is reducible, ask the patient to reduce the hernia themselves while lying flat. This is less intrusive and less likely to cause them pain.

Inguinal hernia

The swelling of an indirect inguinal hernia appears through the external inguinal ring. It has a cough impulse and is compressible. It appears above and medial to the pubic tubercle and does not transilluminate. A direct inguinal hernia is a bulge through the posterior wall of the inguinal canal.

Femoral hernia

This has the same characteristics as the inguinal hernia, but the bulge lies below the inguinal ligament. It emerges below and lateral to the pubic tubercle and is not tender except in the presence of strangulation.

Lymphadenopathy

The groin lymph nodes lie below the inguinal ligament. They are usually firm and rubbery with normal overlying skin. The lower limb and perineum should be carefully inspected to look for an infective or malignant cause.

Hydrocoele of the cord

This is a smooth rounded swelling that moves on gentle traction of the testis. It is possible to get above the swelling, and the swelling is not reducible but does transilluminate.

Femoral artery aneurysm

The main feature of a femoral artery aneurysm is an expansile swelling in the groin. Pulsatility alone may be present in prevascular femoral hernia or lymphadenopathy.

Saphena varix —dilation of the SFJ.

A saphena varix is only present on standing. It has a cough impulse or fluid thrill and is compressible but refills. Tapping on the long saphenous vein below the varix produces a fluid thrill.

Undescended and retractile testis

The characteristic feature is an empty hemiscrotum on the ipsilateral side. Retractile testes can be milked down into the scrotum, but this is rarely possible for undescended testes.

INVESTIGATION OF PATIENTS WHO HAVE A GROIN SWELLING

An algorithm for the investigation and diagnosis of a groin swelling is given in Fig. 14.2. Usually, the diagnosis has been established by a careful history and examination. Some specialized investigations may help to establish the diagnosis in equivocal cases.

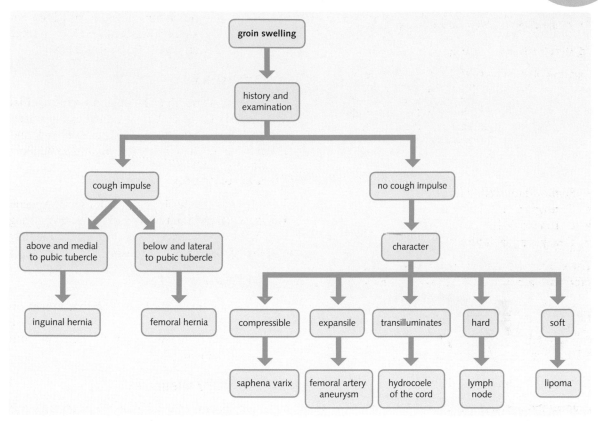

Fig. 14.2 Investigation and diagnosis of a groin swelling.

Doppler duplex scan

This may be useful for demonstrating spheno-femoral incompetence in the case of a saphena varix.

Ultrasound can be useful for differentiating a solid groin lump from a hernia sac containing gut.
Computed tomography (CT) may sometimes be used if the history is suggestive of a hernia but there is no palpable lump in the area and ultrasound has not identified a hernia.

LYMPHADENOPATHY SCREEN

Screening for an underlying cause of lymphadenopathy includes:

- Full blood count.
- Serology for antibodies to cytomegalovirus and *Toxoplasma gondii*.
- Paul–Bunnell or monospot test to detect heterophil antibodies in Epstein–Barr virus infection (infectious mononucleosis).

Scrotal swelling

Learning objectives

You should be able to:

- Give a differential diagnosis for a scrotal swelling.
- Recognize the presenting symptoms and signs of testicular torsion.
- Understand the importance of the relationship of the swelling to the testis and epididymis.
- Understand the importance of transillumination in the assessment of a scrotal swelling.
- Name the tumour markers important in testicular tumours.

Scrotal swellings are another very common presentation to the surgical outpatient department and to the acute surgical emergency department.

DIFFERENTIAL DIAGNOSIS OF A SCROTAL SWELLING

The differential diagnosis of a scrotal swelling is given in Fig. 15.1.

HISTORY TO FOCUS ON THE DIFFERENTIAL DIAGNOSIS OF A SCROTAL SWELLING

Age

The patient's age may be of some help in diagnosis. It is rare for testicular torsion to present in men over 30 years of age. Testicular tumours also occur in particular age groups:

- Teratomas occur in young men (age 20–30 years).
- Seminomas usually present in older men (age 30–50 years).

Pain

Most scrotal swellings give rise to discomfort as a result of compression by clothes, but pain is not usually a feature of epididymal cysts, hydrocoeles, tumours or varicocoeles.

Inguinal hernias can cause moderate discomfort on straining.

Pain is the main feature in testicular torsion and epididymo-orchitis:

- Testicular torsion gives rise to severe scrotal pain of sudden onset and it may be associated with vomiting and suprapubic pain. There may be some preceding episodes of similar but less severe pain due to incomplete torsion owing to the underlying anatomical abnormality (Fig. 15.2).
- Epididymo-orchitis usually has a longer, more insidious onset and there is usually no history of preceding testicular pain.

Always check the testes of adolescent boys who complain of lower abdominal pain—it may be due to torsion.

Fig. 15.1 Differential diagnosis of a scrotal swelling

System involved	Pathology
scrotal swelling	inguinal–scrotal hernia, epididymal cyst, hydrocoele of the cord, haematocoele, varicocoele, epididymo-orchitis, testicular tumour and testicular torsion

Fig. 15.2 Abnormalities leading to torsion of the testis.

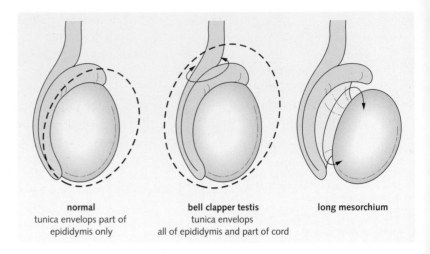

normal
tunica envelops part of
epididymis only

bell clapper testis
tunica envelops
all of epididymis and part of cord

long mesorchium

Any history of trauma?

Scrotal trauma is usually well remembered by the patient and often occurs in sporting injuries. A history of sudden painful swelling after such injury is often indicative of a haematocoele.

Any micturition problems?

Epididymo-orchitis is usually associated with urinary tract infection and there may therefore be a preceding or concomitant history of dysuria and frequency. This may be absent in viral epididymo-orchitis.

EXAMINATION OF PATIENTS WHO HAVE A SCROTAL SWELLING

The scrotal swelling should be examined when the patient is standing up. Clear explanation of what the examination will involve followed by a confident and focused examination keeps patient anxiety and embarrassment to a minimum.

Patients usually have questions they want to ask but are too embarassed. An open question such as 'do you have any questions?' may not help them overcome that embarassment. Commenting that it is common for patients to have questions about how the lump or diagnosis can affect urinary or sexual function and then asking whether the patient has any such queries is usually more successful.

Characteristics of swelling

Testicular tumours are typically hard, non-tender *craggy* swellings that usually occupy the whole testis by the time the patient presents to the clinician.

Hydrocoeles and haematocoeles are usually much softer and fluctuant but, in a chronic haematocoele where the blood has clotted, the appearance can be very similar to that of a testicular tumour.

Varicocoeles are not palpable in the supine patient but, on standing, have a characteristic feel that is often described as 'a bag of worms'.

In torsion of the testis the testis lies horizontally and is exquisitely tender.

The scrotal skin may also be changed. Epididymo-orchitis can give rise to a red swollen scrotum, but this may also occur with prolonged torsion or advanced testicular tumour.

A varicocoele is more common on the left and is described as a 'bag of worms' on palpation.

Is it possible to palpate above the swelling?

Inguinal hernias descending in the scrotum can be easily identified because it is impossible to get above the swelling. All other swellings are confined to the scrotum.

Is the swelling separate from the testis and epididymis?

This is an important diagnostic feature:

- Epididymal cysts are palpable within the epididymis and separate from the testis.
- Encysted hydrocoeles of the cord are also palpable separately from the testis and epididymis.
- The testis is not usually palpable within a vaginal hydrocoele or haematocoele but, occasionally, the surface of the testis can be felt in a lax hydrocoele.
- The testis is palpable through a varicocoele and if the patient is laid flat the scrotal contents feel normal.

Is the swelling transilluminable?

Placing a torch behind the swelling may cause the whole swelling to glow. This indicates the presence of clear fluid in the swelling, as occurs with hydrocoeles and epididymal cysts. Haematocoeles are not transilluminable.

INVESTIGATION OF PATIENTS WHO HAVE A SCROTAL SWELLING

An algorithm for the investigation and diagnosis of a scrotal swelling is given in Fig. 15.3.

Several basic investigations may be useful adjuncts to the clinical examination.

Urinalysis

This establishes the presence of any underlying urinary infection if there is epididymo-orchitis and can guide antibiotic therapy. It may also establish an infective cause for a secondary hydrocoele.

Ultrasonography

This is useful for examining the testis and epididymis. This is especially important if there is a hydrocoele or haematocoele, where the testis is not clearly palpable. It may establish a cause for a secondary hydrocoele.

Specialist ultrasound scanning with Doppler colour flow can establish whether the blood flow to the testis is normal and therefore help in the diagnosis of torsion (but see below).

β-Human chorionic gonadotrophin and α-fetoprotein, LDH.

These tumour markers may be increased in the presence of testicular tumour.

Operative exploration

The differential diagnosis of epididymo-orchitis and torsion can be very difficult clinically and even Doppler ultrasound is not a foolproof way to distinguish one from the other. It is therefore often wise to explore the acutely painful testis, especially in the young patient. Suspected torsion is a ‼ SURGICAL EMERGENCY ‼

‘A scar in the scrotum is better than only one testis in the scrotum’. If in doubt, explore a painful testis.

Fig. 15.3 Investigation and diagnosis of a scrotal swelling.

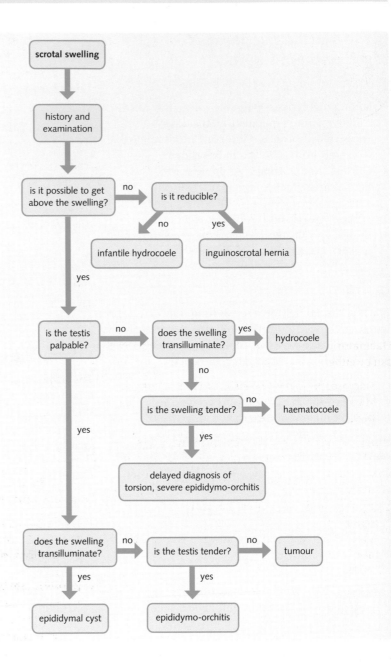

Haematuria

Learning objectives

You should be able to:

- Define haematuria.
- Recognize those pigments that may discolour the urine, mimicking haematuria.
- Give a differential diagnosis for haematuria originating in the different anatomical parts of the urinary tract.
- Understand the significance of the information gleaned from the palpation of the prostate rectally.
- List the radiological investigations available for the assessment of the urinary tract.

Haematuria is the passage of blood in the urine and can be either:

- Macroscopic ('frank')—visible to the naked eye.
- Microscopic—detectable only with urine testing sticks or microscope examination.

Other pigments, including drug therapies (e.g. co-danthramer) or vegetable pigments (e.g. beetroot), may discolour the urine, giving the appearance of haematuria. The urine dipstick also picks up myoglobin and may show a positive reaction in muscle trauma.

It is useful to think of the causes of haematuria in terms of anatomy (Fig. 16.1).

DIFFERENTIAL DIAGNOSIS OF HAEMATURIA

The differential diagnosis of haematuria is given in Fig. 16.2.

Never insert a suprapubic catheter into someone who has haematuria of undiagnosed cause. It may be due to a bladder tumour, which may be seeded into the abdominal wall by the catheter.

HISTORY TO FOCUS ON THE DIFFERENTIAL DIAGNOSIS OF HAEMATURIA

Pain

Painless haematuria is often associated with urothelial tumours of bladder, ureter or kidney.

The characteristics of pain associated with haematuria may suggest the diagnosis:

- Painful micturition indicates inflammation of the bladder or prostate.
- Colicky loin to groin pain is typical of a ureteric calculus.
- Burning pain in the penis or urethral opening in women is associated with urinary infection.
- Pain in the perineum associated with dysuria, fever and rigors is seen in prostatitis.
- Constant dull loin pain can be a sign of renal carcinoma.

Clots

Spindle-shaped clots are usually seen in renal bleeding (e.g. due to renal carcinoma).

Large clots in the urine indicate bladder pathology.

Drug history

Oral anticoagulants are an important cause of haematuria:

Fig. 16.1 (A) An intravenous urogram showing right hydronephrosis and hydroureter. (B) An intravenous urogram showing a filling defect in the left lower ureter (arrow) due to ureteric carcinoma.

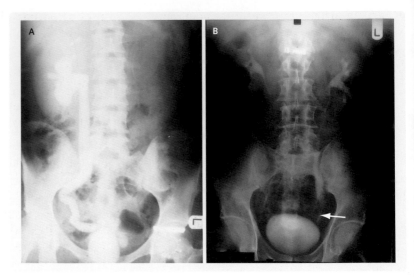

Fig. 16.2 Differential diagnosis of surgical causes of haematuria

System involved	Pathology
kidney	calculus, adenocarcinoma, transitional cell carcinoma, pyelonephritis and trauma
ureter	ureteric calculus and transitional cell carcinoma
bladder	transitional cell carcinoma, cystitis and calculus
prostate and urethra	prostatitis and trauma

infection
exercise - induced
GN, SLE
warfarin, NSAIDs, coagulop.

- Minor bleeding may become quite frank haematuria when the patient takes warfarin.
- Overanticoagulation can present with frank haematuria.

EXAMINATION OF PATIENTS WHO HAVE HAEMATURIA

Abdominal examination

The examination includes a general abdominal examination, but specific features should be looked for.

Bladder

It is unusual for a bladder tumour to be large enough to palpate abdominally, but the bladder itself may be palpable secondary to urinary retention due to infection or clot retention obstructing urinary flow.

Vaginal examination in women may reveal a pelvic mass arising from the bladder or reproductive organs. Before attempting a vaginal examination on a patient who has presented with haematuria, explain the relevance of the examination to the patient as the patient may think it inappropriate otherwise. For example one might say 'The posterior aspect of the bladder is palpable through the vaginal examination and I would like to perform this if you agree'.

Renal mass

Renal tumours may be palpable on bimanual examination and ballottement.

Rectal examination

The prostate is easily palpable on rectal examination:

- An exquisitely tender prostate is a feature of prostatitis.

PR, US, IVP, U+E, FBP, coag, XR KUB, cystoscopy.

- In perineal trauma where the membranous urethra has been ruptured, the prostate rides high.
- A smooth enlarged prostate is benign.
- A hard craggy prostate is probably malignant.

INVESTIGATION OF PATIENTS WHO HAVE HAEMATURIA

An algorithm for the investigation and diagnosis of haematuria is given in Fig. 16.3.

Urine dipstick

This will show minute traces of blood in the urine. It will also indicate the presence of protein and nitrites from bacterial breakdown of urea, suggesting infection.

Microscopy and culture

Microscopy will confirm the presence of red blood cells, white cells and organisms in infection. Culture of the urine will confirm the identity of the organism and help to identify the antibiotic sensitivity.

Urine cytology

Urothelial tumours will shed cells into the urine that can be seen on staining and microscopy.

Early morning specimens of urine (EMUs) have a higher yield of cells and so patients should be asked to provide the first specimen of the day for cytology.

Blood tests

Full blood count

This may reveal:

- Anaemia in severe haematuria.
- Polycythaemia in renal carcinoma (due to erythropoietin secretion).

Urea and electrolytes

These will indicate any degree of renal failure. Remember that renal failure will not occur until 60% of kidney function is lost, and therefore normal urea and creatinine levels do not indicate that there is no renal damage.

Plain radiography and contrast studies

Approximately 90% of kidney stones are radio-opaque and will show up on a plain abdominal film ('KUB' is used to refer to a plain film showing the kidneys, ureter and bladder.)

Radiolucent and radio-opaque stones will show up on an intravenous urogram (IVU), which will reveal delayed excretion or dilatation of collecting systems and indicate the level of any obstruction.

Ultrasonography

Evaluation of the upper renal tracts is necessary in all patients with microscopic and macroscopic

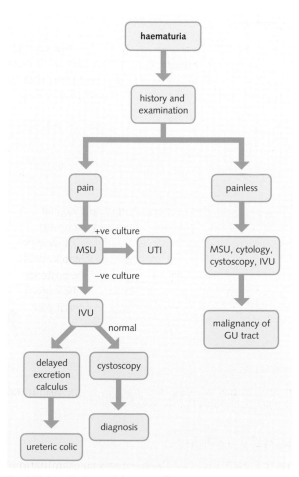

Fig. 16.3 Investigation and diagnosis of haematuria. (GU, genitourinary; IVU, intravenous urogram; MSU, midstream urine; UTI, urinary tract infection.)

haematuria. An ultrasound scan with a KUB radiograph is now preferred instead of an IVU in the initial investigation of the upper urinary tracts.

Ultrasound scans show:

- Dilatation of the collecting systems.
- Intrarenal pathology such as tumours or stones.

Computed tomography

Computed tomography (CT) is used for the evaluation and staging of urological malignancies. Another role is in the assessment of patients with renal trauma. CT urograms are also being used to diagnose renal tract obstruction.

Cystoscopy and biopsy

Direct examination of the urethra and bladder can reveal the pathology causing haematuria, such as a bladder tumour.

Retrograde contrast studies of the ureters can also be performed by cystoscopic insertion of ureteric catheters. Such investigations can reveal small urothelial tumours of the ureters.

Persistent haematuria with a normal initial assessment requires a nephrology opinion to exclude renal parenchymal disease.
GN

Urinary difficulty

Learning objectives

You should be able to:

- List the symptoms of obstructive urinary difficulty and those indicative of detrusor instability.
- Name a common drug that affects bladder emptying.
- Recognize when urethral cathelerization is contraindicated.
- Understand the importance of the neurological examination when assessing a patient with urinary retention.
- Define the investigation of 'urodynamics'.

Urinary difficulty is a very common problem in the ageing population and may be tolerated as part of 'old age' by many for several years before seeking medical help. Often the patient does not present until he or she (most people who have urinary difficulty are male) cannot pass urine at all (i.e. they have urinary retention).

Chronic urinary retention, where the bladder has not emptied completely for a long time, can cause renal failure.

DIFFERENTIAL DIAGNOSIS OF URINARY DIFFICULTY

The differential diagnosis of urinary difficulty is given in Fig. 17.1.

HISTORY TO FOCUS ON THE DIFFERENTIAL DIAGNOSIS OF URINARY DIFFICULTY

Symptoms

The symptoms of urinary difficulty can be broadly split into obstructive and instability symptoms:

- Obstructive symptoms are hesitancy, poor stream, postmicturition dribbling and a sensation of incomplete voiding.

- Detrusor instability symptoms are urgency, urge incontinence, frequency and nocturia.

Often these symptoms are mixed in obstructive disease because chronic obstruction leads to detrusor hypertrophy and instability. Further history should then be obtained to find the cause of the pathology.

Nocturia is the most reliable symptom of urinary difficulty as the patient can accurately remember the number of times they get up during the night.

Penile discharge

Urethritis is often associated with stricture formation (gonorrhoea in particular causes stricture in the bulbous urethra after infection of the periurethral glands) and subsequent micturition problems.

The passage of frank blood through the urethra following perineal trauma is suggestive of urethral injury.

Backache

A history of unrelenting back pain or 'sciatica' may be indicative of metastatic deposits in the spine, as may be seen in prostatic carcinoma. It may also predate

Fig. 17.1 Differential diagnosis of urinary difficulty

System involved	Pathology
prostate	benign prostatic hypertrophy and prostate cancer
bladder neck and urethra	primary or secondary (e.g. due to stricture, carcinoma, calculus)
pelvic mass	uterine and ovarian masses
vaginal wall	cystocoele (due to anterior vaginal wall collapse)
neurological causes	Guillain–Barré syndrome, diabetes mellitus, chronic alcoholism and cauda equina syndrome
colon	constipation

neurological urinary difficulty in cauda equina syndrome.

Radiotherapy

Previous radiotherapy (e.g. for a rectal tumour) can lead to a radiation cystitis.

Instrumentation

Damage from instrumentation may have occurred at a previous operation to the bladder or prostate or result from a traumatic catheterization or self-inflicted trauma.

Trauma

Low back injury may cause compression of the sacral roots, causing cauda equina syndrome.

A history of a fall astride a bar or pole should alert the clinician to the possibility of membranous urethral injury. Any patient who has such a history leading to retention should not be catheterized urethrally. Specialist investigation should be performed under the supervision of the urology team (see below).

Drug history

Any drug that has anticholinergic side effects will affect bladder emptying, the most common drugs being tricyclic antidepressants and pro-pantheline.

EXAMINATION OF PATIENTS WHO HAVE URINARY DIFFICULTY

General examination

Long-standing urinary difficulties can interfere with renal function and such patients may be uraemic. The clinician should look for:

- Anaemia.
- A lemon tinge to the skin.
- Furred tongue.
- Uraemic smell.

Abdominal examination

The most obvious feature in obstructive urinary problems is bladder distension. The bladder may be palpated as a smooth mass arising out of the pelvis that is dull to percussion. Renal enlargement may be present in long-standing obstructive uropathy.

Digital rectal examination

The prostate is easily felt through the rectal mucosa and its character should be noted.

Benign features include smoothness and firmness, with preservation of the median sulcus.

Malignant characteristics include:

- A hard craggy gland.
- A discrete hard nodule.
- Loss of the median sulcus.
- Fixity or erosion through rectal mucosa.

In benign prostatic hypertrophy, the actual size of the prostate and the severity of the symptoms are unrelated.

Vaginal examination

This should be performed in women to exclude a pelvic mass.

Neurological examination

If there is any history of back injury or pain, a neurological examination of the lower limbs and perineum should be performed to elicit any deficit, especially in the sacral dermatomes. A deficit in this distribution may suggest cauda equina syndrome or cord compression.

INVESTIGATION OF PATIENTS WHO HAVE URINARY DIFFICULTY

An algorithm for the investigation and diagnosis of urinary difficulty is given in Fig. 17.2.

Urine dipstick, culture and microscopy

Urine should be sent for analysis to rule out infective causes. Cytology may also be useful (see Chapter 16).

Blood tests

Full blood count

This may show anaemia associated with chronic renal failure. An increased white cell count can indicate underlying infection.

Urea and electrolytes

These are measured to assess renal function.

Prostate-specific antigen

This may be increased in prostatic carcinoma, but can also be falsely increased in prostatitis or after urethral catheterization.

Flow rate

This is a simple test to measure the flow of urine. Obstructive pathology causes a low flow rate and prolonged voiding time. A poor flow rate may be due to passage of a small volume of urine. The patient must pass over 100 mL of urine to obtain an accurate flow-rate recording.

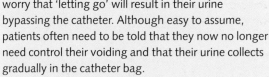

After urethral catheterization, the patient may need further reassurance. Patients often worry that 'letting go' will result in their urine bypassing the catheter. Although easy to assume, patients often need to be told that they now no longer need control their voiding and that their urine collects gradually in the catheter bag.

Urodynamics

This usually incorporates a flow test as above, but also measures bladder pressures using a special catheter. It can demonstrate bladder instability and hypersensitive bladders.

Radiography

Plain abdominal radiography—a KUB view (i.e. showing kidneys, ureters and bladder)—can show urinary calculi.

A contrast study (intravenous urography) may show:

- Renal tract dilatation.
- A prostatic impression on the cystogram phase.
- Trabeculation of the bladder wall.
- Postmicturition residual urine.
- Radiolucent stones.

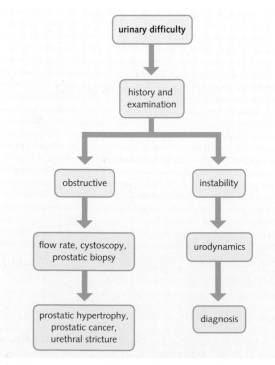

Fig. 17.2 Investigation and diagnosis of urinary difficulty.

Ultrasonography

As well as showing renal tract dilatation, ultrasound may also demonstrate the prostate, bladder wall thickening and residual urine volume.

Cystoscopy

This is the best investigation to show obstructive lesions of the urethra, prostate and bladder neck.

Ascending urethrography

Where there has been a fall astride an object and urethral damage is a possibility, water-soluble contrast may be gently injected into the urethra under fluoroscopic surveillance to ensure that there is no urethral injury before catheterization.

Learning objectives

You should be able to:

- List the symptoms and signs that suggest malignancy when associated with a skin lesion.
- Recognize the difference in the ulcer edges of a basal cell and a squamous cell carcinoma.
- Name common benign skin lesions and recognize their characteristic examination features.

Skin lesions are a common presentation in surgical outpatients. They can range from being non-significant to being life-threatening. It is therefore of paramount importance to be able to distinguish between these lesions.

It is helpful to consider the lesions in terms of anatomical layers.

DIFFERENTIAL DIAGNOSIS OF A SKIN LESION

The differential diagnosis of a skin lesion is given in Fig. 18.1.

HISTORY TO FOCUS ON THE DIFFERENTIAL DIAGNOSIS OF A SKIN LESION

How was it discovered?

Many skin lumps are noted while washing and may have been present for some time. There may be a history of local penetrating trauma preceding the lump, alerting the clinician to the possibility of a foreign body. The lump may have presented because of pain.

Duration and development of symptoms

The duration of a lump may provide some clues about its nature:

- A lump that has been present for years is more likely to be a benign condition.
- A rapidly growing lesion of short duration is more suggestive of a malignant lesion.
- Cystic lesions can grow rapidly and cause pain if they become infected.

When trying to assess level of sun exposure when a lesion is suspicious of a melanoma, it is often more useful to ask about destinations of previous holidays and occupational history. *rem: outdoor jobs.*

Change in size and shape

How a lump changes over time may also be helpful in diagnosis. A rapidly growing lesion may ulcerate through the skin. Rapid change may also be a feature of malignancy.

Itching and bleeding

These are both worrying symptoms in a pigmented lesion and are often associated with malignancy, especially malignant melanoma.

Previous lesions

The patient may have had previous lesions excised. This is of particular importance in malignant melanoma.

Fig. 18.1 Differential diagnosis of a skin lesion

System involved	Pathology
ulcers	arterial, venous, vasculitic, pressure, malignant and neuropathic
in the skin	melanoma, benign naevus, viral wart, seborrhoeic keratosis, pyogenic granuloma, neurofibroma, strawberry naevus, telangiectasia, dermoid cyst, sebaceous cyst, keloid and hypertrophic scar
under the skin	lipoma, implantation dermoid arteriovenous malformation, ganglion, lymph node and bursa cyst.

Characteristics that suggest malignancy:
- Rapid growth.
- Ulceration.
- Colour change.
- Itching.
- Bleeding.
- Halo of pigmentation.
- Satellite nodules.
- Metastases.

EXAMINATION OF PATIENTS WHO HAVE A SKIN LESION

Lump

Position, size, shape, colour, texture, edge and composition of the lesion should be recorded (see Chapter 40).

Specific features may be elicited, as outlined below.

Position

Most lesions can occur anywhere on the body, but some have a preponderance for certain areas of the body:
- Warts—most common on the palmar surface of the hands or on the feet (i.e. verruca).
- Seborrhoeic keratosis—not on areas subject to abrasion.
- Moles—more often on limbs.
- Malignant melanoma—limbs, head and neck.

- Strawberry naevus—usually head and neck.
- Hydradenitis suppurativa—axilla and groin.
- Basal cell carcinoma—upper one-third of the face and forehead.

Surface

Note the surface of the lesion:

- Smooth—any subcutaneous lesion, sebaceous cyst, dermoid cyst.
- Pearly—early basal cell carcinoma.
- Rough—viral wart, papilloma, seborrhoeic keratosis.

Lymph drainage

Lymph nodes may be enlarged in:

- Malignant melanoma—often infiltrated with tumour.
- Squamous cell carcinoma—two-thirds will be enlarged because of malignant infiltration, one-third will be enlarged because of secondary infection of the tumour.
- Pyogenic granuloma—local nodes are only enlarged if there is severe infection.

Local tissues

Melanoma may exhibit a depigmented halo or satellite nodules.

Squamous cell carcinoma may produce a thickened oedematous local reaction.

Special features

Some lesions have pathognomonic features:

- Seborrhoeic keratosis—can be picked off, leaving a pink patch of skin with a few capillary bleeding points only.

- Strawberry naevus—is compressible and the lesion can be completely emptied of blood, leaving a baggy patch of skin which gradually refills on releasing pressure.
- Arteriovenous malformation—may have a thrill or bruit and can be associated with a giant limb.
- Aneurysm—is pulsatile and expansile.

Ulcers

The edges of the ulcer are the most revealing feature of the underlying cause (Fig. 18.2).

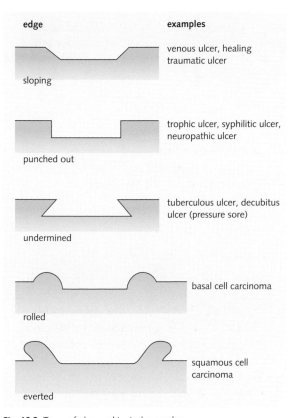

edge	examples
sloping	venous ulcer, healing traumatic ulcer
punched out	trophic ulcer, syphilitic ulcer, neuropathic ulcer
undermined	tuberculous ulcer, decubitus ulcer (pressure sore)
rolled	basal cell carcinoma
everted	squamous cell carcinoma

Fig. 18.2 Types of ulcer and typical examples.

INVESTIGATION OF PATIENTS WHO HAVE A SKIN LESION

An algorithm for the investigation and diagnosis of a skin lesion is given in Fig. 18.3.

Often the diagnosis is made from the history and examination.

Excision biopsy

whole lesion

The only investigation of importance is histology, and this is usually performed as an excision biopsy under local anaesthetic. Occasionally, incisional wedge biopsies are taken of large lesions and further treatment is planned when definitive histology is available.

Any suspicious skin lesion should be excised for precise histology.

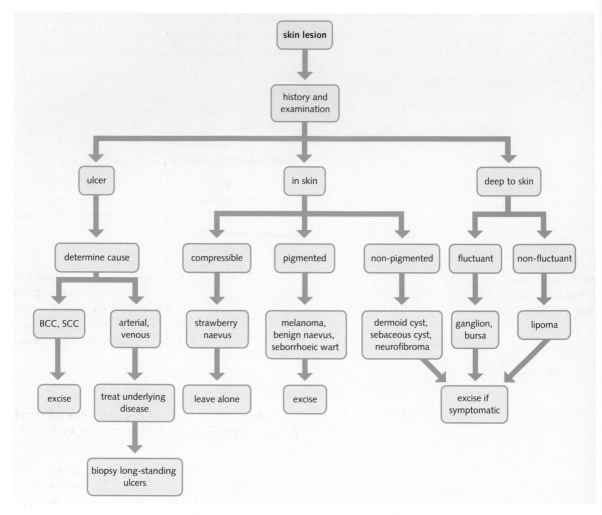

Fig. 18.3 Investigation and diagnosis of a skin lesion. (BCC, basal cell carcinoma; SCC, squamous cell carcinoma.)

You should be able to:

- Understand the classification of anaemia.
- Recognize the clinical signs that suggest anaemia.
- Understand the investigations that are appropriate in the investigation of the different types of anaemia.

Anaemia results from many chronic diseases. In this chapter, we will be concerned only with the causes of anaemia that are relevant to the general surgeon.

DIFFERENTIAL DIAGNOSIS OF ANAEMIA

The differential diagnosis of anaemia is given in Fig. 19.1.

Anaemia is a symptom and not a diagnosis. The underlying cause should be found.

HISTORY TO FOCUS ON THE DIFFERENTIAL DIAGNOSIS OF ANAEMIA

Symptoms

The following symptoms are common for all causes of anaemia:

- Fatigue.
- Headaches.
- Lightheadedness. /dizzy
- Breathlessness (especially on effort).
- Angina.
- Intermittent claudication.
- Palpitations.

However, the severity of symptoms is related not only to the degree of anaemia, but also to its speed of onset. A slow, gradual anaemia will be well tolerated down to very low haemoglobin levels, but a rapid blood loss may produce some profound symptoms.

Gastrointestinal blood loss

A careful history about possible gastrointestinal loss of blood should be obtained. Symptoms include:

- Dyspepsia. ⁻ PUD
- Haematemesis—due to peptic ulceration, oesophagitis, gastric or oesophageal cancer.
- Melaena—due to peptic ulceration, oesophagitis, gastric or oesophageal cancer.
- Fresh rectal blood loss—due to carcinoma of the colon or rectum or inflammatory bowel disease.
- Change in bowel habit—due to carcinoma of the colon or rectum or inflammatory bowel disease.

These symptoms (especially the rectal blood loss) may be very mild but, over the long term can produce profound anaemia.

Common causes of asymptomatic blood loss from the gastrointestinal tract are peptic ulceration and caecal carcinoma.

Fig. 19.1 Differential diagnosis of anaemia

System involved	Pathology
microcytic hypochromic	blood loss from the gastrointestinal or genitourinary tracts and inadequate iron uptake or absorption
normochromic	feature of chronic disease (e.g. chronic renal failure, rheumatoid arthritis)
macrocytic	due to vitamin B_{12} or folate deficiency, pernicious anaemia (an autoimmune condition in which there are autoantibodies to gastric parietal cells or intrinsic factor and as a result vitamin B_{12} cannot be absorbed), anaemia following gastrectomy, anaemia in coeliac disease, anaemia following ileal resection for Crohn's disease involving the terminal ileum, anaemia due to chronic alcoholic liver disease

Menstrual history

A history of the following may be sufficient to cause chronic anaemia in premenopausal women:

- Heavy periods (menorrhagia).
- Intermenstrual bleeding.

Family history

A family history of various conditions may be very informative. Such conditions include:

- Coeliac disease.
- Familial polyposis coli and carcinoma of the colon.
- Bleeding diatheses.
- Haemoglobinopathies.

Drug history

Several drugs may lead to gastrointestinal blood loss, including:

- Non-steroidal anti-inflammatory drugs. NSAIDs
- Corticosteroids. warfarin
- Potassium supplements.

Drugs that cause bone marrow suppression include:

- Cytotoxic drugs

Other drugs cause anaemia by causing folate depletion. These drugs include phenytoin, primidone and methotrexate.

Alcohol

As well a being a risk factor for upper gastrointestinal haemorrhage, alcohol is also associated with chronic liver disease.

Travel

The commonest cause of anaemia worldwide is hookworm infestation of the gastrointestinal tract. Tropical sprue may be another acquired condition leading to anaemia.

EXAMINATION OF PATIENTS WHO HAVE ANAEMIA

General examination

The degree of anaemia can be estimated by looking at the colour of the conjunctivae and mucous membranes.

There may be signs of weight loss and cachexia associated with either malignancy or chronic inflammatory bowel disease.

Cardiovascular system

The following are features of anaemia of any cause:

- Rapid and bounding pulse.
- A systolic flow murmur.
- In severe anaemia, there may be a degree of heart failure.

Mouth

Pale mucous membranes are a non-specific sign of anaemia, but certain features in the mouth may be associated with specific causes:

- Smooth tongue—due to atrophy of papillae is seen in iron deficiency.
- Angular stomatitis—may be present with either iron deficiency or vitamin B_{12} deficiency.
- Glossitis—inflamed tongue seen in vitamin B_{12} deficiency and possibly also in iron deficiency

anaemia with dysphagia or as part of Plummer–Vinson syndrome.

- Telangiectasia on lips—associated with Osler–Weber–Rendu syndrome and pigmentation associated with Peutz–Jeghers syndrome.

Skin and adnexa

There may be skin pigmentation changes:

- Lemon-yellow tint in vitamin B_{12} deficiency.
- Vitiligo occurs in patients who have pernicious anaemia.

Hair and nails may be affected in iron deficiency anaemia, resulting in:

- Brittle hair.
- Brittle nails.
- Koilonychia—spoon-shaped nails.

Abdominal examination

Palpable features in the abdomen that may be associated with iron deficiency anaemia include:

- Tumour of large bowel—especially caecum.
- Fibroid uterus.
- Gastric carcinoma.
- Inflammatory mass due to Crohn's disease.

Examination of the abdomen should include rectal examination for rectal tumours and melaena stool, and a vaginal examination in women.

INVESTIGATION OF PATIENTS WHO HAVE ANAEMIA

An algorithm for the investigation and diagnosis of anaemia is given in Fig. 19.2.

It is important to test patients from the relevant ethnic groups for sickle and thalassaemia *Blacks* traits when investigating anaemia. These two conditions can also present with an acute abdomen secondary to a sickle crisis or splenomegaly. It is often useful to ask about patients' ethnic background, and specifically about their trait status as they may have been tested in the past.

Blood tests

Full blood count

This will tell the clinician the degree and type of anaemia by demonstrating whether it is a hypochromic, microcytic anaemia or macrocytic anaemia.

Reticulocyte count

This reflects the number of immature red cells being produced by the bone marrow. The reticulocyte count is increased in haemolytic anaemias.

Iron studies

Iron studies may help distinguish between iron deficiency and chronic disease anaemias:

- Serum iron level is low in both iron deficiency and anaemia of chronic disease.
- Total iron-binding capacity is increased in iron deficiency.
- Total iron-binding capacity is decreased in anaemia of chronic disease.
- Serum ferritin level is low in iron deficiency.

Serum vitamin B_{12} and red cell folate

These will be low in deficiency states.

Schilling test

This is a test to assess vitamin B_{12} absorption and distinguishes between pernicious anaemia and terminal ileal malabsorption. It is usually not performed in older patients as the most likely cause of B_{12} deficiency is pernicious anaemia. It is much more helpful in younger patients where the likely diagnosis is Crohn's disease.

Fecal occult blood test   *FOB.*

This is a simple test for blood in the feces. The presence of blood suggests that there may be a gastrointestinal source of bleeding, but the test is oversensitive so should be interpreted with caution.

Investigation of gastrointestinal haemorrhage

The upper and lower gastrointestinal tract should be investigated by endoscopy and radiological methods (see Chapters 3 and 6), such as:

Fig. 19.2 Investigation and diagnosis of anaemia.

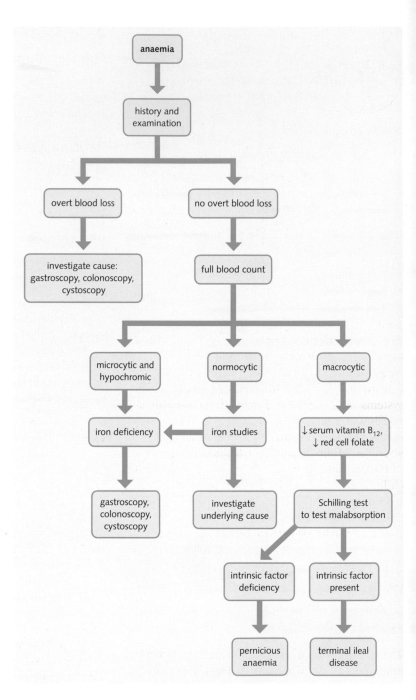

- Oesophagogastroduodenoscopy.
- Colonoscopy.
- Barium meal and follow-through.
- Barium enema.

Colposcopy and hysteroscopy

If there is suspected abnormal vaginal blood loss, the vagina and lining of the uterus should be inspected to look for carcinoma of the cervix or uterus or for causes of menorrhagia such as fibroids.

Midstream urine, intravenous urography and cystoscopy

If there is any blood in the urine, the urinary tract is investigated using intravenous urography and cystoscopy to look for renal carcinoma and urothelial tumours.

Learning objectives

You should be able to:

- Name common causes of abdominal pain in neonates, infants and children.
- Recognize the typical signs of pyloric stenosis and intussusception.
- Understand the signs that help differentiate between mesenteric adenitis and appendicitis.
- Appreciate the often non-specific signs of a sick child and the importance of early senior review.

Young children with acute lower abdominal pain frequently present as surgical emergencies. Assessing the child is difficult as they and their parents are frequently distressed. Young children are poor historians—they also have efficient cardiovascular systems and are therefore able to compensate late into serious illness. Experience is required to diagnose peritonitis and avoid deaths. Neonates and young children are usually admitted under the care of the paediatricians, who assess and resuscitate the child. The child is usually then referred to the surgeon if a surgical cause for the illness is suspected. Ideally, children under 5 years of age should be referred to a specialist paediatric surgical unit.

DIFFERENTIAL DIAGNOSIS OF ACUTE ABDOMINAL EMERGENCIES IN CHILDHOOD

The differential diagnosis of acute abdominal emergencies in children is given in Figs 20.1 and 20.2.

The correct diagnosis is difficult to make in young children. A senior doctor should therefore review the child early.

HISTORY TO FOCUS ON THE DIFFERENTIAL DIAGNOSIS OF ACUTE ABDOMINAL EMERGENCIES IN CHILDHOOD

Young children will be unable to give a history of pain.

A history of a fretful child crying and drawing up the legs is commonly obtained from the parents.

Young children are frequently reluctant to be examined. Kneeling and talking to them at their height helps an adult to appear less intimidating. Offering to perform the examination on a teddy or a doll before examining the child may also make them more cooperative.

Age

The age of the child will give an indication of the underlying pathology:

Fig. 20.1 Differential diagnosis of acute abdominal emergencies in early childhood

Paediatric surgical emergencies (by age)	Pathology
vomiting in infancy	pyloric stenosis, intussusception and malrotation
abdominal pain in childhood	appendicitis, obstructed inguinal hernia and torsion of the testis

Fig. 20.2 Differential diagnosis of medical causes of abdominal pain in early childhood

Medical causes of abdominal pain	Pathology
abdominal pain in childhood	urinary tract infection, mesenteric adenitis, constipation, gastroenteritis, colic, oesophagitis, gastritis, pneumonia and milk allergy

psychological

- Neonate—meconium ileus, atresia in a section of the gastrointestinal tract, pyloric stenosis.
- Infancy—intussusception, obstructed inguinal hernia, malrotation, constipation.
- Childhood—appendicitis, mesenteric adenitis, urinary tract infection, torsion of the testis.

Site

Most young children are unable to localize abdominal pain. Young children with appendicitis tend to present late, with 75% of them found to have a perforated appendix at surgery.

Vomiting

In pyloric stenosis, the baby (usually male) will present at 4–6 weeks after birth with projectile vomiting. The parents may report a visible mass in the right upper quadrant, with the child eager to re-feed after vomiting. The vomitus contains milk and no bile. The condition is due to hypertrophy of the pyloric muscle.

Bilious vomiting suggests bowel obstruction or intussusception. The passage of blood and mucus per rectum (redcurrant jelly stool) increases the suspicion of intussusception.

EXAMINATION OF ACUTE ABDOMINAL EMERGENCIES IN CHILDHOOD

General examination

Physical signs are often lacking. Check for signs of dehydration (e.g. restlessness or lethargy), reduced tissue elasticity and dry mucous membranes.

Vital signs

These are usually preserved until late in the illness. A child with mesenteric adenitis often has a pyrexia of 38°C but looks well and is often running around, whereas a child with appendicitis looks unwell, may have a pyrexia of 38°C and is lethargic.

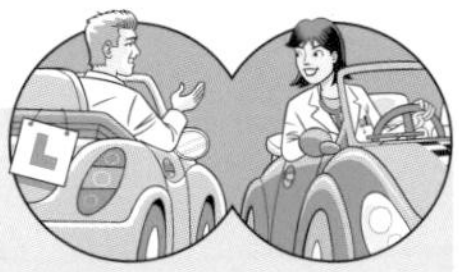

Parents of a sick child are very anxious. Remember to reassure them regularly. Commenting that they did the right thing to bring the child to the surgery or the hospital is often very reassuring because parents often agonize over this decision.

Abdominal examination

A young child with peritonitis may just present as a sick child with few abdominal signs. The omentum is poorly developed in young children, which probably accounts for the high rate of complicated perforated appendicitis in this group. A child with mesenteric adenitis has tenderness in the right iliac fossa but no peritonism.

A palpable lump in the groin leads to the suspicion of inguinal hernia. It is important to question the parents, who may have observed an obvious swelling that has now disappeared. Remember to check the scrotum for a testis on each side. The lump may represent a retractile or undescended testis. A torted testis may present with vomiting and suprapubic pain. The testis usually lies horizontally and is exquisitely tender.

INVESTIGATION OF ACUTE ABDOMINAL EMERGENCIES IN CHILDHOOD

An algorithm for the investigation and diagnosis of acute abdominal emergencies in childhood is given in Fig. 20.3.

Blood tests

Full blood count

This should be requested with a differential white cell count.

- High haemoglobin and haematocrit are seen in dehydration.
- Low haemoglobin can be due to haemolysis in the neonate.
- An increased white cell count is seen in infective conditions. A neutrophilia is seen in bacterial infections.

Blood glucose

The infected starved child is at risk of hypoglycaemia.

Urea and electrolytes

These are measured to assess renal function and dehydration.

Liver function tests

An elevated bilirubin may be due to:

- Infection (e.g. urinary tract infection).
- Poor fluid intake.

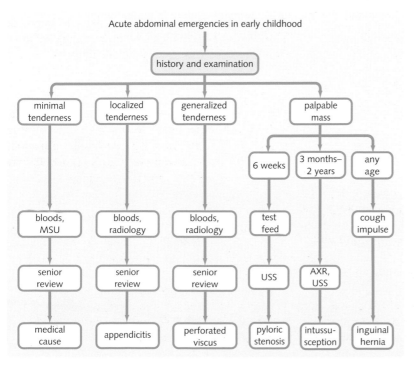

Fig. 20.3 Investigation and diagnosis of acute abdominal emergencies in childhood. (AXR, abdominal radiograph; MSU, midstream urine; USS, ultrasound scan.)

- Haemolysis.
- High gastrointestinal obstruction.

Acute-phase reactants

C-reactive protein is a marker of acute inflammation but is non-specific.

Blood gases

Analysis using a capillary technique can reveal acidosis, alkalosis and hypoxia.

Urine *Always test the urine*

A midstream urine should be tested with a dipstick and the sample should then be sent for urgent microscopy and culture. In children in nappies, urine can be collected by a 'clean catch' into a sterile pot, or into an adhesive plastic bag. Suprapubic aspiration is the method of choice in the severely ill infant under 1 year old requiring urgent diagnosis and treatment.

Microbiology cultures

If septicaemia is suspected, cultures of blood, cerebrospinal fluid and suspected infected sites should be undertaken.

Radiology

Chest radiography

A chest radiograph may show signs of pneumonia.

Abdominal radiology

Plain abdominal radiography may show:
- Dilated loops of bowel (e.g. obstructed hernia) or intussusception.
- Gasless appearance (e.g. volvulus due to malrotation).
- Fecolith (e.g. appendicitis).

50% of children under 2 years of age with appendicitis will have a visible fecolith on plain abdominal radiograph.

Ultrasonography

This may demonstrate:
- Pyloric muscle hypertrophy in pyloric stenosis.
- Free fluid or collections associated with appendicitis.
- Hydronephrosis in pelviureteric junction obstruction.
- A mass in intussusception if not obscured by bowel gas.
- Inguinal hernia.

Contrast studies

These should be performed in suspected malrotation. They will typically show an abnormally placed duodenojejunal flexure, with small intestinal loops located on the right side of the abdomen.

If intussusception is suspected and there is no peritonitis, a contrast enema will confirm the diagnosis and result in reduction in 80% of cases.

Computed tomography

Computed tomography (CT) is performed if a surgical diagnosis is suspected and cannot be identified by other means.

DISEASE AND DISORDERS

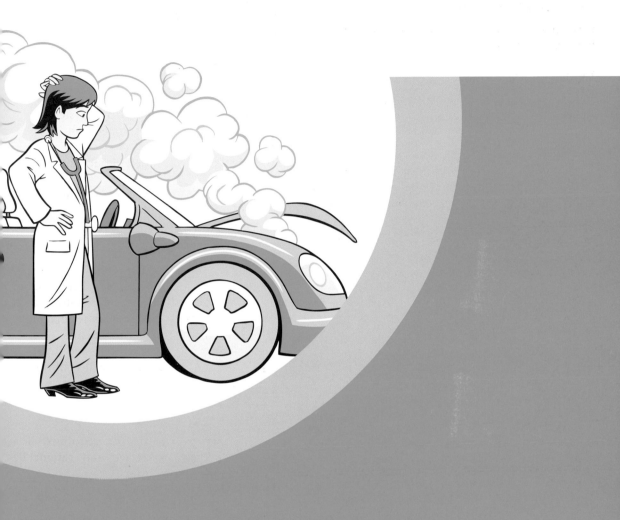

Oesophageal disorders

Learning objectives

You should be able to:

- Describe the normal mechanism that prevents reflux of gastric contents into the oesophagus.
- Define a hiatus hernia and the different types.
- Understand the medical and surgical treatment options in gastro-oesophageal reflux disease (GORD).
- Define the predisposing factors for oesophageal cancer.
- Describe the treatment of squamous cell carcinoma of the oesophagus.
- Name the classic appearance of achalasia on barium swallow.
- Understand the clinical signs of a perforation of the oesophagus.

The oesophagus extends from the pharynx to the gastric cardia and measures 25–30 cm in length. It has an upper sphincter, the cricopharyngeus, which is at the level of the sixth cervical vertebra, and a lower sphincter derived from the inner circular muscle fibres of the oesophagus (40 cm from the incisors on endoscopy). The mucosal lining is squamous epithelium, except for the lowest 2 cm, which is columnar epithelium.

The commonest symptoms of oesophageal disease are reflux and dysphagia.

GASTRO-OESOPHAGEAL REFLUX

Background

Normally, reflux of gastric contents is prevented by:

- The lower oesophageal sphincter.
- The angle of His.
- Crural fibres of the diaphragm.
- The prominent mucosal folds, which act as a plug.
- Positive intra-abdominal pressure acting on the lower oesophagus maintaining a high-pressure zone.

If these mechanisms fail or there is a hiatus hernia (i.e. a weakness in the diaphragm, which allows the stomach into the chest), either a sliding hiatus hernia or a paraoesophageal hernia, then the gastric contents can reflux into the oesophagus, causing oesophagitis (Fig. 21.1).

Clinical presentation

The symptoms of reflux are:

- Retrosternal pain exacerbated by bending over or lying down.
- Regurgitation of acid into the mouth.
- Dysphagia if a stricture develops.

Complications of reflux are:

- Oesophagitis—ulceration of the oesophageal mucosa ranging from mild to severe.
- Barrett's oesophagus—this is metaplastic change of the columnar epithelium to squamous epithelium and may progress to dysplasia and malignant change.
- Barrett's ulcer—this can bleed or perforate.
- Iron deficiency anaemia—chronic blood loss from severe oesophagitis.
- Stricture—when oesophagitis heals it can develop into a fibrotic stricture, which causes dysphagia.
- Oesophageal cancer—this can develop in a long segment of Barrett's mucosa with dysplasia.

Fig. 21.1 Symptoms and complications of sliding and rolling hiatus hernias.

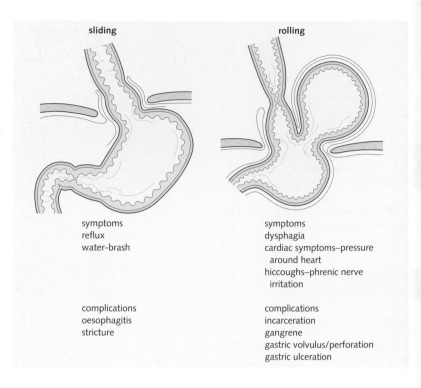

sliding

symptoms
reflux
water-brash

complications
oesophagitis
stricture

rolling

symptoms
dysphagia
cardiac symptoms–pressure
  around heart
hiccoughs–phrenic nerve
  irritation

complications
incarceration
gangrene
gastric volvulus/perforation
gastric ulceration

Management

Investigations include:

- Barium swallow—defines the anatomy of a hiatus hernia or stricture.
- Endoscopy and biopsy—direct visualization of damaged mucosa.
- pH monitoring and manometry—24-hour monitoring of pH and pressure.

Patients who have symptoms of reflux are given simple advice to avoid situations that exacerbate symptoms (i.e. sleep propped up, weight reduction, stop smoking, decrease intake of alcohol, caffeine and spicy foods).

Medical treatment includes antacids and alginates, which provide a protective barrier against the gastric contents (Fig. 21.2).

- Gastric acid production can be decreased by histamine H_2 antagonists or proton pump inhibitors.
- Prokinetic drugs can increase the oesophageal motility and the tone of the sphincter.

Most people respond to medical treatment, but if there are any complications or the patient is young then surgical treatment is appropriate.

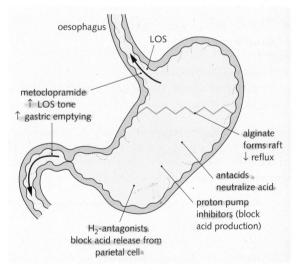

oesophagus

LOS

metoclopramide
↑ LOS tone
↑ gastric emptying

alginate
forms raft
↓ reflux

antacids
neutralize acid

proton pump
inhibitors (block
acid production)

H_2-antagonists
block acid release from
parietal cell

Fig. 21.2 Sites of action of drugs used to treat gastro-oesophageal reflux disease. (LOS, lower oesophageal sphincter.)

If the patient has a stricture it is dilated endoscopically by bougies and then a fundoplication can be performed laparoscopically or by open operation. The hiatus hernia is reduced and the fundus of the stomach is wrapped around the lower oesophagus, and this increases the pressure to prevent reflux.

Patients who have a benign oesophageal stricture usually have a past history of gastro-oesophageal reflux.

BENIGN TUMOURS OF THE OESOPHAGUS

These are unusual, but the commonest is a leiomyoma, which causes dysphagia and can be removed from the submucosa to relieve symptoms.

OESOPHAGEAL CANCER

Background

Carcinoma is increasingly common in the western world. It is more common in men, the male to female ratio being 3 to 1, and patients are usually over 50 years of age. There is a high incidence in China and South Africa.

Predisposing factors are:

- Barrett's oesophagus with dysplasia.
- Corrosive oesophagitis.
- Achalasia. *Tylosis*
- Plummer–Vinson syndrome. *P-K-B syndr.*
- Environmental factors, including smoking, alcohol and dietary nitrosamines. *vit-defic.*

Carcinomas of the upper and middle thirds of the oesophagus are squamous cell carcinomas and those of the lower third are adenocarcinomas. The tumours spread locally and via the lymphatics and bloodstream.

Clinical presentation

The presenting symptoms include progressive dysphagia, iron deficiency anaemia and weight loss (because many cases present late). *Chest pain, dyspepsia.*

Management

Diagnosis and assessment of oesophageal cancer is made by:

- Barium swallow—enables assessment of the position and length of the stricture (Fig. 21.3).
- Endoscopy and biopsy—defines the histological type of tumour.

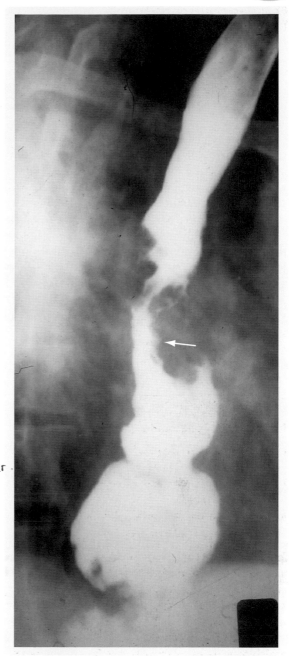

Fig. 21.3 Barium swallow showing oesophageal cancer (arrow).

- Endoscopic ultrasonography *US.*—provides accurate assessment of paraoesophageal disease and operability.
- Computed tomography (CT) scan of the chest and liver—to stage the tumour and assess any metastases.
- Bronchoscopy—may be performed if bronchial involvement is suspected.

• PET•

Accurate assessment helps to plan treatment. If the tumour is operable and the patient is fit for a major thoracoabdominal operation then oesophageal resection with gastric or colonic interposition is the best symptomatic treatment. Neoadjuvant chemotherapy (i.e. chemotherapy before the operation) increases the survival of patients compared to those who have surgery only.

Many oesophageal carcinomas are inoperable, so treatment is palliative. A squamous cell carcinoma of the upper and middle thirds will respond to radiotherapy. All tumours can be intubated with plastic or metal stents, and lasers can be used to destroy the tumour to give some relief of dysphagia. Palliative chemotherapy and radiotherapy improve dysphagia. Intraluminal radiotherapy (brachytherapy) has fewer side effects than external beam radiotherapy and provides good palliation.

The prognosis is very poor. After resection, the 5-year survival is 15% but, overall, the 5-year survival is only 4%. *10% 5yr surviv.*

> Carcinoma of the lower one-third of the oesophagus is usually adenocarcinoma and the rest are squamous cell carcinomas.

ACHALASIA

Background

This condition is due to degeneration of the myenteric nerve plexus so that there is a failure of peristalsis and failure of relaxation of the lower oesophageal sphincter. It can present at any age, but usually between 30 and 60 years of age. It is more common in women, the male to female ratio being 2 to 3, and there is a risk of malignancy in the long term.

Clinical presentation

The usual symptoms are progressive dysphagia, weight loss and aspiration pneumonia.

> In achalasia regurgitation occurs on lying flat and is effortless.

Management

The diagnosis is made by:

- Chest radiography *CxR*—may show a grossly dilated oesophagus with a fluid level and signs of aspiration pneumonia.
- Barium swallow—this will show a grossly dilated, tortuous oesophagus with a very narrow segment – 'rat tail' – at the lower oesophageal sphincter (Fig. 21.4). *birds-beak on Barium*
- Manometry—this will demonstrate failure of relaxation of the sphincter.
- Endoscopy and biopsy—to detect malignant change.

Medical treatment is usually ineffective.

Pneumatic dilatation of the sphincter may give temporary relief, but operation (Heller's cardiomyotomy, which divides the lower oesophageal sphincter to the level of the mucosa) provides the best results.

Other motility disorders can produce dysphagia and retrosternal pain, which may simulate a myocardial infarction. Assessment includes a barium swallow and manometry, which will show the typical pattern of oesophageal contractions. These may be diffuse and uncoordinated or produce a corkscrew oesophagus (i.e. high-amplitude wave; Fig. 22.5). Therapy with long-acting nitrates and calcium channel blockers may be beneficial.

PHARYNGEAL POUCH

Background

Pharyngeal pouch (Fig. 21.6) is a condition of elderly people and it is more common in men than women. It is due to a mucosal protrusion between the parts of the inferior pharyngeal constrictor—the thyropharyngeus and the cricopharyngeus (i.e. Killian's dehiscence). It is thought to occur because of increased pressure developing when the upper oesophageal sphincter fails to relax.

Clinical presentation

The symptoms of a pharyngeal pouch are those of dysphagia, but with a characteristic 'double swallow' when the pouch empties. There may be a visible swelling in the neck. Regurgitation of the contents of the pouch may produce halitosis or recurrent aspiration pneumonia.

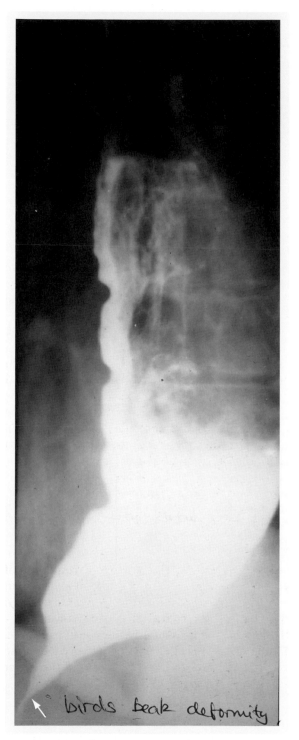

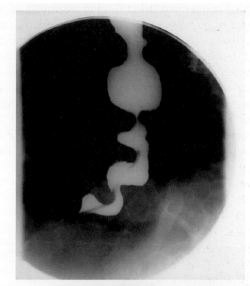

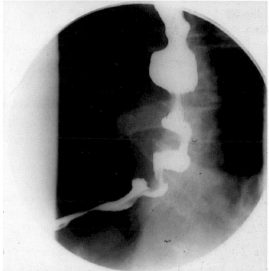

Fig. 21.5 Barium swallow showing typical contractions of a corkscrew oesophagus.

A double swallow is characteristic of a pharyngeal pouch.

birds beak deformity

Fig. 21.4 Barium swallow showing achalasia. The oesophagus is dilated and there is a 'rat-tail' segment (arrow) at the lower oesophageal sphincter.

Management

The diagnosis is made by the classic appearance of the pouch on a barium swallow.

Treatment can be an operative excision of the pouch with a myotomy of the cricopharyngeus.

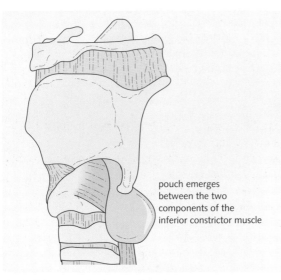

pouch emerges
between the two
components of the
inferior constrictor muscle

Fig. 21.6 Anatomy of a pharyngeal pouch.

However, as the majority of patients with this diagnosis are elderly and frail, endoscopic stapling diverticulotomy is the procedure now most commonly carried out to treat this condition.

PLUMMER–VINSON SYNDROME

This occurs in middle-aged and elderly females. The syndrome consists of dysphagia and iron deficiency anaemia. The dysphagia is associated with hyperkeratinization of the oesophagus with formation of a web in the upper part. The condition is premalignant.

SURGICAL EMERGENCY !

Perforation of the oesophagus

Background
This can occur:
- As a result of swallowing a foreign body.
- During oesophagoscopy and dilatation, especially if there is a malignant stricture.
- Spontaneously, as a result of violent vomiting.

Clinical presentation
The symptoms are sudden onset of pain in the neck, chest and abdomen. The patient may develop circulatory collapse, pyrexia and surgical emphysema in the supraclavicular region of the neck.

Management
Oesophageal perforation is a surgical emergency. The complication of mediastinitis has a very high mortality rate.
A chest radiograph may show mediastinal air, a pneumothorax, or fluid in the pleural cavity. A barium swallow confirms the site of rupture. If the underlying problem is benign then surgical treatment is performed to resect or repair the damaged oesophagus. If the problem is due to malignancy and the patient is unfit for a major operation, the patient is kept nil by mouth and intravenous fluids, antibiotics and parenteral nutrition are prescribed. A chest drain is inserted.

Suspect oesophageal perforation if a patient presents with surgical emphysema in the neck with a history of vomiting.

Further reading

Bennet G in Pounder R (ed.) 1994 *Oesophageal Disorders: Recent Advances in Gastroenterology.* Churchill Livingstone, Edinburgh

Griffin SM, Raimes SA (eds) 2005 *Oesophagogastric Surgery. A Companion to Specialist Surgical Practice*, 3rd edn. Elsevier Saunders, Philadelphia

Scottish Intercollegiate Guideline Network (SIGN) 2006 *Management of Oesophageal and Gastric Cancer.* http://www.sign.ac.uk

Moayyedi P, Talley NJ 2006 Gastro-oesophageal reflux disease. *Lancet* 24; **367**: 2086–2100

Watson A (ed.) 1984 *Disorders of the Oesophagus: Advances and Controversies.* Urban & Schwarzenberg, Wien

Yamada T (ed.) 2003 *Textbook of Gastroenterology*, 4th edn. Lippincott Williams & Wilkins, London

Gastric and duodenal disorders

Learning objectives

You should be able to:

- Name four locations in the gastrointestinal tract where peptic ulceration can occur.
- Describe the mechanism by which peptic ulceration occurs.
- Understand why peptic ulceration is associated with microcytic and macrocytic anaemia.
- Understand the treatment for *Helicobacter pylori*-positive gastritis.
- Understand how the diagnosis of Zollinger–Ellison syndrome is confirmed.
- Describe the symptoms and signs gastric cancer presents with.
- Describe the spread of gastric cancer.

The main function of the stomach is to act as a reservoir for ingested food. The upper part of the stomach is capable of adaptive relaxation to accommodate the food. The antrum acts as a mill and its contractions fulfil two functions:

- To churn the food into chyme.
- To deliver it in graduated amounts into the duodenum.

There is some digestion of the food by hydrochloric acid and pepsin.

Dyspepsia is a very common problem that is often treated by self-medication, but has several different causes, some of which are potentially serious.

PEPTIC ULCERATION

Background

There are several locations where ulceration can occur:

- Stomach.
- Duodenum.
- Oesophagus.
- Meckel's diverticulum in the terminal ileum.

Ulceration occurs where there is a breakdown in the mucosal defence mechanism, and may be associated with increased or inappropriate acid or pepsin secretion. Cytoprotective systems such as mucosal prostaglandin E_2 and mucosal bicarbonate secretion are both reduced in patients who have duodenal ulceration. These circumstances produce the right environment for the proteolytic enzyme pepsin to cause mucosal ulceration. There is also strong evidence for the involvement of the organism *Helicobacter pylori* in the aetiology of peptic ulceration. Other associations with peptic ulceration are:

- Smoking.
- Alcohol.
- Blood group O.
- Non-steroidal anti-inflammatory drugs (NSAIDs).
- Corticosteroids.
- Stress.
- Hyperparathyroidism.
- Zollinger–Ellison syndrome (i.e. gastrinoma).

COX-2 inhibitors have reduced gastric complications compared to traditional NSAIDs. They are, however, linked to an increase risk of thrombotic events (myocardial infarction and stroke) compared to traditional NSAIDs and are contraindicated in patients with ischaemic heart disease or cerebrovascular disease.

Classification of peptic ulceration

Peptic ulcers are classified into the following categories:

- Gastric ulcer type I—generally occurs on the lesser curve of the stomach.
- Gastric ulcer type II—occurs in the pyloric and prepyloric region and has the same features as duodenal ulcer.
- Duodenal ulcer—usually occurs in the first and second parts of the duodenum.

The features and presentation of gastric and duodenal ulcers are outlined in Fig. 22.1.

Complications of peptic ulceration

Complications associated with peptic ulceration are:

- Perforation—⟦ SURGICAL EMERGENCY ⟧ this will produce sudden onset of severe generalized abdominal pain.
- Haemorrhage—⟦ SURGICAL EMERGENCY ⟧ due to erosion of a vessel in the ulcer base causing haematemesis and melaena.
- Pyloric stenosis—when a duodenal or pyloric ulcer heals with scarring it can cause stenosis. The patient presents with progressive vomiting of undigested food, weight loss, dehydration and hypokalaemic hypochloraemic alkalosis.
- Malignancy—only associated with gastric ulcers (1% of cases).
- Iron deficiency anaemia—may be a presentation of peptic ulceration.

Management

Diagnosis is made by gastroscopy. Biopsies are taken to assess for gastritis, malignancy, or *H. pylori*

infection using the 'CLO test' (i.e. rapid urease test). Antibodies to *H. pylori* can be measured, but will reveal present and past infection.

Treatment of peptic ulcers is as follows:

- Duodenal ulcers associated with *H. pylori* are treated with triple therapy (i.e. proton pump inhibitor for 6 weeks and amoxycillin and metronidazole for 1 week). Treatment produces 80% eradication of infection and healing of ulcer.
- Peptic ulcers not associated with *H. pylori* are treated with either H_2-antagonists or proton pump inhibitors, which heal 90% of ulcers after 6–8 weeks of treatment.
- Elective operation for duodenal ulceration is rarely required since the introduction of proton pump inhibitors but, if operation is required, a highly selective vagotomy is performed. An operation may be required if a gastric ulcer fails to heal, and this usually means a partial gastrectomy (i.e. excision of ulcer and antrum and restoration of gastroduodenal continuity).

Operations are required for the complications of peptic ulcers. These often occur in the elderly population and complications include:

- Perforation.
- Bleeding.
- Pyloric stenosis.

Diagnosis of perforation is made from a history of acute abdominal pain, signs of peritonitis and free gas under the diaphragm on a chest radiograph. At laparotomy the perforation is oversewn with an omental patch. A gastric ulcer should be biopsied to exclude malignancy.

Fig. 22.1 Clinical features of gastric and duodenal ulcers (f, female; m, male)

Feature	Duodenal ulcer	Gastric ulcer
age	30–60 years	usually 50 years
sex	m > f	m:f = 1:1
epigastric pain	worse at night	worse after food
associated features	relieved by food and antacids	vomiting and reflux, iron deficiency anaemia
periodic pain	yes—attacks last 4–5 days followed by relief for a few weeks	no periodicity

A diagnosis of bleeding is made at endoscopy and it may be possible to stop the bleeding by injecting the vessel with adrenaline or coagulating the vessel with diathermy or a laser. If the bleeding recurs or continues, the patient requires an emergency operation to underrun the vessel. If it is a duodenal ulcer, this may occasionally be combined with a vagotomy and pyloroplasty (Fig. 22.2). A partial gastrectomy (Fig. 22.2) may be needed to remove a gastric ulcer.

The initial management of pyloric stenosis is to correct the fluid and electrolyte imbalance. A subsequent vagotomy and gastroenterostomy is required to bypass the pyloric obstruction (Fig. 22.2).

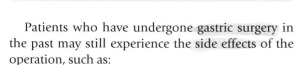

Patients who have a gastric ulcer need a repeat endoscopy 6–8 weeks later to make sure the ulcer has healed.

Patients who have undergone gastric surgery in the past may still experience the side effects of the operation, such as:

- Steatorrhoea and diarrhoea.
- Dumping—the symptoms of fainting, vertigo and sweating, which may be due to the osmotic effect of rapid transit of food from the stomach into the small intestine after pyloroplasty or gastric surgery. Fluid is absorbed into the jejunum, causing temporary hypovolaemia.
- Bile reflux and vomiting.
- Small stomach syndrome.
- Anaemia—may be due to iron deficiency, because hydrochloric acid is required for iron absorption, or due to vitamin B_{12} deficiency, because intrinsic factor is required. Both hydrochloric acid and intrinsic factor are absent after partial gastrectomy.
- Stomal ulceration.
- Malignancy in the gastric remnant.

EROSIVE GASTRITIS

Background

Erosive gastritis is a common problem with several causes, including NSAIDs and critical illness.

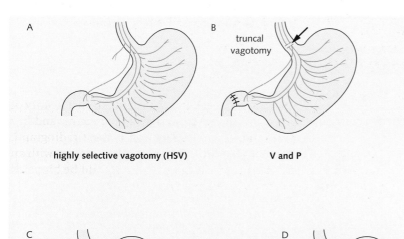

A   B
truncal
vagotomy

highly selective vagotomy (HSV)   V and P

C   D
gastric ulcer

Billroth   gastroduodenostomy   gastroenterostomy
partial gastrectomy

Fig. 22.2 Gastric operations. (A) In highly selective vagotomy the branches of the vagus nerve innervating the parietal cells are divided to decrease gastric acid secretion. (B) In vagotomy and pyloroplasty (V and P) the main vagal trunks are divided (arrow) to reduce gastric acid secretion. Pyloroplasty is required to overcome the impaired gastric contraction that results. (C) Partial gastrectomy for gastric ulcer. (D) Gastroenterostomy.

Clinical presentation

In erosive gastritis there is often diffuse oedema and erythema of the gastric mucosa, with focal mucosal haemorrhage, erosions and ulceration. The condition may present with haematemesis.

CHRONIC ATROPHIC GASTRITIS

Chronic atrophic gastritis may be categorized into two types:

- Type A is associated with achlorhydria, impaired absorption of vitamin B_{12}, the presence of parietal cell antibodies in serum and the development of pernicious anaemia.
- Type B is caused by chronic mucosal damage (e.g. by dietary salts, viral infections, bile reflux, *H. pylori* infection). The gastritis may undergo metaplasia to intestinal-type epithelium and subsequently develop dysplasia, and may progress to carcinoma.

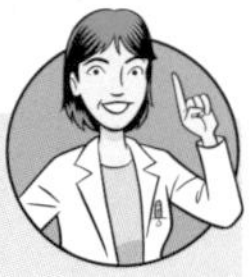

> Chronic atrophic gastritis does not usually bleed.

ZOLLINGER–ELLISON SYNDROME

Background

This is intractable gastroduodenal ulceration caused by:

- Gastrin secretion.
- An amine precursor uptake and decarboxylation (APUD) tumour, which is commonly found in the pancreas and can be benign or malignant.

Management

Diagnosis is made by measuring serum gastrin levels.

Treatment is by use of a proton pump inhibitor or resection if it is a solitary tumour.

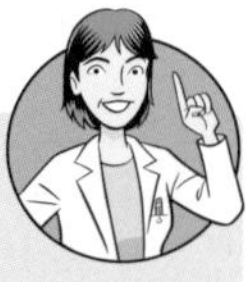

> Zollinger–Ellison syndrome is confirmed by acid secretion tests, which show high levels of resting acid secretion.

GASTRIC CANCER

Background

Gastric tumours can be benign or malignant, but cancer is more common. Benign tumours include:

- Adenomas—epithelial polyps.
- Leiomyoma.
- Fibroma.
- Neurofibroma.
- Haemangioma.

Malignant tumours include:

- Adenocarcinoma (most common).
- Leiomyosarcoma and lymphoma.

Gastric cancer is the third commonest gastrointestinal cancer in the UK. Its incidence is declining, but there appears to be an increasing incidence of cardia tumours subsequent to the introduction of H_2-antagonists. It tends to present late in the UK and has a poor prognosis. The peak age is 70–80 years and it is more common in men than in women.

In other parts of the world (e.g. Japan), there is a high incidence of gastric cancer and there are screening programmes to detect it early. Risk factors for the development of gastric cancer are outlined in Fig. 22.3.

Pathology

The macroscopic morphology of gastric cancer is shown in Fig. 22.4. Early gastric cancer comprises a nodule or ulceration confined to the mucosa and submucosa but, in the UK, most of the gastric cancers have invaded the muscularis propria at the time of presentation to produce any of the following:

- Malignant ulcer with raised everted edges.
- Polypoid tumour (proliferating mucosa protruding into the lumen).

Fig. 22.3 Risk factors for development of gastric cancer

atrophic gastritis
blood group A
pernicious anaemia
adenomatous polyps
diet—spicy, salty foods, excess nitrates
smoking
alcohol
Helicobacter pylori infection

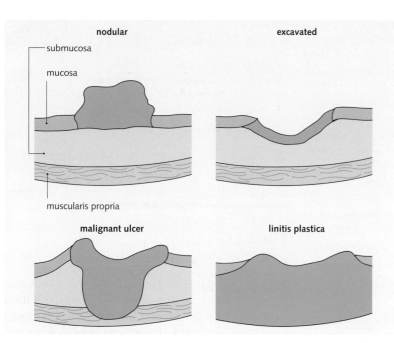

Fig. 22.4 Growth patterns of gastric cancer.

- Colloid tumour (a gelatinous growth).
- Linitis plastica (submucous infiltration by cancer cells, resulting in a marked fibrotic reaction and the stomach is contracted and thickened with little mucosal ulceration).

Most gastric cancers are adenocarcinomas and they are defined as intestinal or diffuse:

- Intestinal cancers arise on a background of atrophic gastritis and are well-circumscribed adenocarcinomas.
- Diffuse cancer arises from a 'normal' stomach and is a poorly localized lesion that infiltrates rapidly into the submucosa. It spreads locally to invade adjacent structures such as the liver, pancreas and transverse colon.

Lymphatic spread is to the nodes along the lesser and greater curvatures of the stomach, to the coeliac axis, hepatic nodes, and then to the supraclavicular nodes via the thoracic duct.

Bloodstream spread is via the portal system to the liver and subsequently to the lungs.

Transcoelomic spread produces peritoneal seedlings and Krukenberg's tumours (i.e. secondary tumours in the ovaries).

Clinical presentation

A diagnosis of gastric cancer should be suspected if there is:

- Recent onset of dyspepsia. *bloating, abdo pain, mass*
- Dysphagia—due to obstruction of the gastro-oesophageal junction.
- Vomiting—may be due to pyloric outlet obstruction. *early satiety*
- Anorexia and weight loss.
- Iron deficiency anaemia.
- Abdominal swelling due to ascites, mass or hepatomegaly.
- Metastatic disease (e.g. jaundice).

The diagnosis is confirmed by gastroscopy and biopsy. Additional assessment and staging can be made by:

- Blood tests (e.g. full blood count, liver function tests).
- Chest radiography. *E·US*
- Hepatic ultrasound—to look for metastases.
- Computed tomography (CT) scan of the abdomen—to assess nodal disease and involvement of adjacent structures.
- Laparoscopy—to assess operability and look for peritoneal seedlings and serosal disease, which is not seen on a CT scan.

Management

If the tumour is resectable and confined to the stomach, gastric resection and radical resection of the drainage lymph nodes gives the best long-term results. Antral tumours are treated by subtotal gastrectomy, but carcinoma of the upper stomach is treated by a total gastrectomy with Roux-en-Y loop reconstruction using small intestine anastomosed to the oesophagus.

If the tumour is unresectable, palliative surgery may be a gastroenterostomy for pyloric outlet obstruction or insertion of a stent for carcinoma of the gastro-oesophageal junction or cardia. The role of chemotherapy is still unproven.

The prognosis is very poor. After 'curative' resection, the 5-year survival rates are only 20% except for early gastric cancer; overall 5-year survival is about 5%.

As our understanding of gastric cancer increases, primary prevention is becoming possible. Preventive measures include:

- Dietary—increased consumption of fruit and vegetables (vitamin C acts as an antioxidant in the stomach and provides protection against potential carcinogens).
- Eradication of *H. pylori*—atrophic gastritis and potentially gastric cancers are closely related to *H. pylori* infections.

GASTRIC LYMPHOMA

The stomach is the commonest site of primary extranodal lymphoma, but gastric lymphoma is still rare. It arises from the mucosa-associated lymphoid tissue (MALT) and *H. pylori* has also been implicated.

Clinical presentation

The symptoms of gastric lymphoma are those of gastric cancer.

Primary gastric lymphomas of the stomach are more common in children.

Management

Treatment is by resection if possible, followed by radiotherapy. Non-resectable tumours can be treated by combination chemotherapy and radiotherapy. The prognosis is better than for adenocarcinoma.

Further reading

Malfertheiner P, Megraud F, O'Morain C *et al*. 2007 Current concepts in the management of *Helicobacter pylori* infection. *Gut* **56**: 772–881

Norton JA, Jensen RT 2004 Resolved and unresolved controversies in the surgical management of patients with Zollinger–Ellison syndrome. *Ann Surg* **240**: 757–773

Yoon SS, Coit DG, Portlock CS, Karpeh MS 2004 The diminishing role of surgery in the treatment of gastric lymphoma. *Ann Surg* **240**: 28–37.

NICE Guidelines 2006 *Dyspepsia*. http://www.nice.org.uk

Clarl CJ, Thirlby RC, Picozzi V Jr, Schembre DB, Cummings FP 2006 Gastric cancer. *Curr Probl Surg* **43**: 566–670.

Shah R. 2007 Dyspepsia and *Helicobacter pylori*. *BMJ* **334**: 41–43

Logan R, Harris A, Misiewicz JJ, Baron JH. 2002 *ABC of the Upper Gastrointestinal Tract*. BMJ Publications, London

Krumholz HM, Ross JS, Presler AH, Egilman DS 2007 What have we learnt from Vioxx? *BMJ* **334**: 120–123

Disorders of the small intestine

Learning objectives

You should be able to:

- Understand the management of small bowel obstruction.
- List five extraintestinal manifestations of Crohn's disease.
- List the causes of acute mesenteric ischaemia.
- Describe where a Meckel's diverticulum is classically found.
- Understand how a Meckel's diverticulum causes rectal bleeding in a child.
- Describe where a mass is typically palpated in a child with intussusception.
- Understand the mechanism by which carcinoid syndrome develops.

The main function of the small intestine is digestion and absorption of nutrients (fats, carbohydrates and proteins). This occurs in the jejunum and the upper ileum. Bile salts and vitamin B_{12} are absorbed from the terminal ileum.

OBSTRUCTION OF THE SMALL INTESTINE

Background

A common cause for acute surgical admission is small bowel obstruction. The speed of onset can be acute, chronic, or acute on chronic.

Clinical presentation

The presenting symptoms are colicky abdominal pain, vomiting, absolute constipation and abdominal distension. The cause may be:

- In the lumen—tumour (e.g. leiomyoma), food bolus, gallstone.
- In the wall—Crohn's disease, radiation stricture.
- Outside the lumen—adhesions, volvulus, hernia, intussusception.

Common causes of small intestinal obstruction are:

- Irreducible hernias.
- Adhesions.

Management

The diagnosis is made from the history and clinical examination, which includes making a note of:

- Hydration.
- Pulse.
- Blood pressure.
- Temperature.
- Mucous membranes.
- Abdominal scars.
- Hernial orifices.
- Distension.
- Presence of high-pitched bowel sounds.

Any signs of tenderness or peritonism imply that the bowel may be becoming ischaemic. This is a ⚡SURGICAL EMERGENCY⚡

Investigations should include:

- Full blood count—may demonstrate an elevated white cell count.
- Renal function.
- Abdominal radiograph—may show small bowel dilatation.

Treatment is by resuscitation with intravenous fluids, and monitoring the pulse, blood pressure and urine output. A nasogastric tube is passed to prevent vomiting and decompress the bowel.

Urgent surgical intervention is required if the patient has a tender irreducible hernia or any signs of peritonism or ischaemia.

If the patient has had a previous operation, adhesions are the likely cause and the patient is initially treated conservatively for 24 hours if they have no signs of peritonism. If the condition fails to resolve, a laparotomy is required.

CROHN'S DISEASE

Background

Crohn's disease is a chronic inflammatory bowel disease. It can affect any part of the alimentary tract from the mouth to the anus, but particularly the small intestine (Fig. 23.1). Its aetiology is obscure. *terminal ileum .*

Crohn's disease occurs more commonly in women, the male to female ratio being 1 to 1.6, and it is usually diagnosed in young adults.

Pathology

Macroscopically, the bowel looks red, oedematous and thickened in Crohn's disease. The mesentery is thickened and the fat encroaches on the bowel wall. The lesions are intermittent (i.e. skip lesions). In the mucosa there are deep ulcers—'rose-thorn ulcer'—which produce a cobblestone appearance. Microscopically, there is transmural inflammation, which may include the presence of non-caseating granulomas.

Fig. 23.1 (A) Pathological features of Crohn's disease, showing mucosal ulceration. Compare this with the features of ulcerative colitis (which affects the colon and rectum, see p. 114) and shown in (B) in which ulceration and inflammation are confined to the mucosa and submucosa.

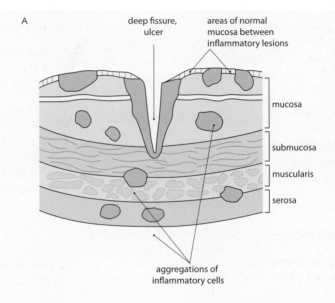

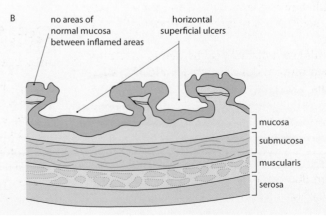

Clinical presentation

The patient may present with:

- Abdominal pain.
- Change of bowel habit and nausea.
- Weight loss.
- Anaemia.
- Malnutrition.

Crohn's disease may cause perianal problems such as perianal sepsis, fistulae, fissures or skin tags.

The initial presentation of Crohn's disease often results from involvement of the terminal ileum and after resection many people have no further problems but, in some people, Crohn's disease is a chronic recurring disease with long-term morbidity.

Extraintestinal manifestations of Crohn's disease include:

- Uveitis.
- Episcleritis of the eye.
- Arthritis.
- Aphthous ulcers.
- Erythema nodosum.

Complications include strictures causing acute or chronic intestinal obstruction. Abscesses may be perianal or intraperitoneal (between the loops of intestine), and fistulae may be enteroenteric, enterocutaneous or vesicocolic.

Management

Diagnosis of Crohn's disease is made by demonstrating:

- Iron deficiency anaemia.
- Elevated erythrocyte sedimentation rate and C-reactive protein.

A small bowel enema will demonstrate Kantor's string sign of a stricture, 'rose-thorn' ulcers and fissures.

An ultrasound scan may be helpful in assessing intraperitoneal abdominal masses related to Crohn's disease.

Crohn's disease usually has an insidious onset, which results in delays in diagnosis.

Treatment is used to prevent acute attacks but has a limited role in preventing relapse. it consists of:

- Corticosteroids.
- Sulphasalazine.
- Immunosuppressants—azathioprine and ciclosporin are used in patients who do not respond to steroids.

Surgical operations are reserved for complications and limited resections are performed because there is a high risk of further problems. If there is a fibrotic stricture, a stricturoplasty is performed.

In the long term, Crohn's disease is chronic so there is a risk of developing short bowel syndrome.

SHORT GUT SYNDROME

This follows massive resection of the small intestine. Common causes are: *ischaemia*

- Mesenteric infarction.
- Crohn's disease.
- Radiation enteritis.

The critical length of small intestine needed to maintain nutrition is 1–2 m. After resection, the remaining intestine adapts by dilatation of the small intestine and villous enlargement to improve absorption. If there is less than 1 m and oral nutrition is inadequate, total parenteral nutrition is necessary.

Resection of the ileum results in malabsorption of vitamin B_{12} and bile salts.

SURGICAL EMERGENCY

Intestinal ischaemia

Background

When not secondary to small bowel obstruction ischaemia of the small intestine can be caused by a fall in cardiac output or vascular occlusion due to embolus or thrombosis of the superior mesenteric artery or vein (Fig. 23.2). These factors may be associated with atherosclerosis or atrial fibrillation.

(Continued)

Fig. 23.2 Mesenteric angiogram—showing abrupt cut-off of the superior mesenteric artery by an embolus.

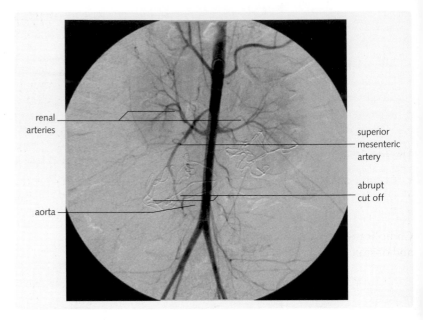

renal arteries

superior mesenteric artery

abrupt cut off

aorta

(*Continued*)

Clinical presentation

There is a history of sudden onset of severe abdominal pain. On examination, the patient is unwell, with increased pulse rate, reduced blood pressure and generalized abdominal tenderness.

Management

The diagnosis is based on:

- Clinical suspicion.
- Elevated white cell count. Do ABG.
- Acidosis.

Treatment is by resuscitation and a laparotomy. If the whole of the small intestine is infarcted in a very elderly patient, it is not appropriate to resect because the patient is unlikely to survive. If part of the bowel is affected then a resection is performed, but it is not anastomosed because of the risk of further ischaemia. The ends of the intestine are brought to the surface as stomas. It is usually not possible to perform an embolectomy.

CHRONIC ISCHAEMIA

Background

Chronic ischaemia is due to atherosclerosis of the superior mesenteric artery.

Clinical presentation

"abdominal angina"

The symptoms of chronic ischaemia are colicky abdominal pain after eating. The patient is afraid to eat, so there is malnutrition and weight loss.

Chronic ischaemia produces an abdominal bruit in 75% of cases.

Management

A diagnosis of chronic ischaemia is made from arteriograms. It may be possible occasionally to insert a stent or to perform a bypass operation.

RADIATION ENTEROPATHY

Background

Radiotherapy may damage the small and large intestine. It causes proliferative endarteritis and vasculitis, resulting in ischaemia and transmural fibrosis. Patients who have diabetes mellitus, hypertension and cardiovascular disease are more prone to the complications of radiotherapy.

Radiation enteritis can present with an acute abdomen during radiotherapy treatment.

Clinical presentation

The symptoms are usually:

- Chronic abdominal pain.
- Diarrhoea.
- Rectal bleeding.

Complications include haemorrhage, perforation and obstruction.

MECKEL'S DIVERTICULUM

Background

Meckel's diverticulum is the remnant of the vitellointestinal duct of the embryo and lies on the antimesenteric border of the ileum. It occurs in 2% of people, 60 cm (2 feet) from the ileocaecal valve and is about 5 cm (2 inches) in length. It may contain heterotopic tissue (gastric, duodenal or pancreatic).

Meckel's diverticulum is a true diverticulum and consists of all intestinal layers.

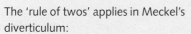

The 'rule of twos' applies in Meckel's diverticulum:

- 2% of population.
- 2 feet from the ileocaecal valve.
- 2 inches in length.

Clinical presentation

The symptoms are usually:

- Chronic abdominal pain.
- Diarrhoea.
- Rectal bleeding.

Complications include haemorrhage, perforation and obstruction. , intussuscept, CA .

INTUSSUSCEPTION

Background

Intussusception in infants and young children may be due to a viral infection causing hyperplasia of the lymphoid tissue, which then acts as the apex of the intussusception. In older children or adults a polyp, carcinoma or Meckel's diverticulum may be the apex. The inner layer of the intussusception has its blood supply cut off by pressure and stretching of the mesentery, so there is a risk of gangrene (Fig. 23.3). A radiograph of intussusception is shown in Fig. 23.4.

Intussusception is the commonest abdominal emergency in the age group 2 months to 2 years.

P172 OHCM

Clinical presentation

In infants, the history of intussusception comprises paroxysms of colic and the child screams. There is associated pallor, vomiting and passage of redcurrant stool. A mass may be palpable in the right iliac fossa. Adults have a history suggestive of intestinal obstruction. sausage-shaped

Management

reduction by air insufflation/enema

If detected early in infants, then the hydrostatic pressure of a barium enema may reduce an intussusception, but if there are signs of peritonism

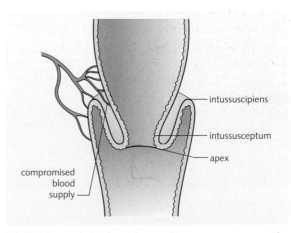

Fig. 23.3 Demonstrating how intussusception can cause gangrene of the bowel.

bowel invagination .

111

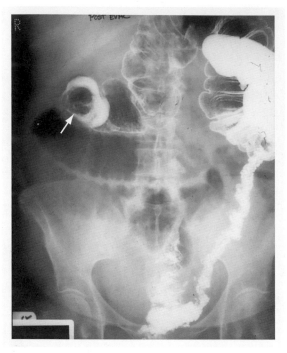

Fig. 23.4 Intussusception. Barium enema showing an ileocolic intussusception (arrow).

or a long history then operative intervention is required. If the bowel is gangrenous, it is resected.

TUMOURS OF THE SMALL INTESTINE

Background

Tumours of the small intestine are rare and the following conditions are benign:

- Adenomas in familial polyposis.
- Gardner's syndrome (familial polyposis and cysts).
- Peutz–Jeghers syndrome (polyps and skin pigmentation).
- Lipomas.
- Leiomyomas.

The malignant tumours include adenocarcinoma, carcinoid tumours, leiomyosarcomas, lymphomas and secondary deposits (e.g. melanoma). Small intestinal tumours tend to present late with intestinal obstruction.

CARCINOID TUMOURS

Background

These are neuroendocrine amine precursor uptake and decarboxylation system (APUD) tumours that arise from Kulchitsky's cells. They can arise anywhere in the intestinal tract and lungs, but commonly in the appendix. The foregut and midgut tumours secrete serotonin (also known as 5-hydroxytryptamine). 5-HT

Clinical presentation

The primary tumour may produce symptoms of:

- Intestinal obstruction.
- Diarrhoea.
- Haemorrhage.

When the tumours metastasize to the liver, the patient develops carcinoid syndrome, which is characterized by:

- Cutaneous flushing.
- Skin rashes.
- Intestinal colic.
- Diarrhoea.
- Bronchospasm.
- Cardiac lesions (tricuspid incompetence).
- Pulmonary stenosis.

Management

The diagnosis is made by urinary estimation of 5-hydroxyindoleacetic acid (5-HIAA), which is a derivative of serotonin.
Treatment is by:

- Resection, if possible.
- Embolization of hepatic metastases.
- Control of symptoms by long-acting somatostatin.

Further reading

Macutkiewicz C, Carlson GL 2005 Emergency surgery. Acute abdomen: intestinal obstruction. *Surgery* **23**: 208–212

Booth CC, Neale G (eds) 1986 *Disorders of the Small Intestine*. Blackwell Science, Oxford

Ellis H 1985 *Intestinal Obstruction*. Appleton-Century-Crofts, New York

Marston A (ed) 1986 *Vascular Disease of the Gut*. Arnold, London

Sagar J, Kumar V, Shah DK 2006 Meckel's diverticulum: a systematic review. *J R Soc Med* **99**: 501–505

Thoreson R, Cullen JJ 2007 Pathophysiology of inflammatory bowel disease: an overview. *Surg Clin North Am* **87**: 575–585

Learning objectives

You should be able to:

- Describe the typical presentation of acute appendicitis.
- Understand how the appearances of Crohn's and ulcerative colitis differ macroscopically.
- Understand how toxic megacolon presents and how it is treated.
- List the complications of diverticular disease.
- Define a vesicocolic fistula and list the symptoms it may present with.
- Understand why sigmoid volvulus develops and in which group of patients it typically occurs.
- Understand how the diagnosis of pseudo-obstruction is confirmed.
- Define a Dukes' C1 tumour by which layers of the bowel it has invaded.
- Understand the electrolyte disturbance that occurs with a villous adenoma.
- Name three complications that can occur with a colostomy.

SURGICAL EMERGENCY

Acute appendicitis

Background

Acute appendicitis is a very common reason for acute surgical admission. It can occur at any age, but is most common in young children and young adults.

Acute appendicitis is thought to be due to luminal obstruction of the appendix with superimposed infection. Obstruction may be by a fecolith or swollen lymphoid follicles after a viral infection. Ulceration of the mucosa occurs and infection with mixed anaerobes and coliforms supervenes. The bacteria proliferate and invade the appendix wall, which is damaged by pressure necrosis.

The blood supply to the appendix is via an end-artery and, when it is thrombosed, gangrene develops. An acutely inflamed appendix may:

- Resolve spontaneously, especially if it is not obstructed, but may recur.
- Become gangrenous and perforate.
- Become surrounded by omentum and loops of bowel to wall off the infection and an appendix mass develops.

Clinical presentation

The illness starts as a mild periumbilical colicky pain followed by anorexia, nausea and vomiting. A few *loss of appetite* hours later, the pain becomes localized to the right iliac fossa. It is a constant pain exacerbated by movement. Diarrhoea may occur if the appendix is retroileal and dysuria may occur if it is pelvic. The symptoms and signs of appendicitis are influenced by the position of the appendix (Fig. 24.1).

On examination, the patient may be flushed and have a pyrexia, tachycardia and fetor.

On abdominal examination, there is peritonism in the right iliac fossa. If the appendix is perforated, the signs of peritonitis are more widespread.

Rectal examination demonstrates right-sided tenderness if the appendix is pelvic. If the symptoms have been present for 4 or 5 days, an appendix mass may be present.

Fig. 24.2 shows the clinical progression of acute appendicitis.

Differential diagnosis

Almost any abdominal condition can be mistaken for acute appendicitis. The differential diagnoses include:

- Mesenteric adenitis—associated with viral sore throats.
- Gastroenteritis.
- Urinary tract infections.
- Gynaecological causes—acute salpingitis, torsion of an ovarian cyst. *, ectopic preg. / rupture*

· Caecal diverticulitis.

(Continued)

(Continued)

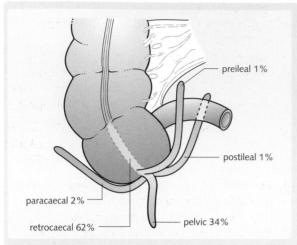

preileal 1%

postileal 1%

paracaecal 2%

retrocaecal 62%

pelvic 34%

Fig. 24.1 Variations in the position of the appendix.

resolution

acute appendicitis

appendix mass

perforated appendix

localized peritonitis

diffuse peritonitis

Fig. 24.2 Clinical progression of acute appendicitis.

Management

Diagnosis of acute appendicitis is made from the history and examination. There is usually a leukoytosis, but this is not specific. An ultrasound examination will demonstrate an appendix mass and ovarian pathology, but does not prove acute appendicitis.

Treatment of acute appendicitis is emergency appendicectomy by either laparoscopic or open surgery.

An appendix mass is treated with intravenous *conservatively.* antibiotics and fluids. The patient is monitored closely in case peritonitis develops.

A normal ultrasound scan does not exclude acute appendicitis.

INFLAMMATORY BOWEL DISEASES

These are ulcerative colitis and Crohn's disease (see Chapter 23, Fig. 23.1). When they affect the colon, these conditions produce similar symptoms, but it is important to distinguish between the two because of their different management and prognoses.

APPENDIX TUMOURS

Background

The appendix is occasionally the site of a tumour, such as adenocarcinoma, mucinous neoplasm or lymphoma. The appendix, however, is the commonest site for a carcinoid tumour. These are usually found incidentally at the tip of the organ and rarely metastasize, and the prognosis is good.

ULCERATIVE COLITIS

Background

Ulcerative colitis affects the colon, commencing from the rectum and proceeding continuously proximally (Fig. 24.3). Its aetiology is obscure, but it may be associated with HLA-B27 and usually presents in people aged 20–40 years. It is more common in women. It is often associated with cessation of smoking.

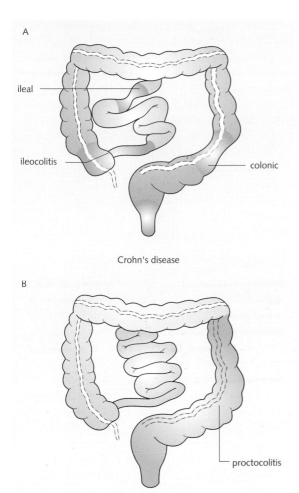

ileal

ileocolitis

colonic

Crohn's disease

proctocolitis

Ulcerative colitis

Fig. 24.3 The distribution of (A) Crohn's disease and (B) ulcerative colitis. Crohn's disease is segmental, involving the ileum or rectum most often. Ulcerative colitis has a continuous distribution, involving the rectum in all cases.

Macroscopically, the mucosa is inflamed, oedematous, ulcerated, bleeding and producing mucous. Pseudopolyps may be seen (i.e. islands of normal mucosa between denuded areas).

Microscopically, there is an inflammatory infiltrate in the mucosa and submucosa. The crypts of Lieberkühn are inflamed and crypt abscesses develop, coalesce and cause ulceration.

Clinical presentation

Ulcerative colitis may have a mild and chronic course if it is confined to the distal colon and rectum. The symptoms are:

- Diarrhoea with passage of blood and mucus.
- Abdominal pain.
- Systemic symptoms of anorexia, low-grade pyrexia and weight loss.
- Non-gastrointestinal symptoms include iritis, arthritis, sacroiliitis, ankylosing spondylitis, pyoderma and erythema nodosum, renal calculi, pyelonephritis, hepatic disease and cholangitis.

Ulcerative colitis may have an acute or acute on chronic presentation as toxic megacolon. The clinical features are:

- Profuse diarrhoea and rectal bleeding.
- Rapid development of hypovolaemia, tachycardia, pyrexia and hypotension.
- Distended and tender abdomen with absent bowel sounds.

Management

A diagnosis of ulcerative colitis is made by:

- Sigmoidoscopy—showing the characteristic appearance of ulcerated, bleeding mucosa, and biopsies are taken to confirm the diagnosis and differentiate from Crohn's disease.
- Barium enema—to assess the extent of the disease—the characteristic changes are loss of the haustrations, and rigidity and shortening of the colon leading to a 'lead pipe' appearance.
- Abdominal radiography in the acute situation—may show signs of perforation or gross dilatation of a toxic megacolon.This is a ‼SURGICAL EMERGENCY‼

The complications of ulcerative colitis are toxic megacolon and carcinoma.

Medical treatment aims to induce and maintain remission and consists of:

- Prednisolone enemas or sulphasalazine orally and by enemas—for mild short-segment disease.
- Systemic corticosteroids—for more severe episodes.
- Immunosuppressants—used in patients unresponsive to steroids (e.g. ciclosporin).
- Surgical operation—if medical treatment fails or complications develop, ulcerative colitis can be eradicated by performing a panproctocolectomy (removing the anus, rectum and colon) and forming a permanent ileostomy. Alternatively, the terminal ileum can be used to create an

ileal pouch, which is anastomosed to the anus at a later stage, when the acute illness has been treated by removal of the colon. Stool frequency is high and continence may be a problem, so the patient needs to be well motivated.

Those patients who have had extensive ulcerative colitis for more than 10 years are at increased risk of developing carcinoma, so should have regular colonoscopy and biopsy to assess for dysplasia.

CROHN'S DISEASE

Background

The pathology of Crohn's disease of the colon is the same as for the small intestine (Fig. 24.1).

Clinical presentation

Crohn's disease of the colon may present with:

- Abdominal pain.
- Diarrhoea.
- Rectal bleeding.
- Mucous discharge.
- Perianal problems.

Management

Treatment of Crohn's disease of the colon is similar to that of ulcerative colitis, except that a panproctocolectomy does not cure the problem and a pouch is not created because of the risk of further disease in the ileum of the pouch (see Chapter 23).

Crohn's disease runs a relapsing and remitting course, and is incurable.

DIVERTICULOSIS

Background

This is common in developed countries, but most people are asymptomatic. The incidence rises with increasing age and it is unusual in people under 40 years of age.

Diverticula develop when the diet is poor in fibre. As a result, the segmental contractions of the colon are more vigorous and prolonged, increasing the intraluminal pressure, which leads to herniation of the mucosa between the taenia coli, giving rise to two rows of diverticula adjacent to the appendices epiploicae. They are pseudodiverticula because they consist only of mucosa and submucosa.

Diverticula are found predominantly found in the sigmoid colon, but they can occur anywhere in the colon, including the caecum, where caecal diverticulitis may mimic appendicitis.

Clinical presentation

Clinical presentations of diverticulosis are:

- Diverticulosis itself—episodes of left iliac fossa pain associated with alternating diarrhoea and constipation.
- Acute diverticulitis—the patient is systemically unwell, with pyrexia, tenderness and peritonism in the left iliac fossa.
- Perforation—diverticulitis may proceed to perforation. If the infection is contained locally, it causes a paracolic abscess but, if not, it may cause generalized peritonitis, which is a ⚠ SURGICAL EMERGENCY ⚠
- Fistula formation—in acute inflammation, the colon may become adherent to the bladder, vagina or small intestine. A vesicocolic fistula causes cystitis and pneumaturia. A colovaginal fistula causes a feculent vaginal discharge.
- Obstruction—acute inflammation may narrow the lumen of the colon, and repeated episodes cause thickening of the bowel wall and a fibrous stricture may develop, which causes episodes of subacute obstruction.
- Haemorrhage—erosion of a vessel at the mouth of a diverticulum may cause significant rectal bleeding. Although many presentations of diverticular bleeding are small volume and self-limiting they can often present with profuse large volume bleeding. This is a ⚠ SURGICAL EMERGENCY ⚠

A perforation maybe identified on a plain abdominal radiograph when both the inside and outside of the bowel wall are outlined by gas (Rigler's sign).

Management

Diverticulosis is usually diagnosed by a barium enema but, if a complication occurs (Fig. 24.4), it may be found at laparotomy. The management of different stages is as follows:

- Diverticulosis—advice about a high fibre diet.
- Acute diverticulitis—most cases settle with intravenous fluids and intravenous antibiotics.
- Peritonitis— ❗**SURGICAL EMERGENCY**❗ resuscitation, intravenous antibiotics and fluids before a laparotomy, resection of the diseased segment of colon, and formation of a colostomy.
- Paracolic abscess—an ultrasound or computed tomography (CT) scan may demonstrate a collection, which may be drained percutaneously or may require a laparotomy.
- Diverticular stricture—if recurrent episodes of subacute obstruction occur, it may be necessary to resect the involved colon with a primary anastomosis.
- Fistula—elective resection of diseased colon, closure of fistula and primary anastomosis.
- Diverticular haemorrhage—the initial management is resuscitation. Most cases settle spontaneously but, if not, an arteriogram is performed to locate the site of bleeding so that the appropriate segment of colon is resected.

Complications of diverticulosis are acute diverticulitis, perforation, fistula formation, obstruction and haemorrhage.

SURGICAL EMERGENCY

Volvulus

This is a twisting of a loop of bowel around its mesentery. It commonly occurs in the sigmoid colon, but can occur in the caecum or small intestine. It causes obstruction of the bowel and the blood supply is obstructed, causing ischaemia and infarction (Fig. 24.5).

In volvulus the bowel twists through 360°, resulting in a closed-loop obstruction.

Sigmoid volvulus

Background

This usually affects elderly patients who may be institutionalized and have a history of chronic constipation.

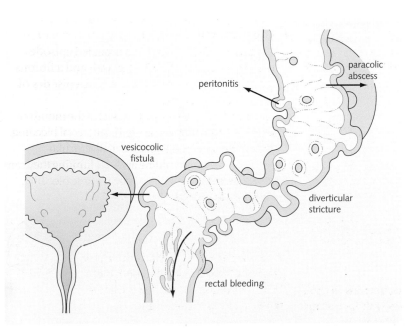

Fig. 24.4 Complications of diverticulosis.

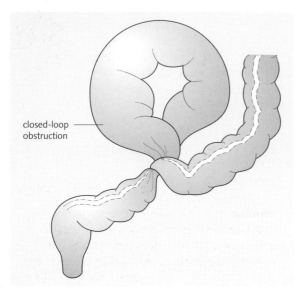

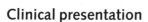

Fig. 24.5 Sigmoid volvulus causing a closed-loop obstruction.

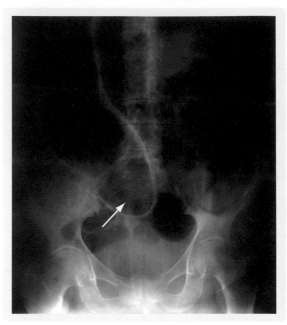

Fig. 24.6 Abdominal radiograph of sigmoid volvulus showing a grossly distended sigmoid loop (arrow).

Clinical presentation

The symptoms are:

- Colicky abdominal pain.
- Absolute constipation.
- Gross abdominal distension.

Management

An abdominal radiograph shows the characteristic appearance of a grossly dilated sigmoid colon (Fig. 24.6). In some cases, it can be decompressed using a rigid sigmoidoscope but, if it is a recurrent problem, it should be resected electively. If it cannot be decompressed or there are signs of peritonism a laparotomy and resection are performed.

Caecal volvulus

Background

Caecal volvulus occurs if there is a congenital abnormality so that the caecum has a long mesentery and the caecum is mobile.

Clinical presentation

The torsion causes an acute closed-loop obstruction so the patient has symptoms of bowel obstruction or peritonitis if the caecum infarcts.

Management

Urgent laparotomy and colonic resection are required.

PSEUDO-OBSTRUCTION

Background

Pseudo-obstruction affects the elderly and infirm and is often associated with prolonged medical illnesses, including:

- Uraemia.
- Chronic lung disease.
- Immobility, especially after orthopaedic surgery.

Management

The X-ray features of pseudo-obstruction are the same as those of mechanical large bowel obstruction and may or may not include dilated small bowel loops. However, if a limited barium enema is performed, it will flow freely into a dilated colon and there will be no signs of an obstructing lesion.

Treatment is conservative and most cases resolve. Electrolyte abnormalities such as hypokalaemia should be corrected because they can exacerbate the problem. Decompression by a colonoscopy is occasionally effective.
The differentiation of pseudo-obstruction and mechanical obstruction can be extremely difficult, and therefore an unprepared barium enema is advised.

COLONIC POLYPS

Background

A polyp projects into the lumen of the bowel and is composed of epithelial and connective tissue elements. They occur anywhere in the bowel, but particularly in the colon and rectum (Fig. 24.7).

Polyps can be:

- Neoplastic (i.e. adenomatous or villous papillomas).

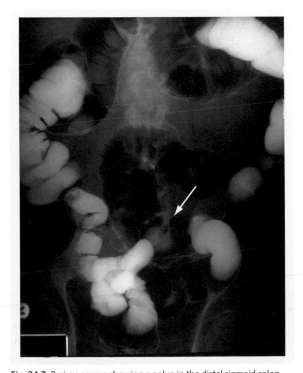

Fig. 24.7 Barium enema showing a polyp in the distal sigmoid colon.

Polyps may be pedunculated (possessing a head and a stalk) or sessile (flat or villous).

- Inflammatory.
- Hamartomatous.

There are several syndromes associated with polyps:

- Familial polyposis coli—an autosomal-dominant condition in which hundreds of adenomas develop through the colon and rectum during the second decade of life. They may be asymptomatic or cause rectal bleeding and diarrhoea, but there is a 100% risk of malignancy within 15 years.
- Gardner's syndrome—multiple colonic adenomas associated with sebaceous and dermoid cysts, osteomas and desmoid tumours of the abdominal wall. There is a high risk of malignant change.

VILLOUS ADENOMA

Background

Villous adenoma is a sessile lesion that secretes large amounts of mucus and may produce diarrhoea and cause hypokalaemia. It carries a risk of developing dysplasia and malignant change.

Villous adenoma can be a cause of hypokalaemia.

COLONIC CARCINOMA

Background

Colonic carcinoma occurs in both sexes and is very common in the UK. Variation in incidence between different countries probably reflects dietary differences, particularly between developed and developing countries. A low-fibre diet causes a long transit time and therefore greater exposure to any carcinogens. Other risk factors include:

- Familial polyposis coli.
- Ulcerative colitis.
- Adenomatous polyps.
- Gardner's syndrome.

Pathologically colonic carcinomas are adeno-carcinomas, which can be:

- Polypoid.
- Ulcerative.
- Annular.
- Diffuse.
- Infiltrating.

The tumour invades the bowel wall and then spreads to the adjacent lymph nodes and the bloodstream. Approximately 3% of tumours are synchronous (i.e. two tumours at the same time) and 3% are metachronous.

Fig. 24.8 shows the modified Dukes' classification of colorectal tumours.

Clinical presentation

The symptoms of colorectal carcinoma depend on its position in the colon and rectum.

Management

A diagnosis of colorectal carcinoma is made by:

- Clinical examination.
- Rigid sigmoidoscopy.
- Barium enema.

A colonic carcinoma has a characteristic appearance of an 'apple core' on barium enema (Fig. 24.9). Colonoscopy can also be used and biopsies can be taken and any other polyps excised.

Blood tests such as a full blood count may show anaemia. Liver function tests and carcinoembryonic antigen are measured to assess and monitor any metastatic disease. A CT scan of the pelvis may be used to assess the operability of a rectal cancer.

Fig. 24.10 shows the different presentations of colonic cancer.

Treatment of colonic cancer is by surgical resection of the colon with its draining lymph nodes. Carcinomas of the rectum can now be resected within 5 cm of the anal margin if the anastomosis is performed with a stapling device (low anterior resection). Different colonic operations are illustrated in Fig. 24.11.

Until recently, radiotherapy and chemotherapy have had a limited role in the management of colorectal cancer, but many patients who have Dukes' C tumours now receive postoperative chemotherapy, which reduces the recurrence rate by 40% and the mortality rate by 30%. Controversy remains over preoperative radiotherapy for resectable tumours of the rectum in which the surgeon is not confident of removing the entire tumour. Patients who have a rectal tumour 'deemed' unresectable may have their tumour downgraded with neoadjuvant chemotherapy. However, there is increased morbidity and mortality following the procedure. Isolated liver metastases may be resected and 25% of patients survive 5 years.

To achieve the best outcomes in colonic carcinoma, a multidisciplinary approach should be adopted and include physician, surgeon, pathologist, radiologist, radiotherapist and medical oncologist.

Screening for colonic carcinoma is worthwhile, although no ideal screening tool is yet available.

Fig. 24.8 Modified Dukes' classification of colorectal tumours

Stage	Definition	5-year survival (%)
A	confined to the mucosa	90
B1	involves part of muscle wall	70
B2	reaches the serosa	60
C1	involves wall, but not completely; local lymph nodes involved	30
C2	involves serosa and lymph nodes	30

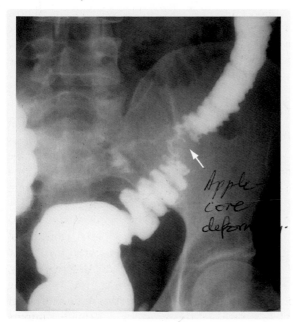

Fig. 24.9 Barium enema showing the 'apple core' appearance (arrow) that is typical of carcinoma of the sigmoid colon.

VASCULAR DISORDERS

Angiodysplasia

Background

Angiodysplasia is a vascular abnormality that occurs in the elderly.

Clinical presentation

Angiodysplasia can cause spontaneous severe rectal bleeding. It usually occurs in the right colon and lesions are identified by arteriography if they are bleeding at a rate of 1–1.5 mL/minute.

Dilated tortuous vessels and 'cherry red' areas are typical of angiodysplasia seen at colonoscopy.

ISCHAEMIC COLITIS

Background

Ischaemic colitis occurs if there is atherosclerosis or increased blood viscosity.

Clinical presentation

The presenting symptom of ischaemic colitis is left-sided abdominal pain, which may be followed by bloody diarrhoea. It may be:

- Acute and cause gangrene and perforation.
- Chronic and cause a stricture, particularly at the splenic flexure of the colon.

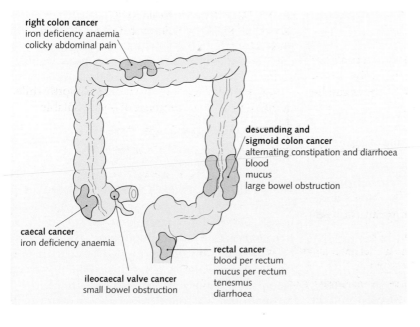

Fig. 24.10 Clinical presentations of colonic cancer. Approximately 70% of colonic cancers are in the left colon.

right colon cancer
iron deficiency anaemia
colicky abdominal pain

descending and
sigmoid colon cancer
alternating constipation and diarrhoea
blood
mucus
large bowel obstruction

caecal cancer
iron deficiency anaemia

ileocaecal valve cancer
small bowel obstruction

rectal cancer
blood per rectum
mucus per rectum
tenesmus
diarrhoea

Fig. 24.11 Different types of colonic operation. Diagram to show the extent of the colonic resection for different operations.

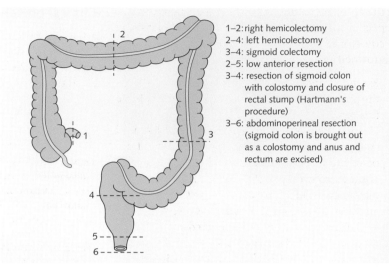

1–2: right hemicolectomy
2–4: left hemicolectomy
3–4: sigmoid colectomy
2–5: low anterior resection
3–4: resection of sigmoid colon with colostomy and closure of rectal stump (Hartmann's procedure)
3–6: abdominoperineal resection (sigmoid colon is brought out as a colostomy and anus and rectum are excised)

A barium enema confirms the diagnosis if there is a narrowed segment with an irregular contour and 'thumb-printing' due to oedema in the mucosa.

Ischaemic colitis usually resolves, although it may progress to gangrene or a late stricture.

Fig. 24.12 Causes of colonic obstruction

Location	Cause
in the lumen	polyploid tumour, constipation
in the wall	malignant, ischaemic, diverticular or radiation stricture
outside colon	hernia, volvulus, intussusception

COLONIC OBSTRUCTION

Background

Colonic obstruction is a common cause for an acute surgical admission.

Clinical presentation

The history of colonic obstruction is:

- Colicky abdominal pain.
- Abdominal distension.
- Increasing constipation progressing to absolute constipation.

There may be a preceding history of change of bowel habit. Vomiting may occur, but this is a late phenomenon. Causes of colonic obstruction are outlined in Fig. 24.12.

Management

Initial blood tests may show an iron deficiency anaemia, suggesting an underlying colonic neoplasm. The patient may be dehydrated and have abnormal electrolytes. If the colon is perforated, there will be free gas on an erect chest radiograph. An abdominal radiograph will show colonic dilatation with a 'cut-off' point. A limited barium enema (on unprepared bowel) is performed to confirm the level of the obstruction. If there is any suspicion of a perforation then Gastrografin is used instead of barium. Double-contrast CT is increasingly used in the acute setting. CT may show:

- Level of obstruction.
- Cause of obstruction.
- Viability of involved bowel.
- Presence of metastases

The ⚠SURGICAL EMERGENCY⚠ is a closed loop colonic obstruction where there is a high risk of bowel perforation, particularly of the caecum. Ischaemia is seen more commonly as a complication of small bowel obstruction though it can occur with large bowel volvulus or a strangulated sliding hernia. Before surgical intervention the patient is resuscitated. At laparotomy a colonic resection is performed.

If the colon is obstructed and there is any associated sepsis, it is not safe to perform an anastomosis, so a colostomy is formed. The operations frequently performed are:

- Extended right hemicolectomy—for lesions of the ascending and transverse colon to the splenic flexure.
- Hartmann's procedure—resection of the sigmoid colon, closure of the rectal stump and formation of an end-colostomy in the left iliac fossa.
- Subtotal colectomy—if the colon is grossly distended it may cause the caecum to perforate and then the whole of the colon is resected and an ileorectal anastomosis is formed.
- Double-barrelled colostomy—if there is a sigmoid volvulus (Fig. 24.5), a sigmoid colectomy is performed and both ends are brought to the surface as a colostomy. This can be easily reversed without a second laparotomy.

Complications of a colostomy are:

- Retraction.
- Prolapse.
- Herniation.   *infection*.
- Stenosis.
- Bowel obstruction.

Colonic obstruction often occurs in the elderly, who have multiple medical problems, and therefore the operation should be performed by experienced anaesthetists and surgeons to reduce the potential risks and any morbidity.

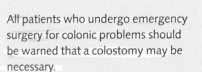

All patients who undergo emergency surgery for colonic problems should be warned that a colostomy may be necessary.

Further reading

Agrawal A, Whorwell PJ. 2006. Irritable bowel syndrome: diagnosis and management. *BMJ* **332**: 280–283

Ahmed I, Deakin D, Parsons SL. 2005 Appendix masss: do we know how to treat it? *Ann Roy Coll Surg Engl* **87**: 191–195.

Anon 2006 Population screening for colorectal cancer. *Drug Ther Bull* **44**: 65–68

Baumgart DC, Sandborn WJ 2007 Inflammatory bowel disease: clinical aspects and established and evolving therapies. *Lancet* **369**: 1641–1657

Janes SEJ, Meagher A, Frizelle FA 2006 Management of diverticulitis. *BMJ* **332**: 271–275

Kapischke M, Caliebe A, Tepel J, Schulz T, Hedderich J 2006 Open versus laparoscopic appendicectomy: a critical review. *Surg Endosc* **20**: 1060–1068

Kerr DJ 2001 *ABC of Colorectal Diseases*. BMJ Publications, London

Madiba TE, Thomson SR 2000 The management of sigmoid volvulus. *J Roy Coll Surg Edinb* **45**: 74–80

Metcalf AM 2007 Elective and emergent operative management of ulcerative colitis. *Surg Clin North Am* **87**: 633–641

Saunders MD 2007 Acute colonic pseudo-obstruction. *Gastrointest Endosc Clin North Am* **17**: 341–60

Scottish Intercollegiate Guideline Network 2003 *Management of Colorectal Cancer*. http://www.sign.ac.uk

Steele RJC 2006 Modern challenges in colorectal cancer. *Surgeon* **4**: 285–291

Learning objectives

You should be able to:

- Define haemorrhoids and describe the positions that they classically occupy in the anal canal.
- List the treatments available to treat haemorrhoids.
- Understand why an anal stretch is no longer recommended in the treatment of anal fissure.
- Name the important aetiological factors in rectal prolapse.
- Understand why a swab is taken for bacteriology when a perianal abscess is incised and drained.
- Define the term 'fistula'.
- Understand why a Seton suture is used in a high anal fistula.
- Describe the lymph nodes that drain the anal canal and understand their clinical significance.

Anorectal problems are common and account for a large number of visits to general practitioners and referrals to surgical outpatient clinics. The common symptoms are:

- Rectal bleeding.
- Perianal swelling.
- Discomfort.
- Pruritus ani.

HAEMORRHOIDS

Background

A haemorrhoid is a venous plexus (anal cushion) that drains into the superior rectal vein accompanying the superior rectal artery. Haemorrhoids occupy the 3, 7 and 11 o'clock positions when looking at the anus in the lithotomy position. The venous plexuses become congested because:

- Straining increases the venous pressure.
- During pregnancy venous return is delayed by the presence of a pregnant uterus.

Haemorrhoids result from straining to pass hard bulky stool that stretches the muscle and causes haemorrhoidal venous plexus engorgement.

Clinical presentation

Symptoms of haemorrhoids are bright red rectal bleeding following defecation, pruritus ani due to mucous discharge, and prolapse. The stages of 'piles' are outlined in Fig. 25.1.

If the haemorrhoids cannot be reduced, it may be because the anal sphincter has gone into spasm. This is acutely painful and causes strangulation and thrombosis of the haemorrhoids.

Management

Haemorrhoids are diagnosed from the history and from examination of the anal canal with a proctoscope. General advice is given about a high-fibre diet to prevent constipation. *+ straining* First- and second-degree haemorrhoids can be treated by:

- Injection sclerotherapy—submucosal injection of phenol in almond oil into the base of the 'pile'. The injection is given using a proctoscope and should be painless because it is given above the dentate line.
- Barron's bands—rubber bands applied to the base of the haemorrhoid to constrict it so that it sloughs off 10 days later.
- Cryotherapy and infrared coagulation.
- Haemorrhoidectomy—if there is recurrent prolapse or the piles are acutely thrombosed. Each haemorrhoid is defined and its pedicle is transfixed and ligated. Complications of the operation include secondary haemorrhage at 10 days and

Fig. 25.1 Features of first-, second- and third-degree haemorrhoids

Stage	Appearance
first degree	small and do not prolapse
second degree	small and prolapse, but reduce spontaneously
third degree	prolapsing 'piles' that have to be reduced manually

haemorrhoidopexy

anal stenosis. Recently, stapling devices have been used to perform haemorrhoidectomies, in the hope of reducing postoperative pain.

ANAL FISSURE

Background

This is an acutely painful condition caused by straining, causing a superficial tear in the mucosa of the anal canal, usually posteriorly. There is secondary spasm of the external anal sphincter, which exacerbates the situation.

Clinical presentation

An anal fissure may cause some rectal bleeding. There is usually a history of throbbing severe perianal pain, which persists for some time after defecation.

Management

On inspection, the fissure will be visible with a sentinel 'pile' (skin tag) (Fig. 25.2). A rectal examination is often impossible due to spasm of the external anal sphincter.

Treatment options include the use of glyceryl trinitrate paste or local anaesthetic ointments, together with an anal dilator to overcome the sphincter spasm. Other medical treatments include oral nifedipine and botulinum A toxin injections. If this does not relieve the situation, a lateral internal sphincterotomy is performed. This relieves the spasm and allows the sphincter to heal. *which they think causes ischaemia*

> Treatment of anal fissure is aimed at reducing the anal sphincter resting tone.

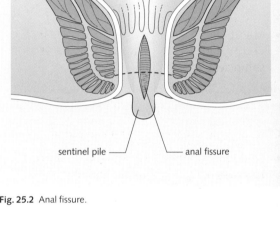

sentinel pile — anal fissure

Fig. 25.2 Anal fissure.

An anal stretch was previously performed, but is no longer recommended due to the risk of causing permanent sphincter damage, resulting in partial incontinence.

PERIANAL HAEMATOMA

Background

Perianal haematoma is an acutely painful condition and results from rupture of a small blood vessel beneath the perianal skin.

Clinical presentation

Perianal haematoma presents as a bluish tender swelling that cannot be reduced. It is usually precipitated by constipation and straining.

Management

Most perianal haematomas resolve spontaneously in a few days. Alternatively, the clot can be evacuated under local anaesthetic.

RECTAL PROLAPSE

Background

Rectal prolapse can occur in children, in whom it is a mucosal prolapse that resolves spontaneously.

A partial prolapse in adults can be treated with a submucosal injection of phenol but, in adults, the prolapse is usually full thickness.

Important aetiological factors are:

- Chronic constipation.
- Multiparity in women, which may damage the pudendal nerves, resulting in weakness of the sphincters.

Clinical presentation

Clinical presentations of rectal prolapse are:

- Discomfort of the prolapse, which may occur spontaneously or follow defecation.
- Rectal bleeding.
- Mucous discharge.
- Incontinence.

Management

Treatment is usually surgical. If the patient is fit for a laparotomy, a rectopexy is performed, which lifts the rectum and secures it to the hollow of the sacrum by a mesh or polytetrafluoroethylene sponge.

In elderly, frail patients, local excision of the redundant rectal mucosa (Delorme's procedure) can be performed.

Rectal prolapses must be reduced because there is a risk of gangrene. A rigid sigmoidoscopy must also be performed to exclude a carcinoma.

PERIANAL ABSCESS

Background

Perianal abscess is a very common problem requiring an acute surgical admission. The anal glands occur between the internal and external sphincters. A breach in the mucosa allows infection into the glands. This subsequently develops into an abscess, which then tracks inferiorly to the perianal region or laterally to the ischiorectal fossa, where it can track to the opposite ischiorectal fossa (Fig. 25.3). Pelvirectal abscesses are normally derived from abdominal or pelvic infections (e.g. appendicitis, Crohn's disease, pelvic inflammatory disease).

Clinical presentation

Patients present with a history of increasing discomfort in the perianal region, with associated throbbing pain and swelling.

Management

Inspection reveals a red, tender, inflamed and indurated area, and the patient is pyrexial. Rapid onset of symptoms and spread of the cellulitis must raise suspicion of necrotizing fasciitis. This is a ⚡SURGICAL EMERGENCY⚡ and surgery should be immediate.

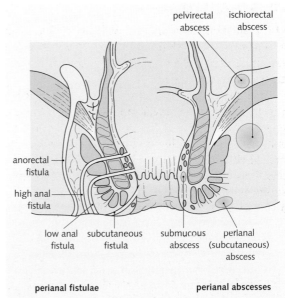

Fig. 25.3 Anatomy of perianal fistulae and abscesses.

Treatment is by incision and drainage under general anaesthesia.

A swab is taken for bacteriology. If skin organisms such as staphylococci are grown, the abscess is a simple skin infection but, if bowel organisms are grown, there is probably an underlying fistula. Endoanal ultrasonography can be used to identify an abscess and/or a simple fistula. In patients who are diabetic or have cancer or any chronic illness associated with a weakened immune system, treatment of any abscess must be prompt.

If a perianal abscess contains bowel flora, an underlying fistula should be suspected.

ANAL FISTULA

Background

A fistula is an abnormal communication between two epithelial surfaces (Fig. 25.2). If a patient has recurrent infections in the same area, or a persistent discharge, then suspect a fistula. Perianal sepsis may also be associated with:

- Crohn's disease.
- Tuberculosis.
- Carcinoma of the rectum.

Management

Magnetic resonance (MR) scanning is a useful investigation for imaging a complex fistula. ELiA

This is followed by examination under anaesthetic. The external opening may be visible and it is probed to find the internal opening:

- If the internal opening is below the level of the internal sphincter the fistula track can be excised and left to granulate.
- If the fistula tracks above and through the sphincters, a Seton suture is used (i.e. a non-absorbable suture is passed along the fistula track). The suture is gradually tightened and causes a fibrous reaction as it cuts its way through the sphincter, so there are no problems with incontinence.

Occasionally, a defunctioning colostomy needs to be formed before exploring a complex fistula.

Goodsall's law—fistulae with external openings posterior to the meridian (east to west) in the lithotomy position usually open on the midline of the anus, whereas those with anterior external openings usually open directly into the anus.

PRURITIS ANI

Background

Pruritus ani may develop secondary to local causes in the rectum and anal canal, causing mucous discharge. Common causes are:

- Haemorrhoids.
- Fistulae.   ← CA
- Fungal infection.
- Thread worms.

Clinical presentation

Pruritus ani is irritation of the perianal skin.

Management

Treatment of pruritus ani comprises:

- Good hygiene.
- Treatment of the underlying cause.

If fecal incontinence is suspected to be the cause of pruritus ani, anorectal manometry and endoanal ultrasound should be performed.

ANAL CARCINOMA

Background

Anal carcinoma is a rare malignancy and usually occurs in elderly people. It is a squamous cell carcinoma that originates in the squamous mucosa of the lower anal canal. Rarer tumours include melanoma of the anal canal.

Most cases of squamous cell carcinoma arise de novo, but it may develop from an area of Bowen's disease (i.e. squamous carcinoma in situ) or it may be related to human papillomavirus infection (some women who have cervical intraepithelial neoplasia have similar changes in the mucosa of the vulva and anal canal).

Clinical presentation

Presenting symptoms of anal carcinoma are:

- Perianal pain.
- Rectal bleeding.
- Discharge.
- Inguinal lymphadenopathy.

Management

A diagnosis of anal carcinoma is made by examination and biopsy.

Treatment is a combination of:

- Chemotherapy.
- Radiotherapy.
- Occasionally, surgical excision of the rectum and anal canal by an abdominoperineal resection.

The prognosis of anal carcinoma is poor.

Further reading

Darling JR, Weiss NS, Hislop TG et al. 1987 Sexual practices, sexually transmitted diseases, and the incidence of anal cancer. *N Engl J Med* **317**: 973–977

Grace RH, Harper IA, Thompson RC 1982 Anorectal sepsis: microbiology in relation to fistula in ano. *Br J Surg* **69**: 401–403

Whitehead SM, Leach RD, Elkyn SJ et al. 1982 The aetiology of perianal sepsis. *Br J Surg* **69**: 166–168

Keighley MRB, Williams NS 2007 *Surgery of the Anus, Rectum and Colon*, 3rd edn. WB Saunders, Philadelphia

Kocher HM, Steward M, Leather AJM et al. 2002 Randomized clinical trial assessing the side-effects of glyceryl trinitrate and diltiazem hydrochloride in the treatment of chronic anal fissure. *Br J Surg* **89**: 413–417

Nisar PJ, Scholefield JH 2003 Managing haemorrhoids. *BMJ* **327**: 847–851

Rousseau DL Jr, Thomas CR Jr, Petrelli NJ, Kahlenberg MS 2005 Squamous cell carcinoma of the anal canal. *Surg Oncol* **14**: 121–132

Stoker J, Rocin E, Wiersma TG, Lameris JS 2000 Imaging of anorectal diseases. *Br J Surg* **87**: 10–27

Hepatobiliary disorders

Learning objectives

You should be able to:

- Describe the important functions of the liver.
- List the complications of portal hypertension.
- Understand why people with portal hypertension develop oesophageal varices.
- Describe the mechanism by which humans become infected by the hydatid parasite.
- Understand why young women are at risk of developing focal nodular hyperplasia of the liver.
- Compare the clinical presentations of biliary colic and acute cholecystitis.
- Name the triad of signs found in the surgical emergency of ascending cholangitis.
- Identify the group of patients at risk of developing acalculous cholecystitis.
- Describe the signs that would lead you to think a patient was developing severe necrotizing pancreatitis.
- Define pancreatic pseudocysts and understand their treatment.

The liver is the largest gland in the body and has two lobes and eight segments. Its functions include:

- Metabolism.
- Synthesis.
- Detoxification.
- Defence (see: Cheshire, *Crash Course Gastrointestinal System*, Chapter 4).

The liver:

- Consumes approximately 20% of total body oxygen, and about 90% of the total hepatic blood flow is from the portal system.
- Produces about 600–1000 mL/day of bile and is responsible for secreting almost all the body's bilirubin (i.e. a breakdown product of haem).
- Is an important site of hepatic protein synthesis and catabolism, so albumin and protein levels are indicators of liver function.

ACUTE LIVER DAMAGE

Background

The liver can be damaged by a number of agents, such as:

- Viruses (e.g. hepatitis A, B or C).
- Drugs (e.g. alcohol, paracetamol).

Other causes of cirrhosis are cryptogenic or auto-immune (e.g. primary biliary cirrhosis) or secondary to biliary obstruction.

Jaundice is the retention of bilirubin in the tissues and is caused by:

- Haemolysis—(prehepatic) when breakdown of red blood cells overwhelms hepatic conjugating capacity.
- Liver cell dysfunction—(hepatic) where there is defective metabolism of bilirubin by the liver.
- Obstruction—(posthepatic) see obstructive jaundice.

Management

Diagnosis of acute damage is based on the presence of high levels of serum transaminases and positive serology for hepatitis viruses. AST.

Assessment of clotting function is another indicator + albumin. of hepatic function because factors II, VII, IX and X are manufactured in the liver with vitamin K.

Acute liver damage may progress to chronic liver damage, cirrhosis, portal hypertension and liver failure.

> Hepatitis serology should be checked for all patients who have jaundice of unknown cause.

PORTAL HYPERTENSION

Background

Portal hypertension develops if there is an elevated portal pressure of more than 15 mmHg, which can result from:

- Inflow or outflow obstruction.
- More rarely, increased portal blood flow into the portal venous system due to an arteriovenous fistula between the portal vein and hepatic artery.

Causes of portal hypertension are:

- Prehepatic—portal vein thrombosis or occlusion by extrinsic compression.
- Intrahepatic—cirrhosis, periportal fibrosis, schistosomiasis.
- Posthepatic—veno-occlusive disease or Budd–Chiari syndrome.

> Remember that the causes of portal hypertension may be prehepatic, intrahepatic or posthepatic.

Complications of portal hypertension

Portal hypertension is associated with the following complications:

- Splenomegaly—causes thrombocytopenia.
- Collateral circulation—demonstrated by the presence of oesophageal and gastric varices (which can bleed) or by caput medusae (i.e. dilated veins around the umbilicus).
- Ascites—resulting from a low serum albumin concentration, increased aldosterone activity and sodium retention, and increased portal pressure leading to transudation of fluid.

Management of bleeding oesophageal varices

The management of bleeding oesophageal varices may include:

- Resuscitation.   *safe alway* / - *Pass ET tube*
- Endoscopic injection sclerotherapy and banding of varices.
- Tamponade with a Sengstaken–Blakemore tube (Fig. 26.1).
- Intravenous vasopressin or somatostatin—to lower the portal venous pressure.
- Transjugular intrahepatic portosystemic shunt—a new technique in which a stent is passed under radiological control from the internal jugular vein through the vena cava into the hepatic vein and into a portal radical in the liver to create a shunt to decrease the pressure.

Risks from a variceal bleed

Patients who bleed from oesophageal varices already have an increased bleeding tendency because of impaired clotting and a reduced number of platelets. Hypovolaemia further damages liver function. Blood in the bowel is broken down by bacteria to release ammonia, which is absorbed and can cause hepatic encephalopathy. Oral lactulose and neomycin are used to reduce ammonia formation and absorption. Following treatment, complications include perforation, ulceration and stricture.

> Enzyme-linked immunosorbent assays (ELISA) can be performed to confirm *Echinococcus granulosus* or *Echinococcus multilocularis* in suspected hydatid disease.

HEPATIC CYSTS

Background

The different groups of hepatic cysts are:

- Simple cysts—usually an incidental finding on ultrasound scan and asymptomatic.
- Cysts of polycystic disease—usually related to polycystic kidneys.
- Hydatid cysts—due to infection with *Echinococcus granulosus* or *Echinococcus multilocularis*. The

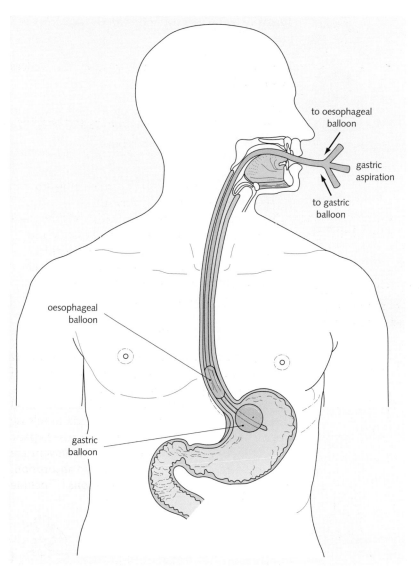

Fig. 26.1 A Sengstaken tube in position. It is used to control bleeding from oesophageal varices.

to oesophageal balloon

gastric aspiration

to gastric balloon

oesophageal balloon

gastric balloon

infection is found in sheep and dogs, and humans are the secondary host. It is endemic in sheep-rearing areas. The cysts can become infected or rupture into the biliary tract or intraperitoneally. Treatment involves medication with albendazole together with surgical excision.

HEPATIC ABSCESSES

Background

Hepatic abscesses can be intrahepatic or in the subphrenic or subhepatic spaces:

- Intrahepatic abscesses may be secondary to cholangitis or due to spread of infection via the portal circulation from infections such as diverticulitis or appendicitis.
- Extrahepatic abscesses develop secondary to intra-abdominal sepsis.

Clinical presentation

The clinical features of hepatic abscesses are:

- Swinging pyrexia.
- Rigors.
- Jaundice.

- Vomiting.
- Right hypochondrial pain.
- Malaise.

> HIV/AIDS should be considered in any unexplained liver abscess.

Management

A diagnosis of hepatic abscess is made by an ultrasound scan, which is used to guide percutaneous drainage. This is combined with systemic antibiotics. Occasionally, surgical drainage is required for multiloculated abscesses containing debris.

HEPATIC TUMOURS

Worldwide, primary hepatoma is a common cause of death but, in the UK, most hepatic tumours are secondary tumours.

Primary benign hepatic tumours

Background

Primary benign hepatic tumours are rare, but include adenoma and focal nodular hyperplasia.

> Adenoma and focal nodular hyperplasia of the liver may be associated with oral contraceptive use.

Clinical presentation

Primary benign hepatic tumours may be asymptomatic, but they may cause pain and can rupture spontaneously and cause intraperitoneal bleeding.

Haemangiomas are common, but are usually asymptomatic.

Primary hepatoma

Background

Primary hepatoma can develop de novo in a cirrhotic liver. It is associated with hepatitis B infection and aflatoxins and is very common worldwide. Most cases present late.

Management

Diagnostic tests include the presence of elevated α-fetoprotein in the serum, ultrasound scan and computed tomography (CT). Most tumours are not resectable and the prognosis is poor.

Cholangiocarcinoma

Background

Cholangiocarcinoma is a malignant tumour of the bile ducts.

Clinical presentation

Usually cholangiocarcinoma presents with painless obstructive jaundice.

Management

Cholangiocarcinoma is rarely resectable, but may be amenable to percutaneous or endoscopic stenting to give symptomatic relief.

Metastatic tumours

These are the commonest type of liver tumour. They are secondary deposits, particularly from:

- Breast.
- Colon.
- Stomach.
- Pancreas.
- Lung.
- Prostate.

Most are multiple and therefore not resectable.

Management

Palliative treatments can include systemic chemotherapy or via the hepatic artery, embolization, cryotherapy or interstitial laser hyperthermia.

CHRONIC LIVER DISEASE

The clinical signs of chronic liver disease are shown in Fig. 26.2.

Fig. 26.2 Stigmata of chronic liver disease

jaundice
ascites
caput medusae
spider naevi
gynaecomastia
palmar erythema
liver flap (hepatic encephalopathy)
Dupuytren's contracture
leukonychia
splenomegaly
clubbing
bleeding tendency — *bruising*
hepatomegaly
muscle wasting

GALLBLADDER DISEASE

Most gallbladder problems are secondary to gallstones, which are very common. There may be a familial tendency, and gallstones are more common in women than men. Other predisposing factors are:

- Obesity. *fat, female, 40, > 4 children,*
- Multiparity. *FHx*
- Chronic haemolytic disease.
- Ileal disease or resection.
- Drugs such as oral contraceptives, diuretics and clofibrate.

Gallstones are formed of cholesterol or bile pigments or are mixed stones.

> Over 90% of gallstones are not calcified and so do not show up on a plain abdominal radiograph.

Pathogenesis of gallstones

Cholesterol stones

Normally, cholesterol and phospholipids are held in solution by being surrounded by bile salts. When there is an imbalance, cholesterol crystals form and lead to the formation of stones.

Bilirubin and pigment stones

These may occur in patients who have chronic haemolytic disorders in which there is excessive production of bile pigments.

Alternatively, certain bacteria contain an enzyme, glucuronidase, which splits bilirubin and then combines with calcium to form calcium bilirubinate.

> In Caucasians, gallstones are composed predominantly of cholesterol, whereas pigmented stones are more common in Orientals.

Clinical presentation

Problems from gallstones are often triggered by ingestion of fatty food because it stimulates the production of cholecystokinin, which stimulates the gallbladder to contract to release bile to digest the fat.

When gallstones are contained within the gallbladder, the clinical presentation may include:

- Biliary colic—a severe episode of pain in the right hypochondrium that radiates to the tip of the scapula. Pain makes the patient restless, may last several hours, and may be associated with vomiting and sweating. Biliary colic is due to a gallstone temporarily obstructing the cystic duct or Hartmann's pouch.
- Acute cholecystitis—this may be preceded by biliary colic, but the pain then becomes localized and persistent in the right hypochondrium. It is associated with vomiting and, on examination, the patient will have a pyrexia and a positive Murphy's sign. It is due to chemical inflammation and secondary bacterial infection of an obstructed gallbladder. It may resolve with antibiotics for Gram-negative organisms.
- Chronic cholecystitis—the gallbladder is thick-walled and shrunken. The symptoms are chronic and non-specific, such as upper abdominal discomfort, flatulence, fatty food intolerance, epigastric or right hypochondrial pain and nausea. *— risk g/bl. CA.*
- Mucocoele—this forms if the gallbladder remains obstructed and the contents are sterile.
- Empyema—this forms if the gallbladder is obstructed and infection persists despite antibiotics.

Gallstones may exit the gallbladder and cause several problems (Fig. 26.3), including:

- Obstructive jaundice—a stone may lodge in the common bile duct (choledocholithiasis), preventing the drainage of bile, so the patient has symptoms and signs of obstructive jaundice.
- Ascending cholangitis—if infection develops in an obstructed biliary system the patient is seriously ill with fever, rigors and jaundice (Charcot's triad), and is at risk of developing septicaemia. Cholangitis is a ⚠SURGICAL EMERGENCY⚠. To differentiate this emergency from other common gallstone-related diagnoses, see Fig. 26.4.

- Pancreatitis—a stone in the common bile duct may travel further down, obstruct the pancreatic duct and cause pancreatic inflammation.
- Gallstone ileus—an inflamed gallbladder may become adherent to adjacent structures such as the duodenum. Persistent inflammation may cause a fistula to develop between the structures so that a large gallstone can pass through the wall of the gallbladder directly into the small intestine and present with small bowel obstruction (i.e. gallstone ileus).

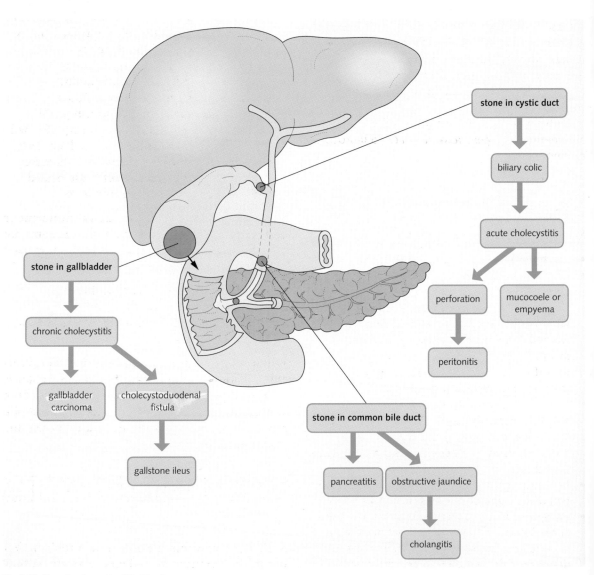

Fig. 26.3 Complications of gallbladder disease.

Fig. 26.4 Differentiating between the four common gallstone-related diagnoses

	Pain	Sepsis	Jaundice
biliary colic	yes	no	no
cholecystitis	yes	yes	no
choledocholithiasis (common bile duct stone)	yes	no	yes
ascending cholangitis	yes	yes	yes

- Perforated gallbladder—occurs if the obstructed gallbladder becomes overdistended and the fundus is ischaemic. Peritonitis develops.

An uncommon complication of chronic gallstone disease is the development of carcinoma of the gallbladder. It is usually discovered late when it has already invaded adjacent structures, so the prognosis is poor. Occasionally, carcinoma of the gallbladder is an incidental finding after cholecystectomy.

Pathologically, 90% of gallbladder carcinomas are adenocarcinomas and 10% are squamous cell carcinomas.

Management

Gallstones are usually diagnosed by ultrasound scan. Management plans are as follows:

- Asymptomatic—no treatment required.
- Chronic cholecystitis—patients are given advice about a low-fat diet and advised to have a cholecystectomy, which is usually performed laparoscopically. Patients should always be warned that it may be necessary to convert to an open cholecystectomy if it is not possible to perform a safe operation due to gross inflammation or technical difficulties.
- Acute cholecystitis—patients are treated with analgesia, intravenous fluids and antibiotics. If this does not resolve, cholecystectomy is required urgently, otherwise it is performed at a later date.
- Perforated gallbladder—peritonitis requires an emergency laparotomy and cholecystectomy.
- Empyema—if the patient is fit for an operation a cholecystectomy is performed but, if the patient is unfit, a cholecystostomy (i.e. percutaneous drainage of the abscess) can be performed instead.

- Gallstone ileus—this is usually diagnosed during a laparotomy for small bowel obstruction. The diagnosis may be suspected if a preoperative abdominal radiograph shows gas in the biliary tree. The gallstone is removed from the ileum by an enterotomy, but the choleduodenal fistula is left because it will seal spontaneously.
- Common bile duct stones—patients are jaundiced clinically and biochemically. The ultrasound scan will show a dilated bile duct and urgent endoscopic retrograde cholangiopancreatography (ERCP) is performed to remove the stones so the bile can drain freely to decrease the risk from infection. If there are signs of cholangitis, the patient is also treated with intravenous fluids and antibiotics.

Some patients are not fit for surgical treatment or decline an operation. Non-surgical treatments are available, but are not very effective and have marked side effects. For the treatments to be effective:

- The gallbladder needs to be capable of contractions.
- The stones should be radiolucent and less than 15 mm in diameter.

Non-surgical treatments include the use of extracorporeal shock-wave lithotripsy. This shatters the stones into small pieces, which are then passed out of the gallbladder, but the patient also has to ingest bile salts such as chenodeoxycholic acid to prevent the stones reforming.

ACALCULOUS CHOLECYSTITIS

Background

Acalculous cholecystitis is a rare problem, but occurs in seriously ill patients who are already requiring intensive treatment (e.g. following cardiac surgery, multiple trauma or burns). Acute inflammation of the gallbladder may result from stasis and secondary infection. Cholecystectomy may be required.

Other acalculous conditions are:

- Cholesterolosis (strawberry gallbladder, i.e. cholesterol deposits in the gallbladder wall).
- Adenomyomatosis (cholecystitis glandularis proliferans).
- Porcelain gallbladder (calcification of the gallbladder).

Acute acalculous cholecystitis requires urgent treatment with percutaneous drainage or immediate cholecystectomy if the patient is fit for surgery.

SURGICAL EMERGENCY

Pancreatitis

Background

This is an acute inflammatory condition of the exocrine pancreas. Acinar injury occurs, releasing pancreatic enzymes into the circulation and the peritoneal cavity. It is a surgical emergency, as although it can be a mild disease it may also present or develop into a very severe illness with life-threatening complications.

Common causes are:

- Duct obstruction—due to gallstones, tumours, abnormal anatomy of the pancreas. *GET SMASH-ED*
- Acinar cell injury—due to alcohol, steroids, diuretics, hypothermia, hypercalcaemia, hyperlipidaemia, viruses (e.g. coxsackievirus and mumps) or trauma.

Clinical presentation

Patients present with an acute onset of severe constant epigastric pain, which often radiates to the back. There may be associated symptoms of nausea or vomiting. The history may give clues about the likely aetiology. Clinical signs may include:

- Tachycardia.
- Hypotension.

- Pyrexia.
- Jaundice.
- Upper abdominal tenderness.
- Peritonism.

If the symptoms have been present for a few days, there may be bruising of the abdominal wall due to tracking of a bloodstained exudate:

- Grey Turner's sign in the flank.
- Cullen's sign in the periumbilical region.

If the patient is developing severe necrotizing pancreatitis, there may be signs of:

- Hypotension due to septicaemia.
- Respiratory depression.
- Diffuse abdominal tenderness with distension because of ascites.
- Absent bowel sounds due to an ileus.

Management

Effective management of pancreatitis is by:

- Diagnosis—this is made by detecting an elevated serum amylase (i.e. 1000 IU/mL). An abdominal radiograph may show a sentinel loop of small intestine in the region of the pancreas. The important differential diagnosis is a perforated peptic ulcer, and this diagnosis is confirmed by the presence of free subdiaphragmatic gas on an erect chest radiograph. Other investigations are performed to assess the severity of the condition according to the Imrie–Ransom criteria (Fig. 26.5). A score of 3 or more suggests severe disease and the patient may need to be treated on an intensive care unit.
- Resuscitation—intravenous fluids, oxygenation.
- Intensive monitoring—pulse, blood pressure, oxygen saturation, temperature, urine output, renal function, glucose and calcium levels.
- Analgesia.
- Imaging of pancreas—an ultrasound scan is useful to diagnose gallstones and pancreatic pseudocysts but, if the patient has severe haemorrhagic or necrotizing pancreatitis, a CT scan is essential to assess the extent of necrotic tissue, which may require surgical debridement.
- ERCP—this is performed to clear the bile duct of any gallstones if this is the cause.
- Cholecystectomy—if the pancreatitis is caused by gallstones a cholecystectomy is necessary to prevent further episodes.

Other causes should be treated appropriately (e.g. complete abstinence from alcohol).

(Continued)

(Continued)

Complications of acute pancreatitis

Complications that can be associated with acute pancreatitis are:

- Pancreatic pseudocyst—this may follow mild or moderate pancreatitis. It is a collection of fluid in the lesser sac (i.e. between the stomach and the pancreas). It may be asymptomatic or cause gastric compression or an abdominal swelling. It is diagnosed by ultrasound scan. If small it may resolve, or it can be drained percutaneously. Large or recurrent cysts require surgical drainage into the stomach (i.e. cystgastrostomy) or into the small intestine (Fig. 26.6).
- Pancreatic necrosis, abscess or intra-abdominal sepsis—these follow severe pancreatitis. They are diagnosed by CT scan and the poor condition of the patient. Urgent laparotomy with radical operative debridement of necrotic tissue is required. The patient requires intensive monitoring in the intensive care unit.
- Pancreatic haemorrhage.
- Acute respiratory distress syndrome. *ARDs*
- Renal failure.

Gallstones and alcohol cause 95% of cases of pancreatitis.

Fig. 26.5 Investigations to assess the severity of pancreatitis (Imrie–Ranson criteria) *only after 48hrs* *valid for alcohol-induced.*

Type of investigation	Parameter
clinical	hypotension
	respiratory difficulty
laboratory	white cell count >16 × 10⁹/L
PaO₂ <8kPa	pO₂ 7.98 kPa (60 mmHg)
Age >55	blood glucose 11.2 mmol/L
Neutr >15x10⁹	serum lactate dehydrogenase (LDH) 350 IU/L
Ca <2mmol/L	aspartate transaminase (AST) (also known as serum glutamic oxaloacetic transaminase (SGOT)) 250 IU/L
Renal Urea >16mmol/L	packed cell volume (PCV) ↓ 10%
E-LDH ~600 *AST-200*	blood urea 18 mmol/L
Albumin <32g/L	serum calcium 2.0 mmol/L
Sugar >10 mmol/L	

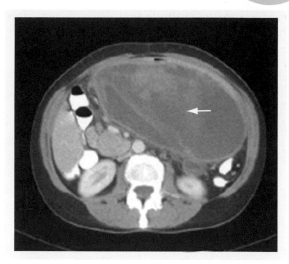

Fig. 26.6 Abdominal CT showing a large pancreatic pseudocyst (arrow).

CHRONIC PANCREATITIS

Background

Recurrent episodes of acute pancreatitis cause permanent damage to the pancreas, which becomes fibrotic and unable to fulfil its exocrine or endocrine functions. The commonest cause is alcohol abuse.

Clinical presentation

The symptoms of chronic pancreatitis are chronic, severe epigastric and back pain associated with the development of steatorrhoea, malnutrition and diabetes mellitus. Other presentations may include obstructive jaundice or duodenal obstruction, which may require treatment with a bypass procedure.

Constant upper abdominal pain is the hallmark of chronic pancreatitis.

Management

Treatment of chronic pancreatitis is aimed at controlling symptoms and comprises:

- Strong analgesics.
- Pancreatic enzyme supplements.
- Diabetic regimens.

A pancreaticojejunostomy is occasionally performed for chronic pain.

PANCREATIC TUMOURS

Background

These can arise from the exocrine or endocrine cells of the pancreas. The commonest tumour is an adenocarcinoma of the pancreas. The incidence of pancreatic carcinoma is increasing and it usually occurs in people over 50 years of age. Predisposing factors may include alcohol, diabetes mellitus and chronic pancreatitis. *smoking.*

Clinical presentation

Most pancreatic tumours present late with symptoms such as:

- Obstructive jaundice if the head of the pancreas is involved.
- Vomiting if there is duodenal obstruction.
- Severe intractable back pain if the body and tail are involved.
- Unexplained weight loss.

Occasionally, a small periampullary tumour presents early with obstructive jaundice.

> Pancreatic tumours tend to present late and are therefore usually inoperable.

Management

Effective management is by:

- Diagnosis—based on clinical suspicion. An ultrasound scan may show a dilated biliary tree and pancreatic mass. CT and endoscopic ultrasonography will provide more accurate information about the extent of tumour and operability. An ERCP may demonstrate a periampullary tumour and enable biopsies to be taken from it, or brush cytology from the pancreas. Tumour markers such as CA19-9 allow disease progress to be assessed.
- Treatment—most patients present late when the tumour is inoperable, so treatment is palliative in the form of analgesia, insertion of a stent to relieve obstructive jaundice or gastroenterostomy for duodenal obstruction.

The prognosis is poor and 90% of patients die within 1 year.

Periampullary tumours may be small and resectable by a pancreaticoduodenectomy (Fig. 26.7). The prognosis of these tumours is better and 50% of patients are alive at 5 years.

ENDOCRINE TUMOURS OF THE PANCREAS

Background

Endocrine tumours of the pancreas are uncommon, but are detected by the recognition of clinical syndromes.

> Suspect a gastrinoma if a patient presents with intractable peptic ulceration.

Management

A diagnosis of endocrine tumour of the pancreas is made by the detection of abnormal serum hormone levels by radioimmunoassay. The tumours are localized and staged by CT scans.

The commonest tumour is an insulinoma, and 90% of these are benign and solitary so they should be surgically resected. The other tumours are more likely to be malignant and may only be suitable for symptomatic treatment.

Fig. 26.8 summarizes the different types of endocrine tumours and their clinical effects.

OBSTRUCTIVE JAUNDICE

Clinical presentation

A diagnosis of obstructive jaundice is based on a clinical history of jaundice, pale stools, dark urine and pruritus, with or without pain.

140

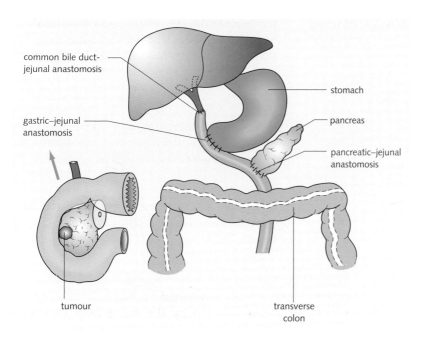

Fig. 26.7 Pancreaticoduodenectomy—Whipple's procedure. The distal stomach, duodenum, common bile duct and the head of the pancreas are removed. The stomach, pancreas and proximal common bile duct are then joined to a loop of jejunum.

Fig. 26.8 Endocrine tumours of the pancreas

Tumour	Hormone secreted	Effects
insulinoma	insulin	hypoglycaemia
gastrinoma	gastrin	Zollinger–Ellison syndrome, intractable peptic ulceration
glucagonoma	glucagon	diabetes mellitus, necrotic migratory erythema, weight loss, weakness, stomatitis
somatostatinoma	somatostatin	diabetes mellitus, gallstones, malabsorption

Management

Investigations include:

- Full blood count.
- Clotting screen.
- Urea and electrolytes—for baseline renal function.
- Liver function tests—show increased bilirubin, alkaline phosphatase and γ-glutamyltransferase. ↑ALP
- Ultrasound scan—shows a dilated biliary tree and may reveal the cause (e.g. gallstones or pancreatic tumour).
- ERCP—can be used to define the level of the obstruction, take biopsies, remove gallstones or insert a stent.
- Percutaneous transhepatic cholangiography—can be used to define the level of obstruction if

unable to do an ERCP, and a stent can also be inserted percutaneously to bypass an obstruction.
- Magnetic resonance cholangiopancreatiography (MRCP) is now rapidly replacing diagnostic ERCP.
- CT scan—can be used to stage and assess the operability of a tumour.

↑ALP
Raised conjugated bilirubin and alkaline phosphatase are seen in obstructive jaundice.

The causes of obstructive jaundice are given in Fig. 26.9.

Fig. 26.9 Causes of obstructive jaundice

Location	Cause
in the lumen of the bile duct	*CBD* gallstones, *Clonorchis sinensis* (liver fluke)
in the wall of the bile duct	cholangiocarcinoma, benign strictures, sclerosing cholangitis, carcinoma of ampulla of Vater
outside the bile duct	porta hepatis nodes, pancreatic cancer, gallbladder cancer, chronic pancreatitis

Complications of obstructive jaundice

Before any invasive procedure, either radiological or surgical, precautions should be taken to prevent complications of obstructive jaundice, such as:

- Cholangitis—infection manifested as rigors, pyrexia and hypotension.
- Renal failure—this may be precipitated by septicaemia or may be due to the absorption of endotoxins from the bowel and their reduced hepatic clearance. Endotoxins can cause acute tubular necrosis and peritubular fibrin deposition.
- Disseminated intravascular coagulation.
- Delayed wound healing and gastrointestinal haemorrhage.

To prevent these complications patients should be resuscitated and well hydrated to maintain renal perfusion. Abnormal clotting is corrected by administering vitamin K and other clotting factors. Administration of oral lactulose decreases the risk of endotoxaemia. Any infection is treated and prophylactic intravenous antibiotics are given before an invasive procedure.

The treatment of jaundice is:

- Use of a stent for inoperable malignant tumours.
- Removal of gallstones by ERCP.
- Laparoscopic or open cholecystectomy with common bile duct exploration.

Fig. 26.10 illustrates Courvoisier's law, which states that in the presence of jaundice, if the gallbladder is palpable then the jaundice is unlikely to be due to a

Fig. 26.10 Courvoisier's law.

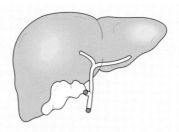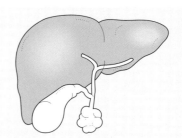

if the gallbladder is palpable in the presence of jaundice the jaundice is unlikely to be due to a stone because in the presence of stones the gallbladder is usually shrunken and fibrotic

exception

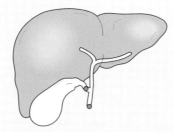

a stone stuck in Hartmann's pouch causing a mucocoele with another stone in the common bile duct

stone because the gallbladder is usually shrunken and fibrotic with gallstones. The exception to this rule is a stone stuck in Hartmann's pouch with another stone in the common bile duct.

Further reading

Beger HG, Warshaw AL, Büchler MW *et al.* 1998 *The Pancreas*. Blackwell Science, Oxford

Beckingham I 2001 *ABC of Liver, Pancreas and Gall Bladder*. BMJ Publications, London

Sanders G, Kingsworth AN 2007 Gallstones. *BMJ* **335:** 295–199

Millward-Sadler GH, Wright IR, Arthur MPJ (eds) 1992 *Wright's Liver and Biliary Disease: Pathophysiology, Diagnosis, and Management*, 3rd edn. WB Saunders, London

Sherlock S 2001 *Diseases of the Liver and Bilary System*, 4th edn. Blackwell Scientific, London

Smith R, Sherlock S (eds) 1981 *Surgery of the Gall Bladder and Bile Ducts*. Butterworths, London

United Kingdom guidelines for the management of acute pancreatitis 2005 British Society of Gastroenterology. *Gut* **54** (Suppl 3): 1–9

Takhar AS, Palaniappan P, Dhingsa R, Lobo DN 2004. Recent developments in diagnosis of pancreatic cancer. *BMJ* **329:** 668–673

Werner J, Feuerbach S, Uhl W, Buchler MW 2005 Management of acute pancreatitis: from surgery to interventional intensive care. *Gut* **54:** 426–436

Gynaecological disorders

Learning objectives

You should be able to:

- Name three types of benign ovarian cyst.
- Understand complications that may occur with ovarian cysts and tumours.
- Describe the management of inoperable disseminated ovarian tumours.
- Name the organisms associated with pelvic inflammatory disease.
- Understand the possible complications associated with pelvic inflammatory disease.
- Name the factors that predispose to ectopic pregnancy.
- Understand the important factors in the management of ectopic pregnancy.
- Define a fibroid and describe how they usually present.

Women who present with lower abdominal pain may have a gynaecological problem. It is usually a benign condition and may be part of the normal menstrual cycle (e.g. mittelschmerz or midcycle pain) due to ovulation. Another common cause of pain is dysmenorrhoea (i.e. pain due to menstruation) and this can be of variable severity. It may be associated with:

- Excessive uterine contractions.
- Endometriosis.
- Pelvic inflammatory disease.

Other symptoms may be menorrhagia, dyspareunia or infertility.

Torsion of an ovarian cyst results in vascular ischaemia and causes pain. The pain is usually located in one of the iliac fossae. An abnormally large ovary such as a polycystic ovary can lead to torsion of the entire ovary. This is a ⚠SURGICAL EMERGENCY⚠

OVARIAN CYSTS AND NEOPLASMS

Many cysts are asymptomatic and are detected by pelvic ultrasound scan. The different benign cysts are:

- Follicular cysts—simple thin-walled cysts, which are asymptomatic and resolve spontaneously.
- Corpus luteum cysts—form after ovulation.
- Endometriosis cysts—these are due to bleeding into a deposit of endometriosis and the blood becomes thick and tarry to form a 'chocolate cyst'.

OVARIAN TUMOURS

Background

Ovarian tumours usually have solid and cystic elements. They are classified as benign or malignant, and as serous, mucinous or endometroid tumours.

An unusual type of benign tumour is a teratoma or dermoid cyst, which usually occurs in women aged between 20 and 30 years, and 20% are bilateral. It is a cystic tumour and may contain a variety of structures such as hair, teeth, skin or cartilage.

Ovarian cancer often presents with vague symptoms and is initially painless.

Clinical presentation

Ovarian tumours may be asymptomatic, or they may present with abdominal distension from a large benign cyst, or from ascites if the tumour is malignant. Pressure symptoms may cause frequency of micturition. Abdominal pain is a symptom if a complication occurs.

If the tumour is malignant, there may be systemic features of malignancy such as weight loss.

Complications

Complications associated with ovarian cysts and tumours are:

- Torsion—this causes severe lower abdominal pain with vomiting. There may be a history of preceding episodes that resolved.
- Rupture—if the cyst is small and benign, it is probably asymptomatic. If a malignant tumour ruptures, this causes severe lower abdominal pain with vomiting and circulatory collapse.
- Haemorrhage into a cyst—this causes similar symptoms to torsion.

Management

Diagnosis is usually made by pelvic ultrasound. If a complication has occurred to a benign cyst or tumour then laparoscopic or open surgical intervention is required.

If malignancy is suspected, the tumour marker CA125 may be elevated and computed tomography or magnetic resonance scan can be used to assess stage and operability:

- If operable, bilateral oophorectomies, a hysterectomy and omentectomy are performed.
- If technically inoperable due to widespread intraperitoneal disease, the tumour is debulked as much as possible and any residual disease is treated with chemotherapy, which has dramatically improved the prognosis of ovarian cancer.

PELVIC INFLAMMATORY DISEASE

Background PID

Pelvic inflammatory disease can be an acute condition or have a more chronic course. Infection may follow delivery or abortion, or commonly it is sexually transmitted. The causative organisms are:

- *Streptococcus* or *Staphylococcus* spp. after operative intervention.
- *Neisseria gonorrhoeae* and *Chlamydia trachomatis* are implicated in sexually transmitted infection.

Clinical presentation

The symptoms of acute infection are:

- Lower abdominal pain.
- Dyspareunia.
- Vaginal discharge.
- Malaise.
- Fever.

Management

Clinical examination will produce tenderness of the lower abdomen and on vaginal examination. A high vaginal swab is taken to find the causative organism. A pelvic ultrasound scan is done to look for complications (Fig. 27.1) such as:

- Hydrosalpinx—an obstructed swollen fallopian tube.
- Pyosalpinx—an obstructed fallopian tube containing pus.
- Tubo-ovarian abscess—an inflammatory process involving the fallopian tube and ovary, which may rupture to cause peritonitis.

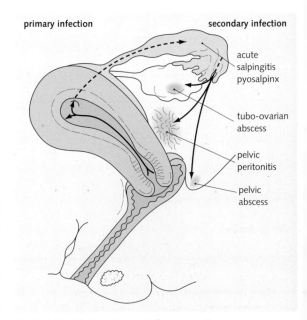

Fig. 27.1 Complications of pelvic inflammatory disease.

Most cases of pelvic inflammatory disease are managed conservatively with analgesia and appropriate antibiotics. Surgical intervention is required for a complication suggesting ongoing sepsis.

> Pelvic inflammatory disease should be treated with broad-spectrum antibiotics. Infection left untreated may result in a tubo-ovarian abscess.

Some patients develop chronic pelvic inflammatory disease due to subacute recurrent infections. This causes chronic pelvic pain, dyspareunia, infertility and an increased risk of an ectopic pregnancy.

SURGICAL EMERGENCY

Ectopic pregnancy

Background
A diagnosis of pregnancy should be excluded in all women of reproductive age who present with lower abdominal pain in case they have an ectopic pregnancy. This is a fertilized ovum which implants outside the uterus, usually in the fallopian tube.
 Predisposing factors are pelvic inflammatory disease and the presence of an intrauterine contraceptive device.

Clinical presentation
The symptoms of ectopic pregnancy occur about 6–8 weeks after conception. There is usually a history of a missed period and possibly a positive pregnancy test. The patient will complain of lower abdominal pain, which is due to distension of the fallopian tube, and there may be some vaginal bleeding.
 If the pain becomes more severe and there is circulatory collapse, the pregnancy has ruptured into the peritoneal cavity.

Management
The diagnosis is made from the history, together with a positive pregnancy test and an ultrasound scan, which demonstrates the swollen tube.
 If the patient presents with acute collapse, an emergency laparotomy is required.

All ectopic pregnancies have to be removed either laparoscopically or at open surgery to prevent rupture. If possible, efforts are made to preserve the fallopian tube.

> Pregnancy should be excluded in young women who have lower abdominal pain because of the risk of an ectopic pregnancy.

ENDOMETRIOSIS

Background

Endometriosis is a common uterine disorder and is due to ectopic deposits of endometrial cells in the lower part of the peritoneal cavity.

Clinical presentation

The main symptom of endometriosis is premenstrual pain that reaches a peak during menstruation and then gradually subsides.

> Endometriosis results in acute abdominal pain when an ovarian 'chocolate cyst' ruptures.

Management

Endometriosis is initially treated by suppressing ovarian function. If complications occur, division of adhesions, laser ablation or surgical excision of the affected organs is required.

LEIOMYOMA

Leiomyoma is a benign tumour of the myometrium.
 Most fibroids are asymptomatic, but they may cause menorrhagia. Pelvic pain may occur if a pedunculated submucous fibroid undergoes torsion or infarcts during pregnancy.

Further reading

Bhoola S, Hoskins WJ 2006 Diagnosis and management of epithelial ovarian cancer. *Obstet Gynaecol* **107**: 1399–1410

Grudzinskas G, O'Brien P M S (eds) 1997 *Problems in Early Pregnancy: Advances in Diagnosis and Management*. Royal College of Obstetricians and Gynaecologists, London

Hammond R 2005 Gynaecological causes of abdominal pain. *Surgery* **23**: 228–231.

Hare MJ 1986 Pelvic inflammatory disease. *BMJ* **293**: 1255–1258

Lathe P, Mignini L, Gray R, Hills R, Khan K 2006 Factors predisposing women to chronic pelvic pain: systematic review. *BMJ* **332**: 749–755

Mishell D, Goodwin T, Brenner P 2002 *Management of Common Problems in Obstetrics and Gynaecology*, 4th edn. Blackwell, Oxford

Seeber BE, Barnhart KT 2006 Suspected ectopic pregnancy. *Obstet Gynaecol* **107**: 399–413

Abdominal hernias

28

Learning objectives

You should be able to:

- Define a hernia.
- Understand why it is necessary to repair hernias.
- Describe the difference between a direct and indirect inguinal hernia.
- Understand how to differentiate between a femoral and an inguinal hernia.
- Define a Richter's hernia.
- Describe the repair of a paraumbilical hernia.
- List the factors that predispose to the formation of an incisional hernia.
- Describe the X-ray appearance of a diaphragmatic hernia diagnosed in a newborn baby.
- Identify a group of patients in whom an obturator hernia classically occurs.
- List the factors that predispose to the formation of a rectus haematoma.

A hernia is a protrusion of a viscus or part of a viscus through its covering into an abnormal situation. A hernia consists of:

- Contents.
- Sac (e.g. peritoneum).
- External coverings.

Hernias occur at natural points of weakness (e.g. umbilicus, inguinal canal or femoral canal) (Fig. 28.1), but may be caused by nerve damage causing muscle weakness. Such weaknesses may be exacerbated by conditions that increase intra-abdominal pressure, such as ascites, chronic cough, constipation, urinary outflow obstruction and heavy lifting. *dilato Sac* ·

TYPES OF HERNIA

The four major types of hernia illustrated in Fig. 28.2 are:

- Reducible—the contents of the hernia will return easily to the peritoneal cavity.
- Irreducible—adhesions form between the contents and the sac so it is impossible to reduce the bowel or omentum, but it is viable.
- Strangulated—the contents of the sac become stuck through the hernial orifice and the blood supply is cut off so the bowel becomes ischaemic. Patients have symptoms of small bowel obstruction and the hernia is a tender inflamed swelling.

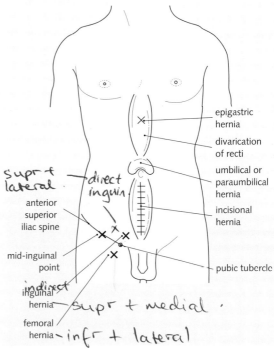

Fig. 28.1 Hernia sites.

Fig. 28.2 Types of hernia.

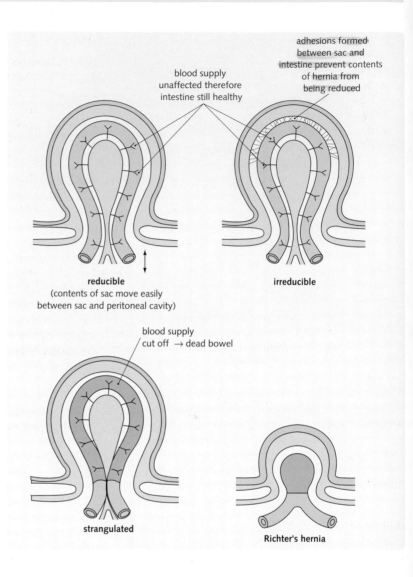

blood supply
unaffected therefore
intestine still healthy

adhesions formed
between sac and
intestine prevent contents
of hernia from
being reduced

reducible
(contents of sac move easily
between sac and peritoneal cavity)

irreducible

blood supply
cut off → dead bowel

strangulated

Richter's hernia

- Sliding—the sac may contain bowel, which is adherent to the sac so it cannot be reduced separately (e.g. sigmoid colon).

Hernias with narrow necks have a high risk of strangulation. The frequency of strangulation for different types of hernia, in descending order, is:
  - Femoral.
  - Indirect inguinal.
  - Paraumbilical.

INGUINAL HERNIA

Background

The anatomy of the inguinal canal and the two different types of inguinal hernia (direct and indirect) are shown in Fig. 28.3.

- Indirect inguinal hernia may be congenital due to failure of obliteration of the processus vaginalis. It can also be acquired later in life when the sac emerges through the deep ring and passes along the inguinal canal together with the vas deferens and acquires the coverings of the cord. It may emerge

    — Risk of strangulation

    — above + medial

indirect inguinal hernia

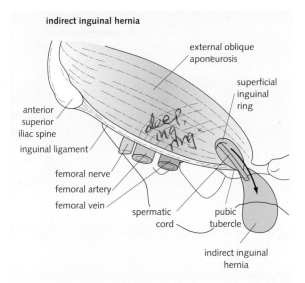

- external oblique aponeurosis
- superficial inguinal ring
- anterior superior iliac spine
- inguinal ligament
- *deep. ing. ring*
- femoral nerve
- femoral artery
- femoral vein
- spermatic cord
- pubic tubercle
- indirect inguinal hernia

direct inguinal hernia

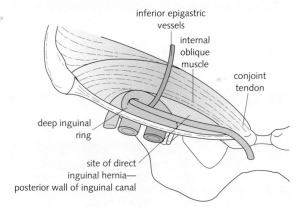

- inferior epigastric vessels
- internal oblique muscle
- conjoint tendon
- deep inguinal ring
- site of direct inguinal hernia— posterior wall of inguinal canal

Fig. 28.3 Anatomy of the inguinal canal to demonstrate indirect and direct inguinal hernias.

through the superficial ring into the upper scrotum.

- Direct inguinal hernia occurs as a result of weakness in the transversalis fascia in Hasselbach's triangle.

  —above & lateral to pubic tubercle.

> Indirect inguinal hernias appear above and medial to the pubic tubercle.

Management

Inguinal hernias should be repaired, especially if indirect. In children, a herniotomy (i.e. excision of the sac) is sufficient but, in adults, a herniotomy is accompanied by repair of the weakness in the posterior wall of the inguinal canal. The darn technique has been superseded by the use of a non-absorbable synthetic mesh (Lichenstein technique), or 'plug', which is used to produce a non-tension repair. This has the lowest risk of recurrence because it does not rely on the strength of the tissues.

A truss is of no significant benefit and many patients can have a hernia repaired under regional anaesthesia rather than a general anaesthetic. Laparoscopic mesh repair causes less postoperative pain and patients return to normal activities earlier. However, it is a difficult technique, which requires a longer anaesthetic and special expertise. It is therefore usually only performed for recurrent or bilateral hernias.

FEMORAL HERNIA

The anatomy of a femoral hernia is shown in Fig. 28.4.

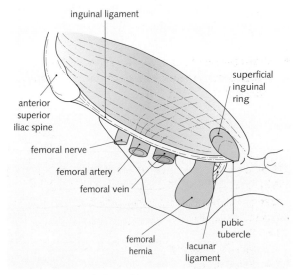

- inguinal ligament
- superficial inguinal ring
- anterior superior iliac spine
- femoral nerve
- femoral artery
- femoral vein
- pubic tubercle
- femoral hernia
- lacunar ligament

Fig. 28.4 Anatomy of a femoral hernia.

Femoral hernias appear below and lateral to the pubic tubercle.

Management

All femoral hernias should be repaired because of the high risk of strangulation. There are several surgical approaches to a femoral hernia—low or high, or via the posterior aspect of the inguinal canal. The sac is identified, the contents reduced and the femoral canal obliterated with non-absorbable sutures.

If the hernia contains small intestine, it may be necessary to extend the incision to allow access to the peritoneal cavity in order to resect the bowel.

Fig. 28.5 compares the features of indirect and direct inguinal hernias, and femoral hernias.

UMBILICAL HERNIA

Background

An umbilical hernia results from a congenital weakness due to persistence of an abdominal wall defect at the site of the umbilicus.

Management

Most umbilical hernias close spontaneously and an operation should not be performed until the child is at least 2 years old, unless the hernia becomes irreducible and strangulates.

PARAUMBILICAL HERNIA

Background

A paraumbilical hernia results from an acquired weakness, especially in obese adults. The defect is just above the umbilicus. The sac often contains omentum or small intestine.

Paraumbilical hernias are acquired and occur in adults due to increased intra-abdominal pressure and are associated with:

- Ascites—malignant/cirrhotic.
- Multiple pregnancy.
- Continuous ambulatory peritoneal dialysis.

Management

A paraumbilical hernia has a marked risk of strangulation and should be repaired by excising the sac and overlapping the edges of the rectus sheath (Mayo repair) with non-absorbable sutures.

EPIGASTRIC HERNIA

Background

An epigastric hernia is a small defect in the linea alba between the xiphisternum and the umbilicus,

Fig. 28.5 Comparison of inguinal and femoral hernias

Feature	Indirect inguinal	Direct inguinal	Femoral
sex	m > f	m > f	f > m
pathogenesis	may be congenital or acquired	acquired	acquired
age	children, adults	adults	middle-aged
descent into scrotum	may descend to scrotum	no	no
reduction	does not reduce immediately	spontaneously on lying down	does not reduce spontaneously
relationship to pubic tubercle	above and medial	above and lateral	below and lateral
controlled by pressure over deep ring	yes	no	no
risk of strangulation	high	very rare	high

which usually contains only extraperitoneal fat, but can be very painful. It does not usually have a sac.

An epigastric hernia can cause marked epigastric pain, mimick ing that of a peptic ulcer.

Management

The defect is closed with non-absorbable sutures.

Weight reduction improves the chances of successful repair in obese patients.

INCISIONAL HERNIA

Background

An incisional hernia occurs through a defect in a scar. It is more likely to occur if there has been a wound infection or haematoma. Patients who are jaundiced, cachexic, on corticosteroids or have a chronic cough have an increased risk of developing this type of hernia. Poor surgical technique also plays a marked role.

Management

Although the defect resulting in an incisional hernia is often large and the risk of strangulation is low, the appearance is unsightly and most patients want the hernia to be repaired. This may be done with sutures if the muscle is strong enough or it may need repair with a synthetic mesh.

UNCOMMON HERNIAS

Richter's hernia

This is an uncommon hernia and is a variant of a strangulated hernia in which only part of the bowel wall is strangulated (Fig. 28.2).

The patient will have some symptoms of abdominal pain and vomiting, but not absolute constipation. The diagnosis may therefore be delayed until the bowel perforates into the hernia sac.

Spigelian hernia

This very rare hernia occurs through the defect at the lateral border of the rectus abdominis muscle after emerging through a defect in the transversus and internal oblique fascia halfway between the umbilicus and the pubic symphysis.

Ultrasound and computed tomography (CT) are useful in confirming the diagnosis of spigelian hernia, especially in obese patients.

Gluteal hernia

This type of hernia crosses the greater sciatic notch.

Sciatic hernia

A sciatic hernia passes through the lesser sciatic notch.

Lumbar hernia

A lumbar hernia passes through the inferior lumbar triangle bounded by the iliac crest, the latissimus (dorsimedially) and the external oblique (laterally).

DIAPHRAGMATIC HERNIA

Background

A diaphragmatic hernia is an internal hernia and may be a congenital defect, which may be evident soon after birth.

The other cause of a diaphragmatic hernia is trauma. The left diaphragm is more commonly injured than the right. Minor tears may not be immediately apparent, but may present several years later with an incarcerated diaphragmatic hernia (i.e. with symptoms of bowel obstruction).

Clinical presentation

The newborn baby has breathing difficulties because the left side of the chest is occupied by the bowel rather than the lung. This is due to incomplete fusion of parts of the diaphragm.

Management

A diaphragmatic hernia requires urgent surgical repair.

OBTURATOR HERNIA

Background

This internal hernia occurs in frail elderly women.

Clinical presentation

The hernia occurs through the obturator canal within the pelvis, so the patient presents with small bowel obstruction. There may be pain along the medial aspect of the thigh because of pressure on the obturator nerve causing referred pain in its area of cutaneous distribution.

Management

Obturator hernia is rare and is usually only diagnosed at laparotomy for obstruction.

RECTUS HAEMATOMA

This abdominal wall swelling develops after abdominal wall straining (e.g. coughing or lifting) and is due to tearing of branches of the inferior epigastric artery. It is common in elderly patients who are being treated with anticoagulants.

Clinical presentation

Rectus sheath haematoma causes severe localized lower abdominal wall pain with a tender mass related to the lower part of the rectus sheath.

Management

A diagnosis of rectus haematoma may be confirmed by an ultrasound scan, and in most cases it is managed conservatively by analgesia and correcting any coagulation problem.

DESMOID TUMOR

This is a slow-growing tumour of the rectus abdominis muscle that usually occurs in young people. It may be related to Gardner's syndrome and may follow pregnancy. It is a tumour of spindle cells and there is a risk of local recurrence after excision.

Desmoid tumours are especially common in postpartum females and are probably due to hormonal change and surgical trauma.

Further reading

Awad SS, Fagan SP 2004 Current approaches to inguinal hernia repair. *Am J Surg* **188**(Suppl 6A): 9S–16S

Davis CJ, Arregui ME 2003 Laparoscopic repair for groin hernias. *Surg Clin North Am* **83**: 1141–1161

Devlin HB, Kingsnorth A 1998 *Management of Abdominal Hernias*, 2nd edn. JB Lippincott Williams & Wilkins, London

EU trialists collaboration 2002 Repair of groin hernia with synthetic mesh: meta analysis of randomized controlled trials. *Ann Surg* **235**: 322–332

Hachisuka T 2003 Femoral hernia repair. *Surg Clin North Am* **83**: 1189–1205

Kingsnorth A 2006 The management of incisional hernias. *J Roy Coll Surg Eng* **88** : 252–260.

Kurzer M, Belsham PA, Kark AE 2003 The Lichtenstein repair for groin hernias. *Surg Clin North Am* **83**: 1099–1117

Muschaweck U 2003 Umbilical and epigastric hernia repair. *Surg Clin North Am* **83**: 1207–1221

Nathan JD, Pappas TN 2003 Inguinal hernia: an old condition with new solutions. *Ann Surg* **238** (Suppl 6): S148–S157

Rutkow IM 2003 The perfix plug repair for groin hernias. *Surg Clin North Am* **83**: 1079–1098

Shouldice EB 2003 The Shouldice repair for groin hernias. *Surg Clin North Am* **83**: 1163–1187

Stephenson BM 2003 Complications of open groin hernia repairs. *Surg Clin North Am* **83**: 1255–1278

Voyles CR 2003 Outcomes analysis for groin hernia repairs. *Surg Clin North Am* **83**: 1279–1287

Learning objectives

You should be able to:

- Undestand why thyroglossal cysts move on swallowing.
- List the causes of a solitary thyroid nodule. Understand how you differentiate between them.
- Name four types of thyroid cancer. Distinguish the different age groups in which they commonly occur.
- Understand the indications for thyroid surgery and the complications that may develop.
- Describe how parathyroid hormone controls the serum calcium concentration.
- List the features seen in primary hyperparathyroidism.
- Describe how a parathyroid gland may be localized preoperatively.

THYROID GLAND

The thyroid gland develops from an endodermal outgrowth from the floor of the pharynx, which subsequently becomes the foramen caecum at the junction of the anterior two-thirds and the posterior one-third of the tongue. The tissue migrates towards the suprasternal notch. Below the larynx, it becomes a bilobed structure and proliferates to form the glandular tissue. The thyroglossal duct atrophies, but remnants may persist to become cysts. Ectopic thyroid tissue may be found anywhere along the route of the thyroid gland.

> The thyroid moves up and down on swallowing due to the investment of the pretracheal fascia.

Physiology

The thyroid gland is responsible for synthesizing thyroid hormones:

- Thyroxine (T_4).
- Tri-iodothyronine (T_3).

These are responsible for maintaining normal metabolism. The gland can become under- or overactive for a number of different reasons, resulting in a range of abnormal symptoms. Tri-iodothyronine and T_4 secretion are controlled by the hypothalamus and the anterior pituitary gland, which releases thyroid-stimulating hormone (TSH).

THYROGLOSSAL CYST

Background

A thyroglossal cyst is a midline swelling of the neck (see Chapter 30, Fig. 30.2). It is usually located below the hyoid bone and, because it is connected to the base of the tongue, it moves up on swallowing and when the tongue is protruded. The cyst may become infected or discharge.

Management

Treatment of a thyroglossal cyst is by surgical excision. The cyst is excised together with its fibrous tract extending to the foramen caecum, and it is often necessary to excise the hyoid bone.

> A radioiodine uptake scan is necessary before excising a thyroglossal cyst, as the cyst may contain some or all of the thyroid tissue.

Infection of a cyst or incomplete excision may produce a fistula track, discharging pus.

THYROID GOITRE

Background

Thyroid goitre is an abnormal swelling of the thyroid gland. Patients who have a goitre can be euthyroid, hypothyroid or hyperthyroid (Fig. 29.1).

Secondary thyrotoxicosis causes predominantly cardiovascular symptoms.

Causes of goitre include:

- Normal physiological change—for example in puberty or during pregnancy.
- Iodine deficiency—a dietary deficiency of iodine results in increased TSH activity to stimulate the gland to produce enough thyroxine, so the gland enlarges.
- Graves' disease—a diffuse smooth vascular swelling of the thyroid gland associated with thyrotoxicosis and eye problems, such as exophthalmos, lid lag and ophthalmoplegia.

Graves' disease is due to the presence of long-acting thyroid-stimulating immunoglobulin (LATS).

- Benign hyperplasia of the thyroid gland resulting in an adenomatous or multinodular goitre—adenomatous and colloid nodules are scattered throughout the gland. The gland may become acutely painful if haemorrhage occurs into a cyst. As the thyroid gland enlarges, it may cause pressure symptoms such as dysphagia and stridor, especially if it is retrosternal.
- Thyroid malignancy.
- Thyroiditis.

SOLITARY THYROID NODULE

Differential diagnosis of a solitary thyroid nodule consists of:

- Thyroid cyst.
- Benign adenoma.
- Thyroid malignancy.

Diagnosis of a solitary thyroid nodule is aided by performing an ultrasound scan, which can differentiate cystic from solid lesions and nodules from diffuse thyroid enlargement. A technetium-99 m pertechnetate isotope scan can be used to differentiate hot and cold nodules. Inactive (cold) nodules corresponding to isolated nodules are indicators of a cyst or a tumour.

Fig. 29.1 Comparison of thyrotoxicosis and hypothyroidism

Feature	Thyrotoxicosis	Hypothyroidism
symptoms	intolerance of heat, weight loss, increased appetite, tremor, palpitations, diarrhoea, sweating, anxiety, oligomenorrhoea	intolerance of cold, weight gain, lethargy, constipation, dry skin and hair, hoarse voice
signs	goitre, tachycardia, atrial fibrillation, warm and moist palms, tremor, Graves' disease (exophthalmos, lid lag, ophthalmoplegia)	pallor, slow pulse, thickened dry skin and hair, periorbital puffiness, loss of outer one-third of eyebrows, peripheral oedema, slow recovery phase to ankle jerk
causes	Graves' disease, secondary thyrotoxicosis in adenomatous goitre	thyroiditis, post-thyroid surgery
diagnosis	↑ T_4 or T_3, ↓ TSH; Graves' disease—presence of LATS	↓ T_4, ↑ TSH; Hashimoto's thyroiditis—↑ levels of antimitochondrial antibody or antithyroglobulin antibody
management	carbimazole or propylthiouracil, propranolol for ↑ heart rate, tremor, radioiodine, subtotal thyroidectomy	thyroxine replacement

If there is a solitary solid lesion, it is investigated by fine-needle aspiration cytology (FNAC). If abnormal cells are obtained then the lesion must be removed to make a precise histological diagnosis in case it is a thyroid cancer. It can be difficult to differentiate benign from well-differentiated cancers by FNAC alone.

Fine-needle aspiration cytology is unable to differentiate between a follicular adenoma and a follicular carcinoma.

THYROIDITIS

Autoimmune Hashimoto's thyroiditis

The patient presents with a diffuse tender goitre.

Diagnosis is made by detecting the presence of thyroid antibodies against thyroglobulin and mitochondria.

The patient is initially euthyroid and then becomes hypothyroid as the gland becomes atrophic and fibrotic. Treatment is by thyroxine replacement therapy.

Riedel's thyroiditis

This very rare condition results in a hard irregular swelling of the thyroid gland because of progressive fibrosis and may produce compression symptoms. Patients are usually euthyroid.

THYROID CARCINOMAS

Thyroid carcinomas are more common in women than men and can occur in young adults. They occur as well-differentiated adenocarcinomas of papillary, follicular or medullary type. These have a relatively good prognosis. Anaplastic carcinomas occur in the elderly and have a very poor prognosis (Fig. 29.2).

Other tumours of the thyroid include:

- Medullary carcinoma—a very rare tumour of the parafollicular or C cells of the thyroid that may arise within the syndrome of multiple endocrine neoplasia. MEN
- Lymphoma of the thyroid—rare, but may be associated with Hashimoto's disease and is responsive to radiotherapy.

THYROID OPERATIONS

Fig. 29.3 shows a diagram of the anatomical relationships of the thyroid gland.

Fig. 29.2 Features of main types of thyroid cancers

Feature	Papillary	Follicular	Anaplastic
proportion of cases (%)	60	25	10
age	children, young adults	middle age	elderly women
location	often multifocal	rarely multifocal	whole gland
growth rate	slow	slow	rapid
spread	lymphatic	blood	local infiltration causing pressure symptoms
management	total thyroidectomy plus lymph node dissection; TSH suppression by thyroxine	thyroid lobectomy, radioactive iodine	usually inoperable; radiotherapy, chemotherapy
prognosis	good	depends upon extent of vascular invasion	very poor

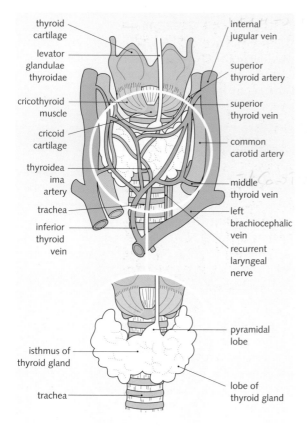

thyroid cartilage

levator glandulae thyroidae

cricothyroid muscle

cricoid cartilage

thyroidea ima artery

trachea

inferior thyroid vein

internal jugular vein

superior thyroid artery

superior thyroid vein

common carotid artery

middle thyroid vein

left brachiocephalic vein

recurrent laryngeal nerve

isthmus of thyroid gland

trachea

pyramidal lobe

lobe of thyroid gland

Fig. 29.3 Anatomy of the thyroid gland.

Curative surgery is not usually possible in anaplastic carcinoma and palliative radiotherapy should be considered.
Dyspnoea may be relieved by dividing the thyroid isthmus or performing a tracheostomy.

Indications for a thyroid operation

The common reasons for surgical intervention include:

- Subtotal thyroidectomy for control of Graves' disease.
- Relief of pressure symptoms from an enlarged multinodular goitre (Fig. 29.4).
- Lobectomy or total thyroidectomy for malignant tumour.

Preoperatively the patient should be rendered euthyroid (if for Graves' disease) by prescribing carbimazole and propranolol to control symptoms.

If the patient is thyrotoxic, Lugol's iodine may be prescribed for 10 days to reduce the vascularity of the gland.

Before operation, the vocal cords should be inspected by direct laryngoscopy to ensure that they are functioning satisfactorily.

Operative procedure

A collar incision is made, skin flaps are elevated, and strap muscles separated to expose the thyroid gland. The middle thyroid vein is ligated and divided, the superior thyroid vessels are ligated, the thyroid lobes are mobilized and the recurrent laryngeal nerves and parathyroid glands are identified and preserved.

Complications of thyroid operations

These are:

- Immediate haematoma—may occur in the first few hours after operation. It can cause laryngeal oedema, stridor and dyspnoea. This is a **⚠SURGICAL EMERGENCY⚠** The wound should be opened immediately, and the patient returned to theatre to control any haemorrhage.
- Recurrent laryngeal nerve injury—manifests as a hoarse voice or a bovine cough if one nerve is damaged. If there is bilateral damage, the patient is unable to speak and any exertion causes airway obstruction. Neurapraxia usually recovers but, if there is unilateral and permanent nerve damage, the cord can be injected with polytetrafluoroethylene. If both nerves are damaged, an emergency tracheostomy is required. This is a **⚠SURGICAL EMERGENCY⚠**
- Superior laryngeal nerve (external branch) injury—produces voice changes such as loss of pitch, but it usually recovers.
- Hypoparathyroidism—this may be temporary or permanent. Signs of hypocalcaemia will be paraesthesia, carpopedal spasm or Chvostek's sign of facial spasm. This is a **⚠SURGICAL EMERGENCY⚠** Immediate treatment is with calcium gluconate intravenously, followed by oral calcium and vitamin D if the response is insufficient.
- Hypothyroidism—if too much thyroid gland is removed then hypothyroidism develops but, if too much remains, there is risk of recurrent symptoms of goitre or thyrotoxicosis.

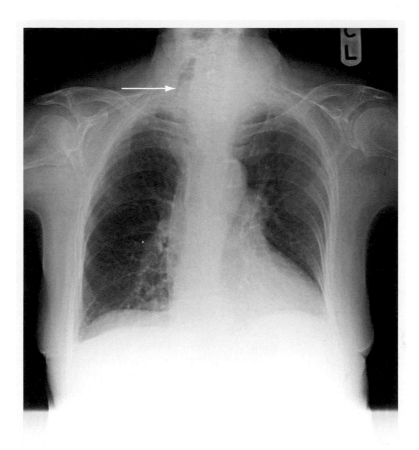

Fig. 29.4 A chest radiograph showing a large multinodular goitre causing tracheal deviation to the right (see arrow).

- Thyroid crisis—rarely seen if the patient is euthyroid preoperatively. It may, however, be precipitated by other illnesses such as pneumonia if the patient is thyrotoxic. Symptoms are pyrexia, agitation, confusion and tachycardia, and medication is given to control the symptoms.

Serum calcium should be measured 48 hours after thyroid surgery.

PARATHYROID DISORDERS

There are four parathyroid glands:

- The superior glands arise from the fourth branchial pouch.

- The inferior glands arise from the third branchial pouch.

The parathyroid glands secrete parathyroid hormone, which:

- Stimulates osteoclastic activity in bones, which releases calcium into the circulation.
- Enhances renal tubular absorption of calcium and inhibits reabsorption of phosphate.
- Facilitates absorption of calcium from the small intestine.

HYPERPARATHYROIDISM

Background

Hyperparathyroidism can be separated into three types as outlined below.

Primary hyperparathyroidism ↑PTH → ↑Ca

Primary hyperparathyroidism is due to a parathyroid adenoma or, rarely, a carcinoma, or due to hyperplasia of the parathyroid glands. Excess production of parathyroid hormone results in:

- Increased serum calcium and alkaline phosphatase concentration.
- Decreased serum phosphate concentration.

Suspect hypercalcaemia in confused, vomiting patients who have malignant disease.

Secondary hyperparathyroidism − ↓Ca → ↑PTH

Secondary hyperparathyroidism is due to hyperplasia of the glands secondary to chronic renal failure. Renal patients have a low serum calcium due to failure of vitamin D production, which is required to absorb calcium from the gut. The resultant serum calcium may be normal or low.

Symptoms of hypercalcaemia are:
- Bones.
- Stones.
- Abdominal groans.
- Psychic moans.

Tertiary hyperparathyroidism

After renal transplantation, most cases of parathyroid hyperplasia regress but, occasionally, the parathyroid glands become autonomous and do not respond to a rising serum calcium concentration.

Clinical presentation

Clinical features of hyperparathyroidism are:

- Renal calculi.
- Bone pain—due to decalcification.
- Pathological fractures—if there is generalized cystic change of bones (i.e. osteitis fibrosa cystica).
- Muscular weakness, anorexia, intestinal atony—because of depressed nerve conduction.
- Polyuria, dehydration.
- Peptic ulceration, acute and chronic pancreatitis.
- Psychiatric disorders.

Management

A diagnosis of hyperparathyroidism is made by measuring the fasting serum calcium concentration on several occasions. It should be corrected for plasma albumin concentration. The differential diagnosis of hypercalcaemia is shown in Fig. 29.5.

Parathyroid hormone concentration is measured by immunoassay techniques. High-resolution ultrasound or computed tomography (CT) or magnetic resonance imaging (MRI) can be used to image the parathyroid glands. A thallium/technetium subtraction scan can also be used.

Parathyroid adenomas and carcinomas are treated by surgical excision.

Hyperplasia of all four glands can be treated by excision of three of the four glands. Localization of the gland at operation may be aided by an infusion of methylene blue immediately preoperatively.

ADRENAL GLANDS

An adrenal gland is found superior to a kidney on each side. The adrenal cortex and medulla are anatomically and functionally separate. The cortex is derived from the mesoderm of the urogenital ridge and has three defined zones (from outside in):

Fig. 29.5 Differential diagnosis of hypercalcaemia

hyperparathyroidism
ectopic parathyroid hormone secretion
(e.g. by small cell lung tumour)
metastatic bone disease
sarcoidosis
multiple myeloma
hypervitaminosis D / vit D intox
familial

- Zona glomerulosa—produces mineral corticoids, principally under the control of the renin-*RAS.* angiotensin system.
- Zona fasciculata—produces glucocorticoids, principally cortisol under the control of adrenocorticotrophic hormone (ACTH). *hypothal-pituitary*
- Zona reticularis—produces sex hormones (e.g. androgens) under the control of the pituitary.

The adrenal medulla is derived from the neural crest and is closely associated with the sympathetic nervous system.

- The medulla produces catecholamines (e.g. adrenaline, (epinephrine) noradrenaline (norepinephrine).

ADRENAL CORTICAL DISORDERS

Cushing's syndrome

Background

Cushing's syndrome is due to an excess of glucocorticoid hormone due to:

- Prolonged oral steroids—most common.
- Cushing's disease—ACTH secreting microadenoma of the anterior pituitary gland.
- Ectopic ACTH secretion (e.g. small cell cancer of the lung).

> Systemic steroids are the commonest cause of Cushing's syndrome.

Clinical presentation

Clinical features of Cushing's syndrome are:

- Abnormal fat deposition.
- Skin changes.
- Abnormal striae.
- Muscular weakness.
- Hormonal and metabolic changes.

Management

There is no single test for the cause of Cushing's syndrome. Cushing's syndrome is diagnosed if the urinary cortisol level is elevated and cannot be suppressed with the low-dose dexamethasone suppression test. The plasma ACTH is measured:

- Low—primary adrenal disease.
- Moderately elevated—Cushing's disease.
- Markedly elevated—ectopic ACTH secretion.

Treatment depends on the cause. Medical treatment is important to provide temporary control of the disease before surgery.

- Unilateral adrenalectomy for adrenal adenomas and carcinomas.
- Pituitary surgery for Cushing's disease.
- Sources of ectopic ACTH secretion are rarely amenable to surgery.

Primary hyperaldosteronism

Background

This is also known as Conn's syndrome and is due to:

- Adenomas.
- Bilateral hyperplasia of the zona glomerulosa.
- Adrenal carcinoma.

Clinical presentations

K excretion

Clinical features are due mainly to hypokalaemia owing to the retention of sodium in exchange for potassium and hydrogen in the distal nephron. The patient usually presents with:

- Moderate to severe hypertension. *Na+ H₂O retent*
- Muscle weakness and cramping.
- Polydipsia.
- Polyuria.
- Nocturia.

> Conn's syndrome is a correctable cause of hypertension.

Management

The diagnosis is made on hypokalaemia, increased urinary potassium, increased plasma aldosterone and *cos RAS already activated.*

decreased plasma renin. If left untreated, it will lead to uncontrolled hypertension and hypokalaemia. Treatment includes:

- Unilateral adrenalectomy for adenomas and carcinomas.
- Other causes can be treated with spironolactone.

Phaeochromocytoma

Background

This is a tumour of the chromaffin cells of the sympathetic nervous system—90% occur in the adrenal medulla. Familial phaeochromocytomas occur in multiple endocrine neoplasia (MEN) types IIa and IIb.

Clinical presentations

The clinical symptoms and signs are due to excess circulating catecholamines. Patients may present with a triad of symptoms:

- Hypertension.
- Severe headaches.
- Palpitations.

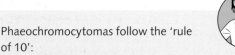

Phaeochromocytomas follow the 'rule of 10':
- 10% are malignant.
- 10% are multifocal.
- 10% are bilateral.
- 10% are extra-adrenal.

Management

The diagnosis is confirmed by finding high levels of breakdown products of catecholamines in the urine and tests include:

- 24-hour urinary free catecholamines.
- 24-hour urinary total metanephrines.
- 24-hour urinary vanillylmandelic acid.

Radiological localization should be performed only after the diagnosis has been confirmed biochemically. CT and MRI are the most reliable methods to localize the tumour. An iodine-131 meta-iodobenzylguanidine (MIBG) scan can also be used.

Incidentalomas

Incidentalomas are small nodules found incidentally within the adrenal gland during investigations (e.g. CT scans) for other problems. These are usually benign and non-functioning, but should be assessed as described.

Phaeochromocytomas require α and β blockade for 2 weeks prior to adrenalectomy. Patients require lifelong follow-up as there is a risk of recurrence.

Further reading

Allolio B, Fassnacht M 2006 Adenocortical carcinoma: clinical update. *J Clin Endocrinol Metab* **91**: 2027–2037

British Association of Endocrine Surgeons 2000 *Guidelines for the Surgical Management of Endocrine Disease*. Royal College of Surgeons, London

Fardon JR (ed.) 2001 *Endocrine Surgery*. Harcourt, London

Friesen SR, Thompson NW (eds) 1990 *Surgical Endocrinology: Clinical Syndromes*, 2nd edn. Lippincott Williams & Wilkins, Philadelphia

Frates MC, Benson CB, William Charboneau J et al. 2005 Management of thyroid nodules detected at US: Society of radiologists in US consensus conference statement. *Radiology* **237**: 794–800

Hall R, Besser M (eds) 1990 *Fundamentals of Clinical Endocrinology*, 4th edn. Churchill Livingstone, Edinburgh

Kaplan EL (ed.) 1983 *Surgery of the Thyroid and Parathyroid Glands*. Churchill Livingstone, Edinburgh

Pollock WF, Stevenson EO 1966 Cysts and sinuses of the thyroglossal duct. *Am J Surg* **112**: 225–232

Wheeler MH, Lazarus JH (eds) 1994 *Diseases of the Thyroid Gland*. Chapman & Hall, London

Neck swellings 30

Learning objectives

You should be able to:

- Distinguish the clinical appearance of infective and malignant cervical lymphadenopathy.
- Understand how the diagnosis is confirmed in suspected lymphoma.
- List the tumours that metastasize to the cervical lymph nodes.
- Describe where a branchial cyst and sinus are typically found.
- Name the salivary glands in which calculi commonly occur.
- Name the organism that commonly causes acute suppurative parotitis.
- Give a common cause of bilateral parotitis.
- Understand when a sialogram is performed.
- Describe the clinical manifestations of Sjögren's syndrome.
- Understand how a salivary gland carcinoma typically presents.

The anatomy of the lymphatic drainage of the neck and triangles of the neck is shown in Fig. 30.1.

CERVICAL LYMPHADENOPATHY

Background

Enlarged cervical glands may be due to a number of different pathologies:

- Primary—disorders of lymph nodes such as lymphoma. Characteristically these glands are 'rubbery', matted and large (i.e. 1–2 cm diameter).
- Secondary—to infection, which may be local or systemic (e.g. due to Epstein–Barr virus, human immunodeficiency virus). These glands are *EBV* smaller, softer and regular. The other common *CMV HIV* cause of cervical lymphadenopathy is metastatic nodes from malignant disease. Characteristically the glands are hard, irregular, and may be fixed.

Management

Any patient who has enlarged cervical nodes should have a full examination to look for other areas of lymphadenopathy or hepatosplenomegaly. Those areas that drain to the cervical nodes should be

examined (including indirect laryngoscopy) to look for a primary lesion.

A full blood count will give information about any abnormalities of the white blood cells. Fine-needle aspiration cytology (FNAC) from the node will produce epithelial cells if it is a metastatic node. If the node is reactive or there is a primary lymph node problem lymphocytes will be non-diagnostic and an excision biopsy is required if a lymphoma is suspected.

If a metastatic node is identified, the primary lesion may be anywhere in the head and neck region, including:

- Larynx.
- Pharynx.
- Floor of the mouth.
- Postnasal space.

If there are hard irregular metastatic nodes, look for a primary lesion before excision. *— virchows node.*

Troisier's sign is an enlarged left supraclavicular node—look for intra-abdominal pathology (due to drainage from the thoracic duct into the left subclavian vein).

163

Fig. 30.1 Lymphatic drainage of head and neck.

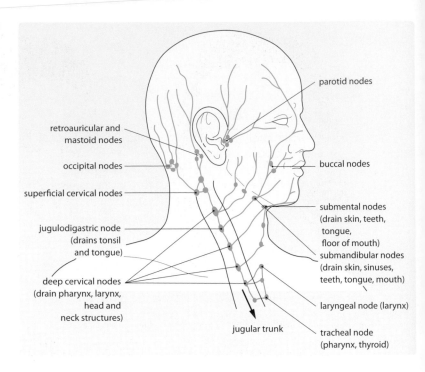

parotid nodes

retroauricular and mastoid nodes

occipital nodes

superficial cervical nodes

jugulodigastric node
(drains tonsil
and tongue)

deep cervical nodes
(drain pharynx, larynx,
head and
neck structures)

buccal nodes

submental nodes
(drain skin, teeth,
tongue,
floor of mouth)
submandibular nodes
(drain skin, sinuses,
teeth, tongue, mouth)

laryngeal node (larynx)

jugular trunk

tracheal node
(pharynx, thyroid)

Treatment may include radical resection of the primary tumour and block resection of the lymph nodes.

OTHER CERVICAL SWELLINGS

Branchial cyst

Background

A branchial cyst arises from a congenital abnormality. In the embryo, the second branchial arch grows down over the third and fourth arches to form the cervical sinus. The sinus usually disappears or may form a branchial cyst. Fig. 30.2 compares the branchial cyst with the thyroglossal cyst discussed in Chapter 29.

Clinical presentation

A branchial cyst is often not apparent until adult life when an infection may precipitate problems. It is a soft swelling arising near the upper, anterior border of the sternocleidomastoid muscle.

Most branchial cysts present as a non-tender, persistent swelling, although some may present as an intermittent swelling.

Management

Aspiration of a branchial cyst shows fluid containing cholesterol crystals. The cyst can be excised to prevent further infection.

Branchial sinus

Failure of obliteration of the cervical sinus causes a discharging sinus anterior to the lower third of the sternocleidomastoid muscle.

Management

If the branchial sinus is excised, the track should be followed up to the side wall of the pharynx to the tonsillar fossa.

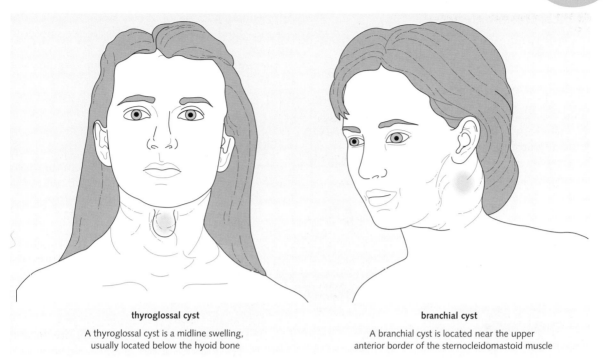

thyroglossal cyst
A thyroglossal cyst is a midline swelling, usually located below the hyoid bone

branchial cyst
A branchial cyst is located near the upper anterior border of the sternocleidomastoid muscle

Fig. 30.2 Clinical appearance of thyroglossal cyst and branchial cyst.

Carotid body tumour

This is a slow-growing tumour arising in the carotid body at the bifurcation of the common carotid artery. The mass transmits the carotid pulsation and may be highly vascular, so it demonstrates pulsation. It may be locally invasive and metastasize.

SALIVARY GLAND DISORDERS

The salivary glands commonly involved in pathological processes are the parotid and submandibular glands; the sublingual glands are rarely affected. The roles of saliva include:

- Facilitation of swallowing.
- Cleansing of mouth, gums and teeth.
- Starch digestion (contains the enzyme ptyalin).

Salivary calculi

Background

Salivary calculi are common in the submandibular gland. The calculi develop on a nidus of debris, with subsequent deposition of mucus, calcium and magnesium phosphate.

Clinical presentation

The classic symptom of salivary calculi is a painful swelling of the gland before and during eating.

Management

On examination, the gland is swollen and tender. Inspection may reveal that the duct orifice is red, with a purulent discharge. Palpation of the duct may reveal the calculus, which may be visible on a radiograph of the floor of the mouth.

The calculus is removed by opening the duct or complete excision of the gland.

Acute suppurative parotitis

Background

Acute suppurative parotitis can occur in postoperative or debilitated patients who have poor oral hygiene and mouth breathing. There is usually an ascending infection caused by a staphylococcal infection.

Clinical presentation

Clinically acute suppurative parotitis is characterized by a tender inflamed swelling of the parotid.

Management

Acute suppurative parotitis is treated with antibiotics. Very rarely, an abscess forms and requires drainage.

Acute parotitis may also be related to the viral infection causing mumps, in which case the swellings are usually bilateral.

Viral parotitis is usually due to mumps, echovirus or coxsackievirus.

Chronic parotitis

This is associated with recurrent episodes of pain and swelling of the parotid glands associated with dilatation of the duct system (i.e. sialectasia).

Sialography demonstrates the changes in the duct system.

Sjögren's syndrome

Background

Sjögren's syndrome is an autoimmune condition associated with dry eyes, xerostomia (i.e. lack of saliva), parotid swelling and rheumatoid arthritis. It may be associated with other autoimmune conditions and it usually occurs in postmenopausal women.

Mikulicz's disease is symmetrical enlargement of the salivary and lacrimal glands caused by a benign inflammatory infiltrate and is characteristic of Sjögren's syndrome.

Management

Treatment of Sjögren's syndrome is symptomatic (i.e. artificial tears and good oral hygiene).

SALIVARY GLAND TUMOURS

There are three types of salivary gland tumour:

- Pleomorphic adenoma.
- Adenolymphoma.
- Carcinoma.

Approximately 90% of the tumours arise in the parotid gland and most of these are pleomorphic adenomas. Most patients are under 50 years of age at presentation and the majority of tumours are benign.

Pleomorphic adenoma

Background

This is usually a slow-growing smooth mass in the lower pole of the parotid gland. The tumour is lobulated with a false capsule and protrusions that go beyond the capsule. It is composed of a variety of epithelial cells with myxoid, mucoid and chondroid elements. The mass usually arises in the superficial part of the gland.

Management

The treatment of a pleomorphic adenoma is a superficial parotidectomy. The 'tumour' should not be shelled out because some of the protrusions may be left behind and predispose to recurrence. The superficial part of the gland is removed after identification and preservation of the facial nerve.

Adenolymphoma

Background

This accounts for 10% of salivary gland tumours. It occurs in men over 50 years of age, and is occasionally bilateral. The tumours are soft and cystic.

Management

Treatment of adenolymphoma is by surgical excision and the prognosis is excellent.

Carcinoma

Background

Salivary gland carcinoma occurs in middle-aged and elderly people.

Clinical presentation

The tumours are hard, irregular, craggy lumps, and the sign of malignancy is facial nerve involvement. It may spread to the local lymph nodes and may ulcerate. The tumours are usually squamous cell carcinomas.

Management

Treatment of salivary gland carcinoma is by radical parotidectomy (when the facial nerve may have to be sacrificed), lymph node dissection and radiotherapy.

Any swelling in the parotid should be treated as a possible parotid tumour.

Further reading

Batsakis JG 1979 *Tumours of the Head and Neck*. Lippincott Williams & Wilkins, Philadelphia

DeBurgh Norman JE, McGurk M (eds) 1995 *Color Atlas and Text of the Salivary Glands Diseases, Disorders and Surgery.* Mosby-Wolfe, London

Donahue BJ, Cruickshank JC, Bishop JW 1995 The diagnostic value of fine needle aspiration biopsy of head and neck masses. *Ear Nose Throat J* **74**: 483–486

McGurk M, Renehan A, Gleave E et al. 1996 Clinical significance of the tumour capsule in the treatment of parotid pleomorphic adenomas. *Br J Surg* **83**: 1747–1749

Paparella MM, Shumrick DA, Meyerhoff WL (eds) 1998 *Otolaryngology: Head and Neck*, 3rd edn. WB Saunders, Philadelphia

Todd NW 1993 Common congenital anomalies of the neck. Embryology and surgical anatomy. *Surg Clin North Am* **73**: 599–610

Gleeson M, Herbert A, Richards A 2000 Management of lateral neck masses in adults. *BMJ* **320**: 1521–1524.

Breast disorders

Learning objectives

You should be able to:

- Understand the roles of oestrogen and progesterone in the development of the breast.
- Describe the lymphatic drainage of the breast and understand the clinical significance.
- Understand the management of cyclical mastalgia.
- List the causes of bloodstained nipple discharge.
- Describe the clinical appearance of a fibroadenoma.
- Understand the management of breast cysts and identify the age group they commonly occur in.
- List the risk factors for breast cancer.
- Define triple assessment.
- List the indications for mastectomy and understand why axillary surgery is performed.
- Understand the different adjuvant treatments available following breast surgery.

Breast problems account for many specialist referrals. Over 90% of them are benign, but the woman's overwhelming concern is about the possibility of breast cancer.

BREAST DEVELOPMENT

The breast develops from a breast bud, which starts to grow at puberty. It is a skin appendage consisting of fat and a major duct system leading to terminal ductolobular units. Oestrogen causes the ducts to sprout and branch at puberty, but progesterone is responsible for lobular development. The breasts increase in size because of fat deposition and connective tissue growth.

During pregnancy, there is a marked increase in the luteal and placental sex steroids and, together with human placental lactogen and chorionic gonadotrophin, these lead to an increase in lobuloalveolar growth in preparation for breast-feeding. Postpartum, the oestrogen levels fall and prolactin and oxytocin stimulate milk production.

The breast arises in the skin and subcutaneous tissues of the chest wall between the second and sixth ribs from the lateral border of the sternum to the midaxillary line (Fig. 31.1).

The blood supply to the breasts is from the perforating branches of the internal thoracic, intercostal, lateral thoracic, subscapular and thoracoacromial vessels. The lymphatic drainage follows the blood vessels to the axillary glands, supraclavicular glands and internal mammary glands.

Axillary lymph nodes are classified into three levels: —in relation to pec. minor.
- Level I—nodes inferior to pectoralis minor.
- Level II—nodes behind pectoralis minor.
- Level III—nodes above pectoralis minor.

Abnormalities of breast development

These include:

- Amastia—absence of the breast.
- Hypoplasia—underdevelopment of the breast.
- Virginal hypertrophy—excessive growth of the breast at puberty.
- Accessory nipples—these are very common, and are found anywhere on the milk line, which extends from the axilla to the groin.

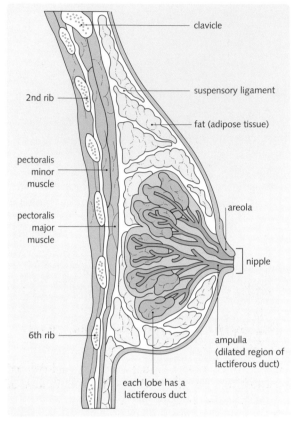

Fig. 31.1 Structure of the mature female breast.

- Accessory breast tissue—this usually occurs in the axilla, and becomes more prominent during pregnancy.
- Poland's syndrome—this is hypoplasia of the breast and chest wall (i.e. absence of the pectoralis major muscle) and the main problem is cosmetic.

BENIGN BREAST DISORDERS

Mastalgia

Background

Mastalgia (i.e. breast pain) is experienced by most women at some time in their reproductive years but, in most cases, it is well tolerated. If the discomfort is cyclical (i.e. worse premenstrually), it is due to cyclical hormonal effects on the breast tissue.

Management

Cyclical discomfort is more likely than other types of mastalgia to respond to treatment such as evening

primrose oil. Other simple measures include a reduction in caffeine intake. If evening primrose oil is not effective, other medications that can be used are danazol and bromocriptine.

If the pain is non-cyclical and localized, it may be musculoskeletal or due to costochondritis—Tietze's syndrome.

> Most women presenting to the breast clinic with mastalgia can be discharged after significant disease is excluded and the patient is reassured.

Breast infections

There are two important types of breast infection:

- Postpartum or puerperal abscess—this is associated with breastfeeding, and is usually caused by staphylococcal infection. Initially it is treated by antibiotics but, if it develops into an abscess, it can be drained by percutaneous aspiration under ultrasound guidance. Occasionally, it requires incision and drainage if it reaches the surface.
- Periductal mastitis—this problem usually occurs in smokers. These women experience episodes of periductal sepsis. The usual bacteria involved include anaerobes, so metronidazole is an appropriate antibiotic. The infection may resolve with antibiotics or develop into an abscess, which requires aspiration or incision, or it may discharge spontaneously to produce a fistula, which discharges intermittently at the areolar margin (Fig. 31.2).

Women who have recurrent episodes of infection need to have a total duct excision and fistulectomy for recurrent discharge.

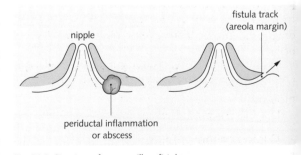

Fig. 31.2 Structure of a mammillary fistula.

Nipple discharge

If the discharge is green, brown, black or cream and occurs from multiple ducts then it is due to duct ectasia (dilatation of the ducts).

Management is reassurance or total duct excision if the discharge is copious.

A bloodstained discharge from a single duct may be due to an intraduct papilloma, duct ectasia or ductal carcinoma in situ. This requires exploration of the duct either by single duct excision (microdochectomy) or by total duct excision.

Nipple and areola change

The areola is prone to skin changes such as eczema, which responds to 1% hydrocortisone.

The nipple may develop an erosive condition associated with underlying malignant change (i.e. Paget's disease). The nipple change is due to malignant cells spreading up the ducts. Women may present with bleeding and discharge from an ulcerated nipple but, in the early stages, the areola is normal. Subsequently, the nipple is destroyed and the condition spreads to the areola.

BENIGN BREAST LUMPS

The breast tissue undergoes considerable change during puberty, pregnancy, and after the age of 35 years when involution starts to occur. There are also cyclical changes due to fluctuating levels in oestrogens and progesterone. Some of the benign breast lumps that occur are just manifestations of these changes (i.e. aberrations of normal development and involution). Fig. 31.3 shows the age distribution of different types of breast lump.

Fibroadenoma

Fibroadenoma arises from the lobules and is seen predominantly during breast development in women in the 15–25-year age group. It may, however, be diagnosed at a later age when involutional changes occur.

The lump is smooth, well defined and mobile. It is also known as a 'breast mouse' because of its mobility.

Diagnosis is made by:

- Clinical examination.
- Characteristic ultrasound appearance.

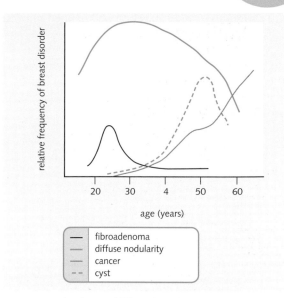

Fig. 31.3 Age distribution of different breast lumps.

- Benign cells on fine-needle aspiration cytology (FNAC) or a core biopsy.

Macroscopically, a fibroadenoma is a well-defined encapsulated structure made up of a combination of epithelial and stromal elements.

Further evaluation is necessary if a breast cyst aspirate is bloodstained or if there is a residual lump.

Phyllodes tumour

This has a similar clinical appearance to that of a fibroadenoma, but develops in older women and tends to be larger (i.e. 3–4 cm in diameter). It has malignant potential, and may develop into a sarcoma.

Breast cysts

Breast cysts are usually found in women over 35 years of age (i.e. when involutional changes occur). Microcysts form as the stroma involutes, and some of these may coalesce to form macrocysts, which may produce a palpable lump. Cysts may be single or multiple and are a feature of fibrocystic change (i.e. painful tender premenstrual nodularity).

Clinically, these cysts may seem to appear suddenly, are tender, and may resolve spontaneously.

On examination, there may be a well-defined smooth mass that is not mobile.

Cysts can be seen on mammograms as well-defined smooth lesions, and on ultrasound scans they have a characteristic appearance.

Diagnosis and treatment of a breast cyst is aspiration to extinction.

Galactocoele

This is relatively uncommon, but is a cystic lump found after breastfeeding and therefore contains milky fluid.

Fat necrosis

Fat necrosis is a common sequel to trauma associated with haematoma formation. Clinically, it produces a hard, irregular lump, and therefore simulates a carcinoma, but is not as common.

BREAST CANCER

Breast cancer is the commonest malignant disease of women in the UK. There are approximately 30 000 new cases of breast cancer diagnosed each year, and approximately 10 000 deaths per year. In the UK, 1 in 10 women will be affected at some time in their life. The risk increases with age, and becomes more common after 50 years of age. It is more common in developed countries.

Only 1% of cases occur in men. Many of these men have female relatives affected by breast cancer, and there is often a genetic link.

Risk factors

Risk factors linked to breast cancer include:

- Genetic factors—the genes of BRCA1 and BRCA2—account for 5% of cases, and are also linked with ovarian cancer.
- A first-degree premenopausal relative who has breast cancer.
- Early menarche.
- Late menopause.
- Nulliparity or late pregnancy.
- Prolonged use (more than 5 years) of hormone replacement therapy.
- Benign breast pathology (i.e. atypical ductal hyperplasia and lobular carcinoma in situ). *sclerosing adenosis.*

Breast screening programme

In the UK, all women aged between 50 and 70 years are invited for screening mammography every 3 years to detect breast cancer at an asymptomatic stage. Since the introduction of breast screening in 1990, mortality has dropped by more than 20%. However, many factors have contributed to this, including earlier diagnosis, better surgery, chemotherapy and radiotherapy.

10% of breast cancers are not seen on mammograms.

Diagnosis of breast cancer

Important aspects in the diagnosis of breast cancer are:

- Clinical features—the obvious features are skin tethering, skin dimple, ulceration, recent nipple inversion, deep fixation, peau d'orange and inflammatory changes. Most breast cancers do not present with advanced clinical signs and may just be a hard irregular mass or an asymmetric change in the breast.
- Imaging—mammographic features of malignancy include spiculated lesions, new mass lesions and microcalcifications (see Fig. 42.7). Mammograms are not so useful in premenopausal women because of their dense glandular breast tissue. Ultrasound is useful for diagnosing benign breast lumps, cysts and breast cancer, particularly for locating asymptomatic impalpable lesions seen on screening mammograms.
- Cytopathology—FNAC from a cancer will produce malignant cells, but core biopsies will give precise pathology.

Frozen section should not be carried out at operation—a diagnosis should be made preoperatively so that women can receive appropriate support and counselling from surgeons and breast care nurses.

Diagnosis of breast cancer is based on triple assessment:
- Clinical.
- Imaging.
- Cytology/ histopathology.

Pathology

Aspects of the pathology of breast cancer to consider are:

- Ductal carcinoma in situ (DCIS) (i.e. preinvasive stage of breast cancer that has not invaded the basement membrane)—after 10–15 years, at least 50% of cases will develop into invasive cancer.
- Invasive ductal carcinoma—this is the commonest type. Pathologists grade the tumours 1–3 depending on the degree of pathological differentiation.
- Invasive lobular carcinoma—this may not be visible on mammograms, and 20% of cases are bilateral. It characteristically infiltrates tissues in a diffuse manner.

- Special pathological types—these are well differentiated and should have a good prognosis (e.g. tubular, colloid, medullary and papillary carcinomas).
- Sarcoma—a very rare malignant tumour of spindle cells that may arise from a phyllodes tumour.
- Paget's disease of the nipple—usually associated with an underlying neoplasm.

Treatment of breast cancer

Fig. 31.4 outlines the staging of breast cancer and 5-year survival rates. All women should have a preoperative diagnosis so that they can be given appropriate information and counselling. Many women can be given a choice of treatment. Being involved in the decision-making process can have a

Fig. 31.4A Staging of breast cancer

Stage	Tumour diameter	Lymph nodes	5-year survival (%)
I	<2 cm	no palpable nodes	80–90
IIA	<2 cm	palpable nodes	60–70
IIB	2–5 cm	± nodes	
III	>5 cm	± nodes	30–40
IV	advanced local disease or metastases	palpable fixed nodes	

Fig. 31.4B TNM (tumour, nodes, metastases) classification of breast cancer

Classification	Criteria
Tis	ductal carcinoma in situ, Paget's disease of the breast
T1	tumour diameter <2 cm
T2	tumour diameter <2 cm
T3	tumour diameter <5 cm
T4	any size tumour with skin changes, fixation
N0	no regional nodal metastases
N1	metastases to ipsilateral nodes
N2	metastases to fixed nodes
N3	metastases to internal mammary nodes
M0	no distant metastases
M1	distant metastases

positive psychological effect. Some women need to be advised about treatment:

- Women are advised to have a mastectomy if there is multifocal disease, widespread DCIS, a large central tumour or a large mass in relationship to the breast size (i.e. 3–4 cm in diameter).
- Women who have a locally advanced tumour or inflammatory cancer may have neoadjuvant chemotherapy in an attempt to downstage the disease before operation.
- Elderly patients who are unfit for operation may be treated with hormonal therapy (e.g. tamoxifen or aromatase inhibitors).
- Some women can have a choice between wide local excision followed by radiotherapy, or a mastectomy. There is no difference in the long-term survival, but there is an increased risk of local recurrence after wide local excision.

- Mastectomy may be combined with a breast reconstruction (either immediately or at a later stage) using tissue expanders or myocutaneous flaps.
- A radical mastectomy (Halsted's operation) with excision of pectoral muscles is only used for locally advanced disease.

Axillary surgery

The extent of operation is controversial, but lymph node status is an important prognostic indicator. Operations range from axillary node sampling to axillary node clearance. The complications of axillary surgery are shoulder stiffness, paraesthesia and lymphoedema. A technique that is increasingly being used is the 'sentinel node biopsy'. The sentinel lymph node is the first axillary node that recieves breast lymph duct drainage. Lymph node mapping identifies this node and it is removed. If the biopsy is positive then the patient needs to have further axillary node surgery. If it is negative, however, there is a very high chance the rest of the axillary lymph nodes are also clear of disease and the patient can avoid axillary surgery. Sentinel node biopsy is becoming widely used because of fewer side effects than with axillary node surgery.

Adjuvant treatment after surgery

Adjuvant treatment reduces the likelihood of relapse. The efficacy of the various treatments depends on:

- Tumour characteristics.
- Age.
- Menopausal status.

Radiotherapy to the chest wall and supraclavicular nodes is given after:

- Breast conservation surgery for invasive breast cancer or DCIS of high or intermediate grade.
- Mastectomy in patients with an increased chance of local recurrence. Significant risk factors are tumour size greater than 4 cm in diameter, vascular invasion and more than four positive lymph nodes.

Hormonal treatments aim to decrease hormonal stimulation of breast cancer cells by oestrogens produced either by the ovaries (premenopausal women) or by peripheral aromatization. Treatments include:

- Tamoxifen — blocks the oestrogen receptors on breast cancer cells. The common side effects are hot flushes and vaginal discharge, but the drug is usually well tolerated.
- Aromatase inhibitors (e.g. anastrazole, letrazole, exemestane)—block the enzyme aromatase which is particularly prevalent in subcutaneous fat. Aromatase converts the androgens that reach the circulation from the ovaries and the adrenals into oestrogens. Aromatase activity increases with age and doubles after the menopause.
- Luteinizing hormone-releasing hormone (LHRH) analogues (e.g. goserelin)—cause a reversible ovarian dysfunction a preferred option for premenopausal women who wish to remain fertile and do not want to undergo surgical oophorectomy or ovarian ablation.

Chemotherapy is recommended to most women with breast cancer after surgery with the exception of:

- DCIS.
- Tumours <15 mm that are node negative where survival is so good the benefits of chemotherapy are outweighed by the adverse effects.

Trastuzumab is a monoclonal antibody against the human epidermal growth factor receptor 2 (HER2). HER2 receptors are present in up to 30% of breast cancers. Overexpression of HER2 correlates with poor prognosis and altered response to hormonal therapy and chemotherapy. Treatment should be given after surgery and chemotherapy for 12 months. It is contraindicated in women with angina or heart failure (ejection fraction <55%).

Prognostic factors for breast cancer are:
- Tumour size.
- Grade of tumour.
- Axillary node status.
- receptor status.

Metastatic disease

Breast cancer cells spread by:

- Lymphatics to the drainage nodes in the axilla, internal mammary chain and supraclavicular fossa.
- Bloodstream to the lungs, liver, bones, adrenals and brain.
- Transcoelomic spread to produce peritoneal and pleural seedlings.
- Local spread to the chest wall, axilla and brachial plexus.

Metastatic disease is treated symptomatically, for example:

- Radiotherapy for painful bone metastases.
- Hormone or chemotherapy for visceral metastases.
- Aspiration of a pleural effusion.
- Dexamethasone and radiotherapy for cerebral metastases.

Bone metastases may be associated with a long period of stable disease, but visceral metastases usually have a very poor prognosis.

GYNAECOMASTIA AND MALE BREAST CANCER

Gynaecomastia is the development of breast tissue in men. Aetiological factors include:

- Puberty—occurs in 30–60% of boys, but 80% regress spontaneously. *testicular failure*
- Kleinfelter's syndrome (XXY)—lack of development of genitalia. *cryptorchidism*
- Chronic liver disease.
- Hormone-secreting tumours—adrenal or testicular malignancy.
- Drugs—anabolic steroids, cimetidine, digoxin, spironolactone, oestrogens, cannabis, zoladex, and other drugs used for the treatment of prostate cancer.

The diagnosis is made by examination and exclusion of a serious underlying cause such as an adrenal tumour. Occasionally, an operation is required for cosmetic reasons.

The differential diagnosis of gynaecomastia is breast cancer, but this usually presents as a hard craggy mass in older men. Diagnosis is made in the same way as for women. Treatment of a breast cancer is by a mastectomy.

Further reading

Barum M, Schipper H 1998 *Breast Cancer*. Health Press, Oxford

British Association of Surgical Oncology: Breast Speciality Group 1998 Guidelines for surgeons in the management of symptomatic breast disease in the United Kingdom. *Eur J Oncol* 24: 464–476

Codd R, Gateley CA 2007 Management of benign disease of the breast. *Surgery* **25**: 264–267

Department of Health 2000 *Breast Screening Programme. England 1998–99*. HMSO, London

Dixon JM 2005 *ABC of Breast Diseases*. BMJ Publications, London

Harris JR, Lippman ME, Morrow M et al. (eds) 2000 *Diseases of the Breast*, 2nd edn. Lippincott Williams & Wilkins, Philadelphia

Hughes LE, Mansel RE, Webster DJ 1987 Aberrations of normal development and involution (ANDI): a new perspective on pathogenesis and nomenclature of benign breast disorders. *Lancet* 2: 1316–1319

Hughes LE, Mansel RE, Webster DJT 2000 *Benign Disorders and Diseases of the Breast: Concepts and Clinical Management*. WB Saunders, Philadelphia

Kontoyannis A Sweetland HM 2007 Adjuvant therapies for breast cancer. *Surgery* 25: 245–279

Kronwitz SJ, Kuerer HM 2006 Advances and surgical decision making for breast reconstruction. *Cancer* 107: 893–907

NICE Guidelines 2006 *Familial Breast Cancer*. http://www.nice.org uk

Rivers A, Hansen N 2007 Axillary management after sentinel lymph node biopsy in breast cancer patients. *Surg Clin North Am* 87: 365–377

SIGN Guidelines 2005 *Management of Breast Cancer in Women*. http://www.sign.ac.uk

Vascular disorders

32

Learning objectives

You should be able to:

- Define 'intermittent claudication' and 'rest pain'.
- Define critical ischaemia.
- Describe the classic appearance of acute limb ischaemia.
- Understand the management of an acutely ischaemic limb.
- Define 'compartment syndrome', describe the clinical features and name the urgent treatment required.
- Name anatomical locations where aneurysms can occur.
- Describe the aetiology of a false aneurysm.
- Describe the differences between an ischaemic and a neuropathic ulcer.
- List symptoms of carotid artery disease and understand the indications for a carotid endarterectomy.
- Describe why varicose veins develop and the treatment options.

Vascular problems include conditions of the veins, arteries and lymphatics. The problems can be acute or chronic.

CHRONIC LIMB ISCHAEMIA

Background

This usually affects the lower limb, rather than the upper limb, but many patients have a history of other ischaemic problems, such as angina, myocardial infarction or a cerebrovascular event. Predisposing factors for all these conditions are:

- Atherosclerosis.
- Diabetes mellitus.
- Hyperlipidaemia.
- Family history.
- Smoking.
- Buerger's disease.

Stages of ischaemia are:

- Intermittent claudication—cramp-like pain in the legs exacerbated by exercise and relieved by rest. Pain develops distal to the obstruction, so blockage of the femoropopliteal segment

causes calf pain, but blockage of the aorta causes buttock pain and impotence (Leriche's syndrome).
- Rest pain—implies that the ischaemia is critical and the viability of the leg is threatened. The pain is severe and requires opioid analgesia.
- Gangrene—in dry gangrene, ischaemia results in death of the tissue. The tissue is black and there is a clear line of demarcation, which may separate. Wet gangrene is brown, moist and ulcerated. The tissue is infected with pathogenic bacteria, so the infection may spread proximally and can cause systemic toxicity.

Management

After the history and full examination of the cardiovascular system, blood tests are taken to:

- Look for anaemia, polycythaemia and hyperlipidaemia.
- Measure blood glucose concentration.
- Assess renal function.

The vasculature is assessed by ankle/brachial pressure measurement, Doppler ultrasound and arteriography (Fig. 32.1). *ABPI*

Fig. 32.1 Arteriogram showing occlusion of the internal iliac artery (arrow) and good flow to the leg. (A) View of external iliac artery. (B) View of superficial femoral artery. (C) Popliteal artery. (D) Distal vessels to lower leg and foot.

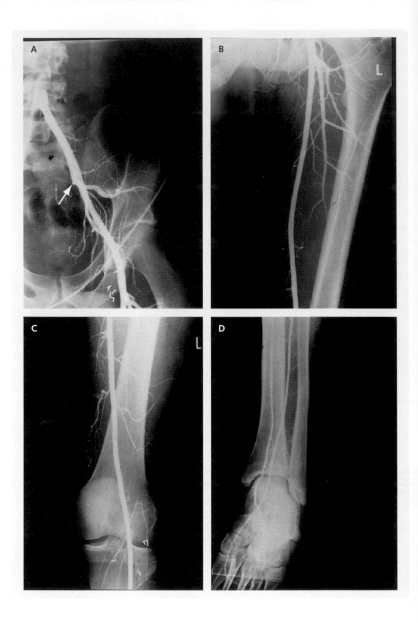

The treatment of chronic limb ischaemia depends on the severity of the condition:

- Intermittent claudication—patients are advised to stop smoking, encouraged to exercise to produce an efficient oxygen extraction from the limited blood supply, and prescribed aspirin 75 mg/day. On this regimen, 60% of patients will improve or remain stable.
- Critical ischaemia—any exacerbating factors such as infection are treated. Arteriography is performed to define the extent and position of the occlusion. A single short segment, less than 5 cm long, can be treated by balloon angioplasty and with a success rate of more than 85% and a 1 year patency of more than 70%. Alternatively, an expandable metal stent can be used.

Critical ischaemia comprises:
- Rest pain for more than 2 weeks.
- Ulceration or gangrene.
- An ankle systolic pressure <50 mmHg.

If the arteriograms show multisegment disease then revascularization is performed by reconstructive surgery. Aortoiliac disease is treated by using a synthetic bifurcated graft from the aorta to both femoral vessels distal to the obstruction (Fig. 32.2).

If the patient is unfit for a major abdominal operation then a graft can be passed from the axillary artery to the femoral vessels under local anaesthetic.

Femoropopliteal disease is bypassed using the patient's own long saphenous vein (reversed) or a synthetic graft.

For grafts to be successful, there should be good inflow and good distal run-off. There is a risk of occlusion in the immediate and later postoperative periods. Aspirin is prescribed to reduce the risk of thrombosis but, if the patient continues to smoke, there is a high risk of graft failure.

SURGICAL EMERGENCY

Acute limb ischaemia

Background

Acute limb ischaemia can occur in the upper or lower limbs and is usually due to an embolus or thrombosis or vascular injury.

Clinical presentation   6 P's

The history is of sudden onset of a painful cold limb. The presence of paraesthesia indicates severe ischaemia, and once mottling occurs this heralds gangrene. Muscle rigidity implies that the damage is irreversible.

If there is no history or signs of previous vascular insufficiency then an embolus is suspected. The common causes of an embolus are:

- From a mural thrombus in the right atrium, associated with atrial fibrillation.
- A thrombus may develop over an area of myocardial infarction.
  Rarer sites of an embolus are from the valves, a ventricular aneurysm, an atrial myxoma or an atheromatous plaque.
  If there is a past history of ischaemia then the problem is probably acute on chronic (i.e. a thrombosis).
  Vascular injury may also occur after trauma or after an intervention such as arteriography.

Management

Once the diagnosis is suspected, the patient is anticoagulated with intravenous heparin to prevent further thrombosis. If the clinical picture suggests an embolus, an urgent embolectomy can be performed under local anaesthetic. A Fogarty balloon catheter is used to extract the embolus (Fig. 32.3). Postoperatively, the patient is anticoagulated to prevent recurrence.

If the history suggests an underlying vascular problem and there are signs of chronic ischaemia, an arteriogram is required to define the problem. Thrombolytic therapy, such as streptokinase, urokinase or tissue plasminogen activator, may be infused locally to lyse the thrombus. It may take 12–72 hours to be effective so cannot be used if the viability of the limb is threatened.

It may be necessary to carry out a reconstructive operation to revascularize the limb.

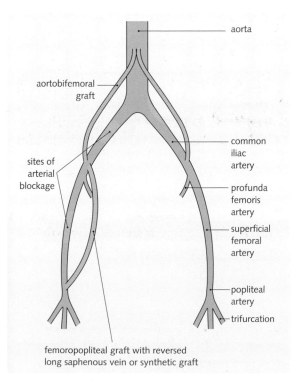

aorta

aortobifemoral graft

sites of arterial blockage

common iliac artery

profunda femoris artery

superficial femoral artery

popliteal artery

trifurcation

femoropopliteal graft with reversed long saphenous vein or synthetic graft

Fig. 32.2 Location of common arterial bypass grafts.

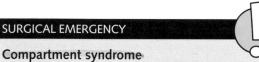

Clinical features of acute ischaemia—the six Ps:

- Pulselessness.
- Pain.
- Pallor.
- Perishing cold.
- Paraesthesia.
- Paralysis.

SURGICAL EMERGENCY

Compartment syndrome

Background
A complication of acute ischaemia is compartment syndrome. Ischaemia and reperfusion of the muscles causes them to swell within their rigid osseofascial compartment. Further increase in pressure exceeds capillary perfusion pressure and thus the blood supply is impaired, causing further ischaemia and swelling.

Clinical presentation
Clinically, the patient has severe pain, especially on moving the muscles of the affected compartment. An urgent fasciotomy is required to open the compartment and allow the muscles to expand. If the muscle is damaged it releases myoglobin, which can cause renal damage, and ischaemia causes lactic acid production and metabolic acidosis.

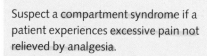

Suspect a compartment syndrome if a patient experiences excessive pain not relieved by analgesia.

ANEURYSM

This is an abnormal dilatation of a vessel, which can occur at several different sites in the body (e.g. abdominal or thoracic aorta, iliac, femoral, popliteal or cerebral arteries; Fig. 32.4). The different types of aneurysm are illustrated in Fig. 32.5. The common causes are:

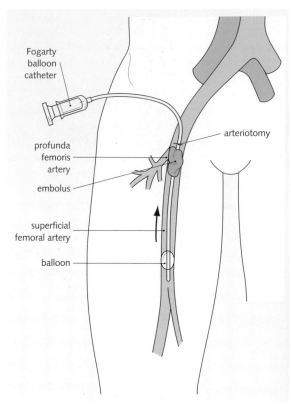

Fig. 32.3 Use of Fogarty balloon catheter to extract an embolus from the superficial femoral artery.

- Congenital—berry aneurysm in the circle of Willis.
- Atherosclerotic—most common.
- Traumatic—after interventional radiology or trauma.
- Inflammatory—mycotic or syphilitic.

SURGICAL EMERGENCY

Abdominal aortic aneurysm

Background
Abdominal aortic aneurysm is the commonest type of aneurysm and the incidence is increasing. Most are associated with smoking, atherosclerosis and hypertension. They usually extend from just below the renal arteries to the bifurcation of the aorta, but some patients also have aneurysms of the iliac vessels.

Fig. 32.4 Locations of common aneurysms

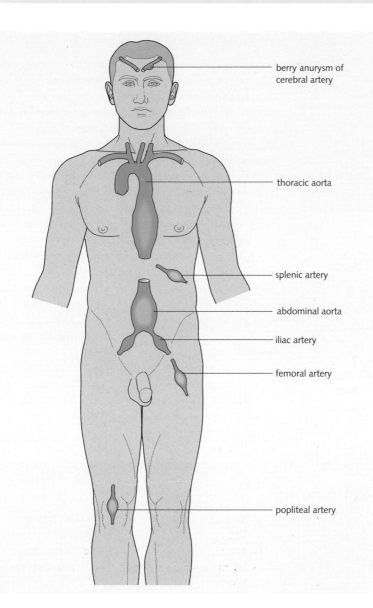

Fig. 32.4 Locations of common aneurysms

- berry anurysm of cerebral artery
- thoracic aorta
- splenic artery
- abdominal aorta
- iliac artery
- femoral artery
- popliteal artery

Clinical presentation

An abdominal aortic aneurysm may present in a variety of ways, as follows:

- It may be asymptomatic—being detected during a routine physical examination, abdominal ultrasound examination or abdominal radiography, because 50% are calcified.
- As an abdominal pulsation.
- With recent onset of severe back pain—may be due to an enlarging aneurysm eroding the vertebrae.
- With back or flank pain (may be similar to ureteric colic) and episodes of hypotension—due to a leaking retroperitoneal aneurysm.

- With circulatory collapse and severe abdominal pain—due to an intraperitoneal rupture.
- With congestive cardiac failure, abdominal bruit, lower limb ischaemia and oedema—due to erosion into the inferior vena cava.

All aneurysms can rupture, thrombose, be a source of embolus, cause pressure symptoms or become infected.

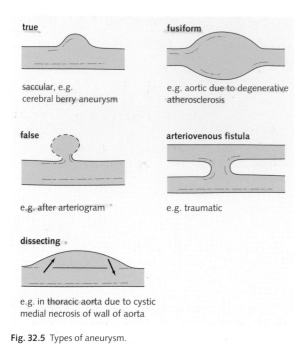

true

saccular, e.g.
cerebral berry aneurysm

false

e.g. after arteriogram

dissecting

e.g. in thoracic aorta due to cystic
medial necrosis of wall of aorta

fusiform

e.g. aortic due to degenerative
atherosclerosis

arteriovenous fistula

e.g. traumatic

Fig. 32.5 Types of aneurysm.

Fig. 32.6 Computed tomography scan
showing an abdominal aortic aneurysm
(arrow).

Management

In the non-acute situation, a diagnosis of abdominal aortic aneurysm is made by an ultrasound scan, but a computed tomography (CT) scan (Fig. 32.6) gives better definition of renal artery involvement, and acutely it may confirm a retroperitoneal haematoma, implying a leak. Aneurysms over 5.5 cm in diameter have a high risk of rupture.

If surgical resection is contemplated, patients should have a detailed cardiorespiratory assessment. If an aneurysm is repaired electively it is replaced with a synthetic graft and 95% of patients survive. If the aneurysm ruptures, many patients do not reach hospital and 50% do not survive the operation, so the overall mortality rate is 85%.

Endovascular aortic aneurysm repair is a modern approach, where a stent-graft is delivered into the aneurysm via the femoral artery under radiological guidance. Less than 50% of aneurysms are suitable for this technique and concerns remain regarding the long-term durability of stent-grafts.

If patients survive the operation, there may be complications related to underlying cardiac, respiratory or renal disease and problems related to clotting abnormalities.

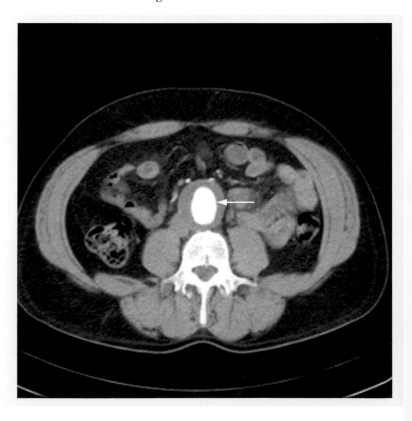

Repair of the aneurysm may cause acute lower limb ischaemia due to embolus or thrombosis, colonic ischaemia or spinal cord ischaemia.

Late complications are graft infection, aortoenteric fistula and development of a false aneurysm at the site of the anastomosis.

SURGICAL EMERGENCY

Thoracoabdominal aneurysm

Background

A thoracoabdominal aneurysm can involve the ascending and descending thoracic aorta, and the abdominal aorta.

Clinical presentation

A thoracoabdominal aneurysm may be asymptomatic, but severe chest, back or abdominal pain indicates expansion and impending rupture.

Management

A chest radiograph shows a widened mediastinum or calcification of the aortic wall. A CT scan defines the extent of the aneurysm:

- Type A dissection of *ascending* aorta—needs aortic arch replacement—very poor outcome.
- Type B dissection of *descending* aorta—treat with conservative control of blood pressure.

Recent onset of back pain or a tender aneurysm is an indication for urgent surgery.

DIABETIC FOOT PROBLEMS

Background

Diabetics have an increased risk of ulceration and infection of the feet because of their predisposition to:

- Atherosclerosis affecting the large vessels.
- Microangiopathy (i.e. thickening of the basement membrane of the small arterioles and capillaries).
- Neuropathy of the sensory, motor and autonomic systems.
- Increased risk of infection because a glucose-rich environment favours bacterial growth.

Management of diabetic's feet

Treatment of a diabetic's foot involves:

- Clinical assessment.
- Radiography to look for osteomyelitis and soft tissue damage.
- Antibiotics to treat bacterial infection after swabs for culture.
- Assessment of arterial circulation—using Doppler scanning or arteriography.
- Good diabetic control.

The best management of a diabetic's foot is patient education and prevention.

Neuropathic ulcers will heal after treatment of infection and debridement of any necrotic tissue.

Ischaemic ulcers will only heal if the arterial supply improves.

Fig. 32.7 gives a comparison of the features of ischaemic and neuropathic ulcers.

AMPUTATION

Despite aggressive surgical intervention, some patients who have atherosclerotic or diabetic problems either present too late or the reconstructive procedures fail and their tissues become ischaemic and die. This causes severe pain and there is often superimposed infection, so amputation is the only treatment left to relieve their symptoms and prevent further complications.

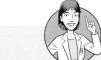

Indications for amputation include:
- Ischaemia/gangrene.
- Malignancy.
- Severe infection.
- Congenital deformity.
- A paralysed 'useless limb'.

The type of amputation depends on the level of an adequate blood supply to allow the wound to heal.

Fig. 32.7 Comparison of features of ischaemic and neuropathic ulcers

Feature	Ischaemic ulcers	Neuropathic ulcers
sensation	painful	sensory impairment
pulses	absent or decreased	present
ulceration	on toes and pressure areas	plantar ulceration—deep, painless
temperature of foot	cold	warm due to autonomic neuropathy
other features	variable sensory changes, intermittent claudication	trophic skin lesions, Charcot's joints

Types of amputation include (Fig. 32.8):

- Above knee.
- Below knee.
- Syme's amputation through the talotibial joint.
- Forefoot amputation.
- Digital amputation.

Following amputation, there should be an active rehabilitation programme of physiotherapy and occupational therapy to encourage the patient to have a prosthesis and return to the community. Many patients, however, experience severe phantom limb pain and their underlying disease progresses so that they require a further operation, and many die within a few years.

CAROTID ARTERY DISEASE

Background

Many patients who have peripheral vascular disease also have atherosclerosis affecting the carotid artery. They usually have hypertension and are smokers. Men are affected more often than women and patients are usually over 65 years of age at presentation.

The commonest cause of ischaemic stroke is thromboembolism of the internal carotid artery.

Clinical presentation

Patients may present with:

- A transient ischaemic attack (TIA) (i.e. transient loss of sensory or motor function) or amaurosis fugax (temporary blindness), which last for less than 24 hours.
- A cerebrovascular event ('stroke').

Management

Clinical examination may demonstrate a bruit over the carotid vessels, but this is not always the case.

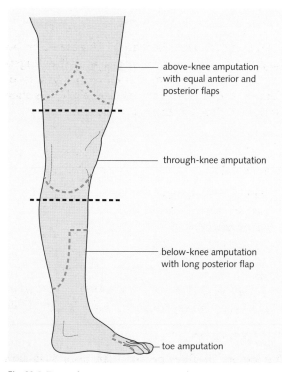

above-knee amputation with equal anterior and posterior flaps

through-knee amputation

below-knee amputation with long posterior flap

toe amputation

Fig. 32.8 Types of amputation.

Duplex scanning of the carotid arteries can detect stenosis, and digital subtraction arteriography will demonstrate the anatomy. If a patient has had a 'stroke', a CT scan can show whether it is due to infarction or haemorrhage.

If there is evidence of carotid artery stenosis, general measures are to stop smoking and control hypertension, diabetes mellitus and hyperlipidaemia.

Antiplatelet drugs such as aspirin decrease the risk of TIA and 'stroke'.

An operation is performed if the patient is symptomatic and the stenosis is over 70%. A carotid endarterectomy is performed to remove the atheromatous plaque. There is a small risk of cerebral damage, but usually the operation is successful.

CORONARY ARTERY DISEASE

Background

This is due to atherosclerosis of the coronary arteries. Risk factors are:

- Smoking.
- Hypertension.
- Hyperlipidaemia.
- Obesity.
- Diabetes mellitus.

Clinical presentation

Coronary artery disease may present with angina or a myocardial infarction.

Management

Coronary angiography is performed to assess the problem. Coronary stents can be used to overcome critical stenosis of a vessel. This procedure is performed in a cardiac catheterization laboratory and insertion is via the femoral artery. If there is triple vessel disease or stenosis of the left anterior descending coronary artery (LAD), coronary artery bypass grafts are required. The internal thoracic artery is anastomosed to the LAD and the long saphenous vein can be used for other grafts. This operation has a 1–4% hospital mortality rate, but only 50% of vein grafts are patent at 10 years and 10% of patients will have a second operation within 10 years.

THROMBOANGIITIS OBLITERANS

Background

Thromboangiitis obliterans (Buerger's disease) is a condition that usually affects young men who are smokers. It is characterized by segmental thrombotic occlusions of small and medium-sized vessels in the upper and lower limbs. There is an associated inflammatory infiltrate, which affects the arteries, veins and, occasionally, the nerves.

Clinical presentation

Patients present with symptoms of peripheral vascular disease, which is progressive unless they stop smoking.

The increased incidence of smoking in women has resulted in an increase in Buerger's disease.

RAYNAUD'S DISEASE

Background

This occurs in young women who have no underlying vascular disease.

Clinical presentation

Patients who have Raynaud's disease have an exaggerated response to the cold. The fingers become white because of ischaemia, blue because of cyanosis, and then red from hyperaemia. This is often associated with pain and paraesthesia.

Management

Treatment is:

- Avoidance of the cold.
- Stop smoking.
- Reassurance.

Nifedipine may be useful.

RAYNAUD'S PHENOMENON

Background

This occurs in older people than does Raynaud's disease and is associated with:

- Autoimmune conditions, such as polyarteritis nodosa and rheumatoid disease.
- Malignancy.
- Myeloproliferative disorders.
- Vibration tools.
- Scleroderma.

Late-onset Raynaud's phenomenon is associated with an underlying cause.

Unilateral Raynaud's phenomenon

This may be associated with subclavian embolic disease or thoracic outlet compression syndrome and there may be neurological signs. This problem is due to a cervical rib compressing the axillary vascular bundle and lower brachial plexus.

Clinical presentation

The neurological symptoms of unilateral Raynaud's phenomenon are worse when the arm is abducted and externally rotated.

Management

Treatment of unilateral Raynaud's phenomenon is excision of the cervical rib and resection of the subclavian aneurysm.

Vasodilators should be considered in Raynaud's phenomenon if symptoms are severe.

VARICOSE VEINS

Background

Varicose veins are tortuous, dilated, superficial veins that have incompetent valves. The long and short saphenous veins in the legs are usually involved. Varicose veins are common, but most are relatively asymptomatic.

Some people have a congenital malformation of the veins (Klippel–Trenaunay syndrome), which comprises varicose veins, limb hypertrophy and a port wine stain.

Most cases of varicose veins are idiopathic or familial, but some are secondary to a previous deep vein thrombosis. In women the veins get worse with each pregnancy because of impaired venous return and progesterone-induced dilatation of the veins.

Normally, blood drains from the superficial to the deep veins by the action of the contracting muscles. At several points there are perforating veins with valves, which regulate one-way flow (see Chapter 40, Fig. 40.8). If the valves become incompetent, especially at the junction of the long saphenous vein and femoral vein, the blood refluxes back into the superficial veins and they become varicose.

In the postphlebitic limb the deep veins are thrombosed, so all the blood returns via the superficial veins, and if there is recanalization the valves are damaged.

Clinical presentation

Many patients are asymptomatic, but others are aware of aching discomfort and swelling of the legs, and are concerned about the appearance. Complications of the veins are:

- Varicose eczema.
- Ulceration secondary to poor capillary circulation.
- Oedema of the skin and therefore poor nutrition to the skin.

At the point where the perforators and the superficial veins meet, there are often blowouts (i.e. bulbous dilatation of the vein). In the groin, this is called a saphena varix. These dilatations may bleed if traumatized. Thrombophlebitis can occur.

Management

Clinical examination will define the extent of the problem, the veins affected and the levels of the incompetent valves. If there is a history of thrombosis, a venogram must be performed to ensure that the deep veins are patent. A duplex scan is also used to demonstrate the level of incompetent valves.

Many patients are advised about support hosiery. Indications for operation are complications such as bleeding and ulceration.

The saphenofemoral junction is the main point of incompetence, so the long saphenous vein and the associated tributaries are disconnected from the femoral vein (high tie). The thigh segment of the long saphenous vein may be stripped, other perforators are ligated and other segments of the vein can be avulsed. Postoperatively, the patients wear support hosiery for several weeks and exercise.

Injection sclerotherapy is only suitable for small veins. The veins are injected with a sclerosant, which causes a chemical thrombophlebitis to occlude the vein.

SUPERFICIAL THROMBOPHLEBITIS

This is local inflammation of a superficial vein and may develop secondary to prolonged cannulation or infusion of an irritant substance, or it may occur in varicose veins.

Thrombophlebitis migrans comprises recurrent episodes of superficial thrombophlebitis and may precede clinical manifestations of malignancy or be associated with connective tissue disease.

SUBCLAVIAN OR AXILLARY VEIN THROMBOSIS

Background

Prolonged arm exercises may precipitate subclavian or axillary vein thrombosis as a result of repetitive venous occlusion, or the thrombosis may develop spontaneously or secondary to cannulation.

Deep vein thrombosis and superficial thrombophlebitis may precede the clinical presentation of a cancer, especially pancreatic cancer.

Clinical presentation

The arm is painful and swollen and there are prominent superficial collateral veins.

Management

Treatment is systemic anticoagulation.

LYMPHATIC DISORDERS

Lymphoedema

Background

A complex system of lymphatic channels drains the subcutaneous tissues. The channels from the legs pass via the lymph node groups to the cisterna chyli and the thoracic duct to return to the venous system. If this transport system fails the protein-rich fluid accumulates in the subcutaneous tissues:

- Primary lymphoedema is a congenital abnormality and may present at birth, in adolescence or in middle age, depending on the degree of the abnormality of the lymphatic system.
- Secondary lymphoedema occurs after interruption or blockage of the lymphatic channels by surgical excision, infection, tumour infiltration or radiotherapy. Filarial worm is the commonest cause worldwide.

Clinical presentation

Whether the lymphoedema is primary or secondary, the limb is swollen and heavy. Initially, the oedema is pitting, but then it becomes fibrosed. The situation is worsened by recurrent episodes of infection (i.e. lymphangitis).

Management

Treatment comprises advice about exercise, massage, compression hosiery and external pneumatic compression to control the swelling.

A rare event is the development of a malignant tumour within the lymphoedema after more than 10 years. This is a lymphangiosarcoma that presents with reddish-blue discoloration or nodules and has a very poor prognosis.

Further reading

Fay D, Wyatt MG, Rose J 2007 Endovascular stent grafting of aortic aneurysms. *Surgery* 25: 346–349

Khan N, McCall J 2007 Imaging in vascular disease. *Surgery* 25: 333–337

London N, Adu D, Bath PMW, Beard JD 2000 *ABC of Arterial and Venous Disease*. BMJ Publications, London

Naylor RA 2007 Carotid artery disease. *Surgery* 25: 350–353

Tai N, Raj JP, Walsh M 2007 Vascular trauma. *Surgery* 25: 323–326

Tambyraja AL, Chalmers RTA 2007 Aortic aneurysms. *Surgery* 25: 342–345

Learning objectives

You should be able to:

- List the organisms that commonly cause urinary tract infections.
- Describe the clinical presentation of acute pyelonephritis and the treatment.
- List the complications that can occur with ureteric calculi.
- Explain how a renal cell carcinoma spreads. Describe the possible chest X-ray features.
- Understand the treatment of a ureteric transitional cell carcinoma.
- Understand the treatment of transitional cell carcinomas of the bladder.
- Describe the scoring system used to grade prostate cancer.
- Identify the age group in which testicular seminoma commonly occurs.
- Understand the options available to treat a patient with benign prostatic hypertrophy unfit for surgery.
- Describe the management of a young boy presenting with acute onset of unilateral scrotal pain.

URINARY TRACT PROBLEMS/ DISORDERS

Urinary tract infection (UTI) is seen in many medical disciplines and in all age groups:

- In children, it may be due to a congenital abnormality or vesicoureteric reflux and needs to be investigated to prevent long-term damage.
- In young adults, women are affected more than men because of a short urethra.
- At all ages, strictures and stones predispose to infection.
- In elderly men, infection is secondary to outflow obstruction. *BPH/prostate*

Diagnosis is confirmed by midstream urine (MSU) and culturing more than 10^5 organisms/mL. Usual organisms are:

- *Escherichia coli*—80% of cases of cystitis and pyelonephritis.
- *Enterobacter* and *Klebsiella* spp.—hospital-acquired infections.
- *Pseudomonas* and *Candida* spp.—immunosuppressed patients or after antibiotics.
- *Proteus* spp.—often associated with urinary calculi.

Recurrent urinary tract infections require investigation to exclude an underlying anatomical or functional abnormality of the urinary tract.

Acute cystitis

Patients who have acute cystitis have symptoms of:

- Frequency.
- Urgency.
- Dysuria.
- Suprapubic pain.
- Malaise.
- Haematuria.

Treatment is oral antibiotics.

Acute pyelonephritis

Clinical presentation

The symptoms of acute pyelonephritis are:

- Pyrexia.
- Loin pain.

189

- Dysuria.
- Rigors. vomiting.
- Malaise.

Management

On examination, the patient is pyrexial and has loin tenderness.

Diagnosis is by MSU and blood cultures. An ultrasound and intravenous urogram (IVU) are used to look for any underlying cause.

Treatment of acute pyelonephritis is with intravenous antibiotics because of the risk of septicaemia. If the infection is inadequately treated it may form a renal abscess, which may develop into a perinephric abscess.

The urine bacterial count in pyelonephritis maybe low (e.g. 10^2–10^3 organisms/mL).

Chronic pyelonephritis

Recurrent infections of the kidney cause chronic inflammation and glomerular fibrosis and may present as hypertension and renal impairment.

Xanthogranulomatous pyelonephritis

This is an extreme form of chronic pyelonephritis. There is an excessive inflammatory response, with lipid-laden macrophages and multiple parenchymal abscesses. Renal function is poor and treatment is often a nephrectomy.

Acute bacterial prostatitis

The symptoms of acute bacterial prostatitis are those of a UTI with low back pain and perineal discomfort. On examination, the prostate is tender.

Treatment is with intravenous antibiotics and then a prolonged course of oral antibiotics to prevent development of an abscess.

Chronic bacterial prostatitis

Chronic bacterial prostatitis may follow acute infection. The symptoms are painful micturition with perineal pain. An MSU should be taken after prostatic massage. Treatment is long-term oral antibiotics.

RENAL TRACT CALCULI

Background

Factors predisposing to renal tract calculi are:

- Inadequate drainage—such as pelviureteric junction (PUJ) obstruction, bladder diverticulum, abnormal anatomy of renal tract.
- Excess of normal constituents—increased calcium (as a result of hyperparathyroidism, sarcoidosis, immobilization), uric acid (after chemotherapy), hyperoxaluria, cystinuria, hyperuricosuria.
- Abnormal constituents—UTI, foreign body, hyperkeratosis of epithelium (e.g. vitamin A deficiency), renal tubular acidosis, medullary sponge kidney.

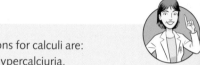

Common reasons for calculi are:
- Idiopathic hypercalciuria.
- UTI.

Clinical presentation

Ureteric calculi may be asymptomatic, or cause haematuria and ureteric colic, which is a severe colicky pain radiating from the loin to the groin and penis or labium. The haematuria may be macroscopic or microscopic.

Management

A diagnosis of ureteric calculus is based on the typical history, detection of haematuria and an IVU, which defines the level of obstruction. Blood tests and a 24-hour urine collection are performed to look for underlying biochemical abnormalities.

Initial treatment is with analgesia, and non-steroidal anti-inflammatory drugs (NSAIDs) such as diclofenac sodium have been found to be effective.

Most calculi less than 6 mm in diameter in the lower urinary tract pass spontaneously. If they do not and there are any signs of infection, urgent intervention is required to extract the calculus. An obstructed urinary tract with superimposed infection is a **SURGICAL EMERGENCY**. Calculi tend to lodge at the PUJ, pelvic brim and vesicoureteric junction, and may cause hydronephrosis and hydroureter with a risk of pyonephrosis.

Treatment of calculi

Renal stones can be fragmented by extracorporeal shock-wave lithotripsy (ESWL) so that they will pass down the ureter. Occasionally, the stone is too large and does not respond to ESWL, so it is removed by percutaneous nephrolithotomy. Under general anaesthetic, a nephroscope is inserted to fragment and remove the stone. The kidney is drained by a nephrostomy tube and a nephrostogram is performed to ensure that the ureter is clear of calculi before the tube is removed.

Open operation may be necessary to remove a staghorn calculus, which is usually seen in women who have had recurrent UTIs. The calculus consists of calcium, ammonium and magnesium phosphate. *Proteus* spp. split urea to form ammonium salts. The problem may be asymptomatic until renal damage occurs. If the stone is large, it may have to be removed by pyelolithotomy or nephrolithotomy, or nephrectomy if renal function is severely impaired.

Ureteric calculi can be removed using a ureteroscope. The calculus can be pushed back to the renal pelvis and then undergo ESWL or be disintegrated by a lithotrite. The stone may be retrieved using a dormia basket. Occasionally, a ureterolithotomy (open surgery) is necessary.

Bladder calculi

Bladder calculi form in a neuropathic or obstructed bladder and diverticula. Schistosomiasis and UTI predispose to their formation. They may cause acute retention. Treatment is stone retrieval by cystoscopy and cystolithotomy.

A filling defect on an IVU may be due to:
- Radiolucent stone.
- Ureteric malignancy.

RENAL CARCINOMA

Background

Renal cell carcinoma is an adenocarcinoma arising from the proximal convoluted tubules. Macroscopically, it is yellow because of its lipid content. It spreads locally through the capsule and along the vein, metastasizes to lymph nodes, and blood-borne metastases are distributed to the lungs and bones.

Clinical presentation

This includes:

- Haematuria.
- Loin pain.
- Abdominal mass.

Systemic effects include anaemia, pyrexia of unknown origin, metabolic disturbances of calcium, ectopic adrenocorticotrophic hormone or antidiuretic hormone secretion, polycythaemia and coagulopathy.

Renal carcinoma may also be an asymptomatic discovery on an ultrasound scan or present with metastases.

Renal carcinoma can cause a left varicocoele if the renal vein is obstructed.

Management

If a diagnosis of renal carcinoma is suspected, the kidney is imaged by computed tomography (CT) scan and this will stage the tumour. The function of the opposite kidney is assessed. A chest radiograph may show cannonball metastases. *to lungs*

The staging of renal carcinoma is:

- I—tumour confined to the kidney.
- II—tumour extends through the capsule.
- III—tumour extends to the renal vein, nodes or fascia.
- IV—distant metastases or local invasion.

Renal cell metastases are often large and solitary, and are commonly referred to as 'cannonball'.

Treatment is by radical nephrectomy. It may be possible to resect solitary lung metastases. Hormone and chemotherapy are not effective, but immunotherapy is under investigation. Overall survival is 40% at 5 years.

NEPHROBLASTOMA (WILMS' TUMOUR)

This is a malignant tumour occurring in children under 5 years of age. It may present as an abdominal mass or pain.

Consider a Wilms' tumour if a child presents with failure to thrive and/or an abdominal mass.

Diagnosis is made by ultrasound or CT scan.
    Treatment is a combination of surgery, chemotherapy and radiotherapy to produce a cure rate of 90%.

TUMOURS OF THE RENAL PELVIS AND URETER

Transitional cell carcinomas of the renal pelvis and ureters are rare. They can present with painless haematuria, clot colic or loin pain, or be associated with transitional cell carcinoma of the bladder.
    Diagnosis is made from urine cytology, IVU, CT scan and ureteroscopy.
    Treatment is nephroureterectomy.

BLADDER CANCER

Background

The incidence of bladder cancer is increasing. It is predominantly a transitional cell carcinoma. Aetiological factors include smoking, and there is an association with the dye and rubber industries (e.g. naphthylamine).
    Squamous cell carcinoma is rare except where schistosomiasis is endemic.
    Adenocarcinoma is very rare and is associated with a persistent urachal remnant. Fig. 33.1 shows the staging and prognosis of bladder cancer.

Most bladder cancers are transitional cell carcinomas, except where schistosomiasis is endemic.

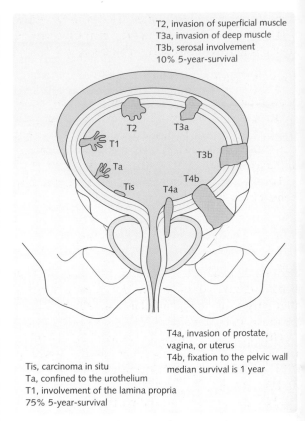

T2, invasion of superficial muscle
T3a, invasion of deep muscle
T3b, serosal involvement
10% 5-year-survival

T4a, invasion of prostate, vagina, or uterus
T4b, fixation to the pelvic wall median survival is 1 year

Tis, carcinoma in situ
Ta, confined to the urothelium
T1, involvement of the lamina propria
75% 5-year-survival

Fig. 33.1 Staging of bladder cancer and prognosis.

Management

Bladder cancer usually presents with painless haematuria (95% of cases). Carcinoma in situ may produce symptoms similar to those of a UTI, but no haematuria. Investigations include:

- MSU and urine for cytology.
- IVU.
- Cystourethroscopy.

CT scan and transvesical ultrasound scanning can be used to assess the depth of the tumour.

Superficial tumours—T0 and T1

These are diagnosed by multiple biopsies to assess the depth. The tumour is resected via a cystoscope (i.e. transurethral resection of bladder tumour; TURBT) and patients are reviewed regularly to look for further tumour. Recurrence occurs in 50%. Risk factors for local recurrence are smoking and large and multiple tumours.
    If there is evidence of carcinoma in situ or there is a high-grade superficial tumour or frequent recurrence, treatment with intravesical chemotherapy may be

used. Intravesical BCG (attenuated *Mycobacterium bovis*) reduces recurrence and progression rates more than traditional intravesical chemotherapy.

Invasive tumours—T2 and T3

More radical treatment, such as radical radiotherapy or a radical cystectomy with formation of an ileal conduit, is required for these tumours. Radiotherapy may result in the side effects of cystitis and proctitis, and make later operation more difficult.

Locally advanced and metastatic tumours may benefit from chemotherapy.

PROSTATE CANCER

Because the population is ageing, prostatic cancer is becoming more common. This is an adenocarcinoma that arises in the glandular epithelium at the periphery of the gland.

Histologically, prostatic cancer is classified using the Gleason grading system for the degree of differentiation. It spreads locally via the lymphatics and bloodstream.

The symptoms of prostatic cancer are those of bladder outflow obstruction or of metastatic bone disease. Screening for prostate cancer is a controversial area but, in many patients, the condition is being detected by an elevated prostatic-specific antigen (PSA) level when they are asymptomatic.

Management

Clinical examination reveals a hard, irregularly enlarged prostate with obliteration of the median sulcus. Blood tests are used to check the renal function and measure PSA.

Transrectal ultrasound can be used to image the prostate and to guide a Tru-cut biopsy. Abdominal ultrasound will reveal signs of bladder outflow obstruction, such as hydronephrosis and residual urine volume. A bone scan can be carried out to look for bone metastases, which are usually sclerotic deposits on plain radiographs.

Treatment is as follows:

- Bladder outflow obstruction—transurethral resection.
- Localized tumours (T1 or T2)—radiotherapy or radical prostatectomy.
- T3 or T4 tumours—radiotherapy, which may produce complications of prostatitis or cystitis.

- Metastatic disease—hormonal manipulation because the tumour is androgen dependent. Methods of treatment include bilateral subcapsular orchidectomy, luteinizing hormone - releasing hormone agonists, or antiandrogens such as cyproterone or flutamide.

Prostatic cancer tends to produce sclerotic metastases.

Fig. 33.2 shows the staging and prognosis of prostatic cancer.

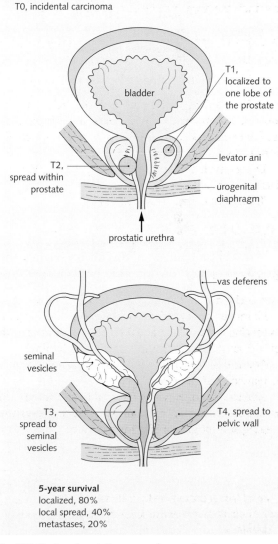

5-year survival
localized, 80%
local spread, 40%
metastases, 20%

Fig. 33.2 Staging of prostatic cancer and prognosis.

TESTICULAR CANCER

Primary testicular cancer develops in young men. Risk factors include cryptorchidism or undescended testis, even after fixation.

Teratoma and seminoma account for 90% of testicular tumours:

- Teratomas occur in 20–30 year olds.
- Seminomas occur in 30–50 year olds.

Both types metastasize to the para-aortic nodes because the testes originate from that area.

Testicular lymphoma may occur in older men and treatment is as for lymphoma in other sites.

Management

Testicular cancer usually presents as a painless, irregular, hard swelling of the testis.

The diagnosis is made by ultrasound scan of the testis and measurement of the tumour markers α-fetoprotein and β-human chorionic gonadotrophin. Lactate dehydrogenase is also measured as an indicator of the amount of tumour. A chest radiograph is taken to look for metastatic disease and abdominal CT is used to stage the disease and look for para-aortic nodes.

Once the diagnosis has been made, an orchidectomy is performed using an inguinal approach so that the cord and vessels are clamped before handling the testis, in order to prevent dissemination. Further treatment depends on the tumour stage.

With improvement in diagnosis, staging and treatment overall cure rates can be as high as 90% and, if the patient is node negative, it can be 100%.

Fig. 33.3 shows the staging and management of testicular tumours.

α-Fetoprotein or β-human chorionic gonadotrophin is raised in 90% of men with teratomas.

PENILE CANCER

This is rare in the UK, but is most likely to occur in uncircumcised elderly men. It is a squamous cell carcinoma that spreads to the inguinal nodes. It presents as a painful ulcerating lesion on the penis or enlarged nodes.

Penile cancer is associated with poor hygiene and is thought to be due to human papillomavirus.

The treatment depends on the size of the lesion at presentation:

- Surgical treatment can range from a circumcision to partial or complete amputation of the penis.
- Radiotherapy may be used for small lesions on the glans.
- A block dissection of the nodes is the best treatment for involved nodes.

Fig. 33.3 Staging of testicular tumours and management

Stage	Definition	Management of teratoma	Management of seminoma
I	confined to testis	orchidectomy and observe or RPLND	orchidectomy and radiotherapy to para-aortic nodes
II	retroperitoneal nodes	chemotherapy and RPLND to residuum	radiotherapy to nodes
	bulky disease		radiotherapy plus chemotherapy
III	nodal disease above diaphragm	chemotherapy	radiotherapy to nodes plus chemotherapy
IV	visceral metastases	chemotherapy	chemotherapy

(RPLND, retroperitoneal lymph node dissection.)

LOWER URINARY TRACT OBSTRUCTION

Fig. 33.4 shows the causes of lower urinary tract obstruction.

Obstructive symptoms are:

- Weak stream.
- Hesitancy.
- Intermittent stream.
- Dribbling.
- Straining.

Irritative symptoms are:

- Frequency.
- Urgency.
- Nocturia.
- Urge incontinence.

Benign prostatic hypertrophy

Benign prostatic hypertrophy (BPH) develops in the central part of the gland, initially in the periurethral glands. Fig. 33.5 shows the effects of bladder outflow obstruction. Changes occur with advancing years, but the precise reason for these changes is unknown. Patients have a combination of symptoms of obstruction and irritation.

Intermittent stream, terminal dribbling and incomplete emptying occur when the detrusor is unable to maintain sufficient pressure to overcome the obstruction. Chronic retention may develop, with a large residual volume and overflow incontinence.

Acute urinary obstruction may be precipitated by a UTI or drugs, such as α-adrenergic, anticholinergic and psychotropic drugs.

The size of the prostate does not correspond to the degree of symptoms. Benign prostatic hypertrophy develops in the central part of the gland.

Management

Examination of a patient who has lower urinary tract obstruction may demonstrate a palpable bladder and an enlarged smooth prostate.

Investigations include an MSU for infection and haematuria and tests of renal function. An ultrasound scan of the pelvis will reveal a residual volume after micturition and any pressure effects on the kidneys. A urine-flow measurement gives an

Fig. 33.4 Causes of lower urinary tract obstruction

Disorder	Causes
meatal stenosis	congenital in newborn or infant males; balanitis in adults
urethral stenosis	trauma or inflammation in females; instrumentation or venereal disease in males
posterior urethral valves	congenital mucosal folds in young males
spasm of urethral sphincter	spinal cord injury, multiple sclerosis
benign prostatic hypertrophy	elderly males
prostatic cancer	elderly males
bladder neck contracture	usually secondary to trauma or operation
cystocoele	women who have had a vaginal delivery or a pelvic operation
detrusor inhibition	anticholinergic agents such as phenothiazines, antianxiolytic drugs
systemic neurological conditions	Guillain–Barré syndrome, diabetes mellitus, uraemia and chronic alcoholism can affect the autonomic nervous system

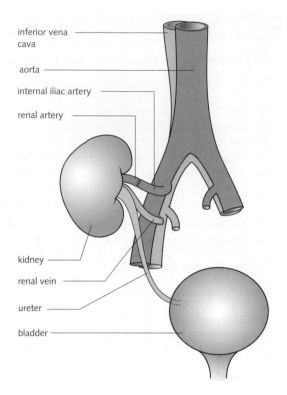

Fig. 33.7 Renal transplantation. (IVC, inferior vena cava.)

Management

A frequency and volume chart should be recorded for 3 days. The patient is examined to look for a cystocoele, palpable bladder or enlarged prostate. A flow rate and ultrasound scan are performed to assess the residual volume in the bladder. Other tests include an MSU, IVU and urodynamic assessment. Videocystometry will show unstable contractions and stress incontinence.

Urge incontinence is managed by:

- Treating any underlying cause.
- Prescribing drugs that relax the smooth muscle.
- An operation may be carried out to distend the bladder or increase the bladder size by augmentation with the caecum.

Stress incontinence is managed by:

- Bladder exercises.
- Drugs that increase the bladder neck closure.
- Operation to lift the bladder neck and urethral suspension.
- An artificial urinary sphincter may be necessary.

TESTICULAR PROBLEMS

Undescended testis

The testis develops on the posterior abdominal wall and descends after the processus vaginalis and gubernaculum into its position in the scrotum. Its progress may be halted or altered so that the testis remains intra-abdominal, inguinal or high in the scrotum. It may not be palpable, and ultrasound or CT scan may be needed to identify it.

If the testis fails to descend by 1 year of age, it should be surgically moved (i.e. orchidopexy). If it remains in an abnormal position the seminiferous tubules are damaged and there are risks of infertility and malignant change and it is more prone to trauma.

SURGICAL EMERGENCY

Torsion of the testis

This is a problem of teenage boys and young adults and may be due to abnormal mesentery on the testis. The history is of an acute onset of scrotal pain, which may be associated with lower abdominal pain and vomiting. There may be a history of preceding episodes that resolved. On examination, the scrotum will be red, and the testis will lie horizontally and be very tender. If diagnosis is delayed, there may be inflammation and a reactionary hydrocoele.

If torsion is a possibility, it requires urgent exploration. If the testis is already infarcted, it is removed. If it is viable after untwisting, both testes are fixed. Even after 4 hours, damage will have occurred to spermatogenesis, but the hormonal function may be preserved.

The differential diagnosis of torsion includes torsion of the hydatid of Morgagni, which is an embryological remnant on the testis.

Epididymitis presents a similar picture, but is unusual in adolescents.

Urgent exploration is essential for suspected torsion of the testis.

Epididymo-orchitis

Sexually transmitted infection or UTI may precipitate epididymo-orchitis. Orchitis may be secondary to viral infection of mumps and appears 3–4 days after parotitis.

Symptoms of epididymo-orchitis are a painful testis and epididymis, with pyrexia, malaise and features of UTI. The scrotum is red, inflamed and tender.

The organisms involved are *Chlamydia trachomatis* or *Neisseria gonorrhoeae* if due to sexually transmitted infection, but Gram-negative organisms if it is secondary to a UTI.

Epididymo-orchitis is treated with appropriate antibiotics.

SCROTAL PROBLEMS

The differential diagnoses for a scrotal mass are described in Fig. 33.8.

Hydrocoele

This is a collection of fluid in the tunica vaginalis surrounding the testis. It may be congenital if seen in boys under 1 year of age and is due to persistent patency of the processus vaginalis. Most close spontaneously.

In adults, it may be primary and idiopathic or develop secondary to infection, tumour or trauma. An ultrasound will reveal any underlying pathology and the hydrocoele should be treated accordingly.

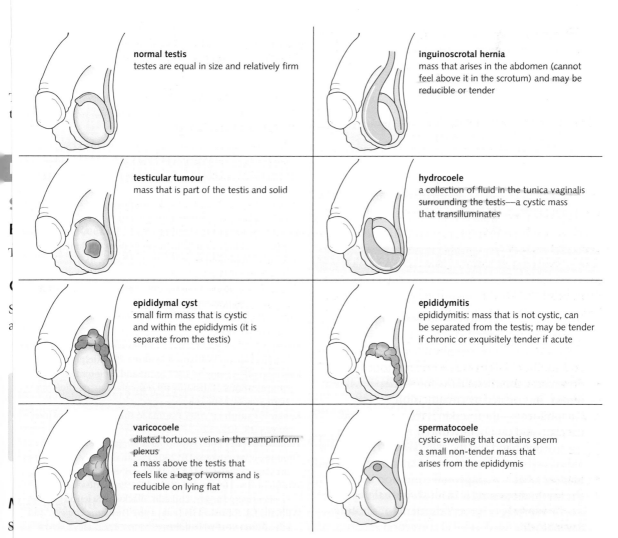

normal testis
testes are equal in size and relatively firm

inguinoscrotal hernia
mass that arises in the abdomen (cannot feel above it in the scrotum) and may be reducible or tender

testicular tumour
mass that is part of the testis and solid

hydrocoele
a collection of fluid in the tunica vaginalis surrounding the testis—a cystic mass that transilluminates

epididymal cyst
small firm mass that is cystic and within the epididymis (it is separate from the testis)

epididymitis
epididymitis: mass that is not cystic, can be separated from the testis; may be tender if chronic or exquisitely tender if acute

varicocoele
dilated tortuous veins in the pampiniform plexus
a mass above the testis that feels like a bag of worms and is reducible on lying flat

spermatocoele
cystic swelling that contains sperm a small non-tender mass that arises from the epididymis

Fig. 33.8 Differential diagnosis of a scrotal mass.

Fig. 34.1 Types of skin lesion

Type	Examples
benign conditions	sebaceous cyst, lipoma, dermoid cyst, hidradenitis suppurativa
benign skin tumours	papilloma, wart, pyogenic granuloma, histiocytoma (dermatofibroma), neurofibroma, keratoacanthoma, seborrhoeic keratoses, solar keratosis
vascular lesions	strawberry naevus, capillary haemangioma, cavernous haemangioma, lymphangioma, glomus body tumour
malignant skin lesions	basal cell carcinoma, squamous cell carcinoma, Kaposi's sarcoma, Bowen's disease
pigmented lesions	naevi, malignant melanoma

Hidradenitis suppurativa

Background

This is a condition affecting the sweat glands that results in recurrent infections and sinuses, which discharge.

Clinical presentation

Hidradenitis suppurativa occurs in the axilla, groins and perineum.

Management

Minor episodes resolve spontaneously, but abscesses may require incision and drainage. Chronic widespread problems are treated by excision of the affected skin, which is left open to heal by granulation tissue.

BENIGN SKIN TUMOURS

Papilloma

A papilloma is an overgrowth of skin that produces a sessile or pedunculated polyp.

Wart

Background

Warts are caused by viruses that produce papillary hyperplasia and excessive keratinization.

Clinical presentation

Warts are commonly seen on the hands and feet (e.g. verrucas). Sexually transmitted disease of the perineum is due to human papillomavirus.

Management

Wart treatments include salicylic acid, cryotherapy, podophyllin and silver nitrate.

Pyogenic granuloma

Clinical presentation

This lesion usually develops after trauma and is an exuberant mass of granulation tissue, which bleeds easily.

Management

Pyogenic granuloma can be excised under local anaesthetic.

Histiocytoma

Background

Histiocytoma (dermatofibroma) is a very common skin nodule caused by infiltration by lipid-filled macrophages.

Clinical presentation

Clinically, histiocytoma is a firm hemispherical nodule.

Management

Diagnosis and treatment of histiocytoma is by excision.

Neurofibroma

This is a small firm subcutaneous mass. It is a benign nerve sheath tumour.

Multiple neurofibromas with café-au-lait spots are a feature of neurofibromatosis (von Recklinghausen's disease), which is an autosomal-dominant condition.

Keratoacanthoma

Background

The history for a keratoacanthoma is that of a rapidly growing lump over a period of 6 weeks, which ulcerates and then regresses and heals over 2–3 months.

Clinical presentation

Keratoacanthoma is often found on the face and hands. An important differential diagnosis is squamous cell carcinoma.

Seborrhoeic keratoses

Background

These are very common in elderly people, especially on the trunk.

Clinical presentation

Seborrhoeic keratoses are raised and pigmented brown and have a waxy feel. Histologically, they consist of stratified squamous epithelium.

Solar keratosis

Background

/actinic
Solar keratosis is very common in elderly people and arises in areas exposed to the sun.

Clinical presentation

red papules
The lesions consist of hyperkeratosis and are premalignant.

Management

Solar keratosis should be excised and advice given about reducing sun exposure.

VASCULAR LESIONS

Strawberry naevus

Background

Strawberry naevus (capillary cavernous haemangioma) occurs about 10 days after birth and rapidly enlarges to several centimetres in diameter.

Clinical presentation

A strawberry naevus is a vascular lesion that appears red, raised and compressible. It regresses spontaneously over a period of several years to leave a small scar.

Strawberry naevi do not require excision unless the lesion interferes with vision or airway.

Capillary haemangioma

Clinical presentation

Capillary haemangioma (port wine stain) can occur at any site, but may correspond to a sensory dermatome.

Management

Attempts to remove a capillary haemangioma cause scarring, so cosmetic camouflage is required.

Capillary haemangioma may be associated with a central nervous system lesion (i.e. Sturge–Weber syndrome).

Cavernous haemangioma

Background

This is a localized collection of dilated veins.

Clinical presentation

Cavernous haemangioma is a bluish–purple lesion.

Management

Cavernous haemangiomas are excised because of the risk of ulceration and bleeding.

Lymphangioma

Clinical presentation

This consists of lymphatic channels, which contain clear fluid. The largest form is a congenital cystic hygroma of the neck.

Glomus body tumour

Background

A glomus body tumour is an arteriovenous formation that is sensitive to temperature.

Clinical presentation

It is usually seen on the digits as a purplish lesion beneath the nails.

Management

Glomus body tumours are exquisitely tender and should be removed.

MALIGNANT SKIN LESIONS

Over the past 10 years, there has been an increased incidence of malignant skin lesions because of increased exposure to ultraviolet radiation, but also increased public awareness of detecting early change. Predisposing factors for the development of malignant lesions are:

- Exposure to sunlight.
- Radiation exposure.
- Chemical carcinogens (e.g. arsenic, coal tar, oils).
- Inherited disorders (e.g. xeroderma pigmentosa).
- Chronic ulceration (e.g. Marjolin's ulcer).

Any suspicious lesion should be excised for precise histological diagnosis.

Basal cell carcinoma (rodent ulcer)

Background

Basal cell carcinoma is a malignant tumour of the basal cells of the epidermis. It invades locally, but does not metastasize.

Clinical presentation

Basal cell carcinoma is a common lesion, especially on the forehead, nose and face, but can occur in many different sites. The characteristic appearance is of an ulcerated lesion with a rolled, pearly margin and telangiectasia.

Management

Treatment of basal cell carcinoma is surgical excision or radiotherapy.

Squamous cell carcinoma

Clinical presentation

Squamous cell carcinoma is an ulcerated lesion with everted edges. It spreads locally, but also metastasizes to regional nodes.

Management

Diagnosis is by biopsy and treatment is surgical excision or radiotherapy.

Kaposi's sarcoma

Background

This is an angiomatous neoplasm affecting the skin.

Clinical presentation

Kaposi's sarcoma is purple and occurs on the hands and feet. It is now a common presentation of acquired immunodeficiency syndrome (AIDS).

Bowen's disease

Background

Bowen's disease is a premalignant change (i.e. squamous carcinoma in situ).

Clinical presentation

Bowen's disease produces a raised red, hyperkeratotic, well-demarcated lesion.

Management

The lesion can be treated with 5-fluorouracil or cryotherapy, but surgical excision is preferable.

PIGMENTED LESIONS

Naevi are benign pigmented lesions that develop from increased numbers of melanocytes. There are several different types depending on the position of the melanocytes, including:

- Lentigo—the melanocytes are in the basal layer of the epidermis. This is usually seen on the face.
- Junctional—the melanocytes are at the junction of the dermis and epidermis. These arise before puberty, and are smooth and flat.
- Intradermal—the melanocytes are in the dermis. This is an elevated lesion and is the commonest variety.
- Compound—the melanocytes are at the junction and in the dermis. This has a mixed appearance and may become malignant.
- Blue—the melanocytes are deep in the dermis.

The signs indicating malignant changes in naevi are listed in Fig. 34.2.

Malignant melanoma

Clinical presentation

A melanoma is usually a brown–black pigmented irregular lesion and may show evidence of bleeding or ulceration, but can be amelanotic.

Malignant melanomas are commonly found on the lower limbs, feet, head and neck. The two common types are:

- Superficial spreading malignant melanoma.
- Nodular malignant melanoma.

Initially, the malignant cells spread laterally and then they grow vertically and have the potential to metastasize via the lymphatic system or bloodstream to the liver, bone, brain, lungs and gastrointestinal tract.

Fig. 34.2 Signs of malignant change of naevus

new lesion
increased size, colour and pigmentation
bleeding, crusting, ulceration
pain, itching
satellite lesions
lymphadenopathy

Other types of malignant melanoma are:

- Acral lentiginous melanoma, which can occur on the soles of the feet.
- Subungal melanoma.

Management

A melanoma is assessed by pathological assessment of the depth of the tumour according to Breslow's classification or Clarke's levels.

A poor prognosis is associated with melanomas that are ulcerated, more than 4 mm deep, occur on the trunk or in men.

Surgical excision is the main treatment.

Subungal melanoma is treated by excision of the digit.

If there are involved nodes, a block dissection should be performed. Sentinel lymph node biopsy in melanoma cases is currently under evaluation.

Local recurrence or satellite nodules without distant metastases are treated by perfusing the limb with a chemotherapeutic agent (melphalan) at 42 °C (i.e. isolated hyperthermic limb perfusion).

Immunotherapy such as interferon improves survival in patients who have regional metastases successfully removed. Melanoma is not responsive to chemotherapy or radiotherapy.

Fig. 34.3 shows the recommendations for surgical excision margins and the prognosis for different stages of melanoma.

Fig. 34.3 Recommendations for surgical excision margins and prognosis for melanoma

Breslow thickness	Excision margin	5-year survival (%)
in situ	clear margins	100
<1 mm	1 cm	95–100
1–2 mm	1–2 cm	80–95
2.1–4 mm	2 cm	60–75
>4 mm	2–3 cm	50

A melanoma 0.75 mm deep has a very good prognosis but, if it is 4 mm deep, it has a very poor prognosis.

Sites of malignant melanoma that have a poor prognosis are the BANS:

- Back of the arm.
- Neck.
- Scalp.

Further reading

Balch C, Houghton A, Sober et al. 1998 *Cutaneous Melanoma*. Quality Medical Publishing, St Louis

Dvorak VC, Root RK, MacGregor RR 1977 Host-defense mechanisms in hidradenitis suppurativa. *Arch Dermatol* **113**: 450–453

Grey JE, Harding KG (eds) 2006 *The ABC of Wound Healing*. BMJ Publications, London

McKee PH 1989 *Pathology of the Skin*. Lippincott Williams & Wilkins, Philadelphia

Morgan WP, Harding KG, Richardson G et al. 1980 The use of silastic foam dressing in the treatment of advanced hidradenitis suppurativa. *Br J Surg* **67**: 277–280

Multidisiplinary working party of the Australian caner network 1997 *Guidelines for the Management of Malignant Melanoma*. The Stone Press, Australia

Rudolph R, Zelac DE 2004 Squamous cell carcinoma of the skin. *Clin Plast Surg* **114**: 82E–94E

Walter F, Elenitsas R, Jaworsky C et al. 1997 *Lever's Histopathology of the Skin*, 8th edn. Lippincott Williams & Wilkins, Philadelphia

Soft tissue disorders

35

Objectives

You should be able to:

- Define 'ingrowing toenail' and describe how it is treated.
- List the causes of Dupuytren's contracture.
- State the site ganglions are commonly found.
- Describe why certain professionals are more prone to pilonidal sinuses.
- Understand the treatment necessary if a limb soft tissue sarcoma is diagnosed.

HAND AND NAIL PROBLEMS

Ingrowing toenail

Background

Ingrowing toenails are common, especially in adolescents, and they usually affect the hallux of the foot.

Clinical presentation

The nail edge starts to grow into the adjacent soft tissue and there may be superimposed infection, so cellulitis and granulation tissue develop. Simple measures to improve foot hygiene include cutting the nail transversely so that the nail does not grow into the soft tissues. An operation may be needed involving:

- Wedge resection (Fig. 35.1)—removal of the edge of the nail and phenolization of the nailbed to prevent regrowth.
- Zadik's operation—excision of the whole nail and nailbed to stop regrowth.

The presence of the peripheral pulses should be checked before carrying out an operation for ingrowing toenails.

Paronychia

Clinical presentation

Paronychia is an infection of the soft tissue at the edge of the nail and commonly occurs in the fingers.

Management

An abscess develops, which requires incision and drainage.

Onychogryphosis

Clinical presentation

Onychogryphosis is a deformity of the nail, especially the hallux of elderly people. The nail is very thickened and twisted.

Management

If the nail is avulsed, it will regrow in the same way and the only treatment is complete removal and ablation of the nailbed—Zadik's operation.

Dupuytren's contracture

Clinical presentation

Dupuytren's contracture is thickening and contracture of the palmar or plantar aponeurosis. It causes flexion of the digits at the metacarpophalangeal and proximal interphalangeal joints. In most cases it is idiopathic, but it can be familial or associated with liver disease, epilepsy and the use of phenytoin.

207

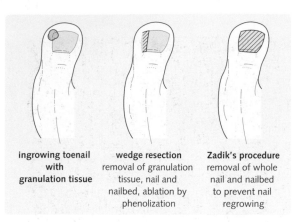

ingrowing toenail
with
granulation tissue

wedge resection
removal of granulation
tissue, nail and
nailbed, ablation by
phenolization

Zadik's procedure
removal of whole
nail and nailbed
to prevent nail
regrowing

Fig. 35.1 Operative treatment for ingrowing toenails.

Management

Treatment is by fasciectomy to straighten the flexed fingers.

Ganglion

Clinical presentation

A ganglion is a benign myxoma of the joint capsule or tendon sheath and is commonly found on the hand or wrist, dorsum of the foot or peroneal tendons of the ankle. It is a soft protrusion from the synovial sheath surrounding a tendon or a joint capsule. It has a synovial lining and contains synovial fluid. It can fluctuate in size, so treatment may not be necessary.

Management

The ganglion can be excised, but will recur if the communication with the capsule or sheath is not identified.

PILONIDAL SINUS

Clinical presentation

A pilonidal sinus ('nest of hairs') occurs in the natal cleft of young hairy males, but it may occur between the fingers of hairdressers. It is due to hairs penetrating into the skin and causing an inflammatory reaction. In the natal cleft, there are central pits with lateral sinuses, which discharge, or an abscess develops.

Management

Abscesses are incised and drained, but the whole sinus and its tracts should be excised to prevent recurrence.

Incision and drainage of pilonidal abscesses results in faster recovery but has a higher recurrence rate than complete excision.

SOFT TISSUE TUMOURS

Clinical presentation

Young people who present with a short history of an intramuscular mass should be suspected of having a malignant tumour (e.g. liposarcoma, rhabdomyosarcoma, chondrosarcoma, lymphoma).

Management

The differential diagnosis includes a lipoma or other benign tumour. Common sites for soft tissue tumours are the limbs, pelvic girdle and retroperitoneum.

Diagnosis is made by imaging by ultrasound, magnetic resonance imaging or computed tomography (CT) to assess the site and extent of the mass (Fig. 35.2).

An image-guided Tru-cut biopsy can be obtained to provide a tissue diagnosis:

- If it is malignant, the patient is assessed for metastatic disease.
- If a solitary sarcoma is identified and it is deemed operable (i.e. it does not invade the neurovascular bundle), it is excised radically (i.e. compartment excision or excision of the whole muscle to completely excise the tumour without breaching its capsule). This may be preceded or followed by radiotherapy or chemotherapy to decrease its size.

The prognosis depends on the size, grade, degree of differentiation and excision margins of the tumour.

A diagnosis of sarcoma should be suspected in any patient who presents with a new intramuscular mass.

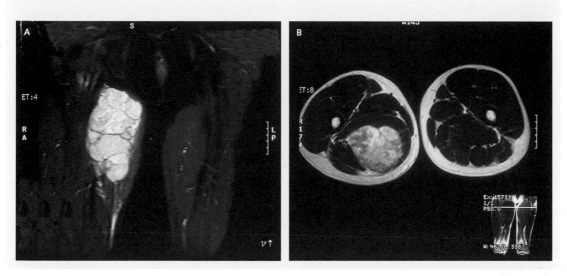

Fig. 35.2 Magnetic resonance images of thigh showing sarcoma of the thigh. (A) Longitudinal view. (B) Cross-sectional view.

Further reading

Green DP, Hotchkiss RN, Pederson WC . (eds) 1999 *Green's Operative Hand Surgery*, 4th edn. Churchill Livingstone, Edinburgh

Jupiter JB (ed) 1991 *Flynn's Hand Surgery*, 4th edn. Lippincott Williams & Wilkins, Philadelphia

Singer S, Demetri GD, Baldini EH, Fletcher CD 2000 Management of soft-tissue sarcomas: an overview and update. *Lancet Oncol* 1: 75–85

Swan MC, Furniss D, Cassell OCS 2004 Surgical management of metastatic inguinal lymphadenopathy. *BMJ* 329: 1272–1276

Varley GW, Needoff M, Davis TR . 1997 Conservative management of wrist ganglia. Aspiration versus steroid infiltration. *Hand Surg* [Br] 22: 636–637

Learning objectives

You should be able to:

- Understand the significance of the golden hour.
- Describe the clinical features of a tension pneumothorax and its treatment.
- Anticipate the percentage of total blood volume lost in a patient with an open femoral fracture, tachycardia, tachypnoea, confusion and hypotension.
- Define 'flail chest' and when it is likely to occur.
- Describe the clininical features suggestive of an oesophageal rupture.
- Understand the principles of liver trauma management.
- Describe how secondary brain damage occurs and how it can be prevented.
- Identify which anatomical structure is injured if an acute extradural haematoma develops.
- Understand the 'rule of nines' with regards to burns.
- Define 'second-degree burn'.

Trauma is the leading cause of death in the first four decades of life. Death may occur at one of three stages:

- Within minutes of the injury—if there is laceration of the brain or brainstem or spinal cord injury, or damage to the heart and major vessels.
- From a few minutes to a few hours after trauma—the 'golden hour'—with rapid assessment and appropriate management deaths can be avoided.
- Several days to weeks after injury—this is usually due to sepsis and organ failure.

The quality of the initial assessment is vital to sustaining life and the quality of life.

The primary survey and management of trauma patients are outlined in Fig. 36.1.

Assessment includes a history of the mechanisms of the injury, because this gives clues about the likely injuries.

Background information on the patient's general health may influence further management.

It is important to assess the vital signs rapidly, and maintain oxygenation and circulation because early death is due to uncontrollable haemorrhage and hypoxia, leading to irreversible organ failure.

Fig. 36.2 shows the areas of possible injury. Once the patient is more stable, a full secondary survey is made to look for non-life-threatening injuries.

A classification of hypovolaemic shock is given in Fig. 36.3.

O-negative blood can be used while awaiting cross-match.

Shock is defined as acute circulatory failure with inadequate tissue perfusion causing cellular hypoxia.

CHEST INJURIES

Tension pneumothorax

Background

This occurs when the lung is damaged by a penetrating injury, which then acts as a one-way valve so that the air escapes from the lung into the

Fig. 36.1 Management of trauma patients

primary survey
A–airway maintenance and cervical spine control
B–breathing and ventilation
C–circulation and haemorrhage control
D–disability and neurological status

resuscitation

secondary survey

definitive care

- Distended neck veins.
- Hypertympanic percussion note.

Treatment is immediate decompression by insertion of a chest drain.

> If you suspect a tension pneumothorax, do not wait for the chest X-ray: treat immediately.

pleural cavity (Fig. 36.4), causing collapse of the lung, mediastinal shift, decreased venous return and decreased ventilation of the opposite lung.

Management

The diagnosis is made clinically based on the following signs:

- Severe respiratory distress.
- Tracheal deviation.
- Unilateral absence of breath sounds.
- Cyanosis.

Open pneumothorax

Background

If there is a large open defect in the chest wall, there is a pneumothorax, but the air is able to escape so the pressure does not increase so rapidly.

Management

The defect in the chest wall should be sealed with dressings and a chest drain inserted.

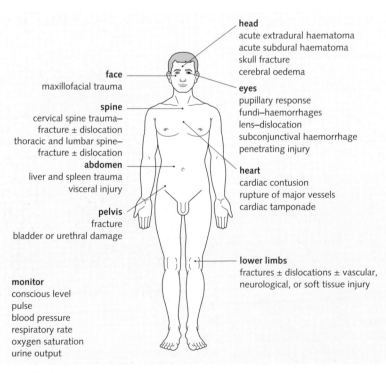

head
acute extradural haematoma
acute subdural haematoma
skull fracture
cerebral oedema

eyes
pupillary response
fundi–haemorrhages
lens–dislocation
subconjunctival haemorrhage
penetrating injury

face
maxillofacial trauma

spine
cervical spine trauma–
fracture ± dislocation
thoracic and lumbar spine–
fracture ± dislocation

abdomen
liver and spleen trauma
visceral injury

heart
cardiac contusion
rupture of major vessels
cardiac tamponade

pelvis
fracture
bladder or urethral damage

lower limbs
fractures ± dislocations ± vascular, neurological, or soft tissue injury

monitor
conscious level
pulse
blood pressure
respiratory rate
oxygen saturation
urine output

Fig. 36.2 Sites of possible traumatic injuries.

Fig. 36.3 Classification of hypovolaemic shock

Class	Blood loss	Clinical features
I	<15%	minimal symptoms and signs
II	15–30% (800–1500 mL)	pulse rate >100, ↑ respiratory rate, ↓ blood pressure and↓ urine output
III	30–40%	tachycardia, tachypnoea, confusion, ↓ blood pressure and ↓ urine output
IV	>40%	life-threatening—skin cold and pale, tachycardia, low blood pressure, oliguria, ↓ consciousness level
	50%	loss of consciousness, pulse and blood pressure

Haemothorax

Background

After blunt or penetrating injury, intrathoracic structures may be damaged, resulting in a haemothorax.

Clinical presentation

There are signs of hypovolaemia and respiratory impairment. A chest radiograph will show fluid in the pleural cavity.

Management

The patient should be resuscitated and a chest drain inserted. If the blood loss is more than 200 mL/hour, a thoracotomy is performed to control haemorrhage.

Flail chest

Background

If there are multiple rib fractures, the normal movement of the chest wall is disrupted (Fig. 36.4).

Clinical presentation

The underlying lung is usually damaged, causing hypoxia. The injured chest wall moves paradoxically (i.e. not with the rest of the chest wall), so the chest movement is decreased and further hypoxia develops.

Management

The patient may need ventilation to maintain oxygenation until the ribs stabilize.

Simple pneumothorax

Background

A fractured rib may penetrate the lung, resulting in a pneumothorax and lung collapse.

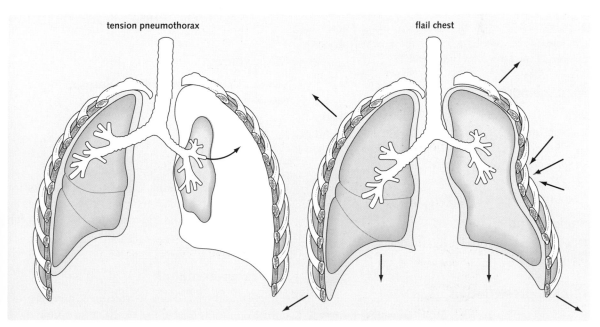

Fig. 36.4 Tension pneumothorax and flail chest. In a tension pneumothorax, air escapes from the lung into the pleural cavity. A flail chest results from multiple rib fractures, which disrupt the normal movement of the chest wall.

Clinical presentation

The patient is breathless. SOB, pleuritic c/pain

Management

A chest radiograph confirms the diagnosis and a chest drain is inserted in the fourth or fifth intercostal space anterior to the axillary line.

Cardiac tamponade

Background

This is usually caused by penetrating injury, but may be due to major blunt trauma.

Clinical presentation

Blood in the pericardium depresses the cardiac output and increases the venous pressure.

Management

The diagnosis is based on the signs of a decreased blood pressure and heart sounds, but increased venous pressure.

Treatment is urgent pericardiocentesis (i.e. aspiration of the pericardial sac).

Traumatic aortic rupture

Background

Approximately 90% of these injuries are fatal at the site of the accident but, if the adventitial layer remains intact, rupture is delayed.

Management

Diagnosis is suspected if there is a widened mediastinum. A computed tomography (CT) scan or aortography confirms the diagnosis and urgent surgical repair is then required.

Oesophageal rupture

Background

Oesophageal rupture is usually due to penetrating trauma.

Clinical presentation

It is suspected by the presence of surgical emphysema in the neck, a left pneumothorax and mediastinal air on chest radiography.

Management

Treatment is urgent surgical exploration.

Diaphragmatic rupture

Background

This is more common on the left side and is caused by blunt trauma, causing radial tears leading to herniation.

Clinical presentation

A diaphragmatic rupture may go unnoticed until the patient develops bowel obstruction many years later.

Pulmonary and myocardial contusion

Background

Trauma to the chest wall usually causes damage to the underlying lung, which may cause respiratory failure 24 hours after injury, even if the ribs are not injured.

Clinical presentation

Myocardial contusion causes chest-wall pain and abnormalities on the electrocardiogram (ECG).

Management

Myocardial contusion may predispose to important arrhythmias. Treatment is supportive.

Rib fracture

Background

Relatively minor trauma can fracture ribs in the elderly. The pain of rib fracture inhibits ventilation, so may cause hypoxia, especially if the patient has underlying lung disease.

Clinical presentation

If the first and second ribs are fractured, there is often marked major injury to the head, neck, spinal cord, lungs and great vessels. In young people, fractures of ribs 4–9 are most common.

Life-threatening thoracic conditions are:
- Tension pneumothorax.
- Cardiac tamponade.
- Open chest wound.
- Massive haemothorax.
- Flail chest.

ABDOMINAL TRAUMA

Background

Blunt or penetrating injuries or compression against the vertebral column can cause marked internal damage. A penetrating injury requires a laparotomy because of the risk of visceral injury.

Management

Patients who have a blunt injury should be carefully assessed and re-evaluated frequently.

An ultrasound or CT scan can be helpful, but cannot exclude some important injuries.

Liver trauma

Background

This is usually associated with other severe injuries.

Clinical presentation

A diagnosis of liver trauma is suspected if the patient is hypovolaemic and there is bruising or fracture of overlying ribs.

Management

A CT scan is useful for assessing the liver. Subcapsular or intrahepatic haematomas are treated conservatively. If there is major liver disruption then an urgent laparotomy to pack or resect the liver is needed.

Splenic rupture

Background

This can occur after minor trauma to a diseased spleen.

Clinical presentation

The presence of left shoulder tip pain, hypovolaemia, abdominal distension and fractures of ribs 9–11 should suggest this diagnosis.

Management

A ruptured spleen is removed, but in children efforts are made to conserve it because of its important immunological functions.

Renal tract trauma

Clinical presentation

A suspicion of renal tract trauma is aroused if the patient has haematuria and fractured lower ribs or a lumbar spine injury. If the kidney is avulsed, the patient is hypovolaemic and there is a flank haematoma, but no haematuria.

Management

Urgent nephrectomy is usually indicated for an avulsed kidney. A renal haematoma causes haematuria and usually resolves spontaneously.

Bladder rupture presents as peritonitis.

Urethral damage occurs in men who have a pelvic fracture or perineal trauma. There will be perineal bruising and the prostate will lie high. If urethral damage is suspected, a urethrogram is performed before catheter insertion.

Suspect a urethral injury if there is perineal bruising and a high prostate. A urethrogram should be performed before attempting to pass a urinary catheter.

HEAD INJURY

Background

Direct or decelerating trauma damages the skull and brain:

- Primary brain damage is directly related to the trauma.
- Secondary brain damage occurs as a result of hypoxia, hypotension, infection and intracranial bleeding.

Clinical presentation

In the conscious patient, the following information should be obtained:

- Mechanism of the injury.
- Duration of time of loss of consciousness.
- Presence of headache, nausea, vomiting, blurred vision, dizziness and retrograde amnesia.

Note that many of these patients are influenced by the effects of alcohol and drugs.

Management

All patients should be evaluated using: *GCS neuro, pupils obs*

- The Glasgow Coma Scale (see Chapter 40, Fig. 40.10).
- Other observations, including blood pressure, pulse, respiration, pupillary response, bruising and presence of rhinorrhoea or otorrhoea.
- Assessment of the tone, power and sensation of the limbs.

Careful examination is made for other injuries. Patients should be carefully and frequently re-evaluated to detect change.

Patients should be resuscitated to prevent secondary brain damage from hypoxia and may require intubation and ventilation.

A skull radiograph is obtained if there has been blunt, penetrating or open injury, and a CT scan is performed if the patient is unconscious or intracranial pathology is suspected.

Fig. 36.5 shows the signs of deterioration following a head injury.

Skull fractures

Background

It is possible to have a fracture, but no intracranial pathology, and vice versa.

Fig. 36.5 Signs of deterioration following a head injury

Glasgow Coma Score decrease >2
headache, nausea, vomiting
↑ blood pressure; ↓ heart and respiratory rate
(i.e. ↑ intracranial pressure)
↓ conscious level
↑ size of one or both pupils
weakness

Management

No action is necessary for a simple linear fracture unless there is intracranial damage. If there is a depressed fracture that is depressed more than the thickness of the skull, operative elevation is required to prevent scarring to the brain and a risk of epilepsy.

Compound fractures need early operative intervention, antibiotics and skin closure to prevent infection.

Basal skull fractures are not evident on skull radiographs, but are suspected if there is cerebrospinal fluid rhinorrhoea or otorrhoea or Battle's sign (i.e. ecchymoses of the mastoid area, haemotympanum and periorbital bruising). Management is conservative, with antibiotics to prevent infection.

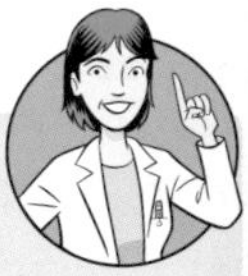

Suspect a basal skull fracture if there is:
- Rhinorrhoea—cerebrospinal fluid (CSF) from the nose.
- Otorrhoea—CSF from the ear.
- Battle's sign—bruising over the mastoid.

A frontal fracture is suspected if the patient has a subconjunctival haemorrhage and the posterior limit is not visible. The patient may also have anosmia or rhinorrhoea.

Acute cerebral injury

Background

A focal injury may be due to a haematoma or contusion.

Acute extradural haematoma

Acute extradural haematoma (Fig. 36.6) usually follows a fall or assault. It is due to a tear in a dural artery (e.g. middle meningeal artery) and is associated with a fracture in the temporoparietal region.

Clinical presentation

The features of acute extradural haematoma are:

- Initial loss of consciousness followed by a lucid interval and later loss of consciousness.
- Dilated and fixed ipsilateral pupil—due to stretching of the oculomotor nerve (third cranial nerve).

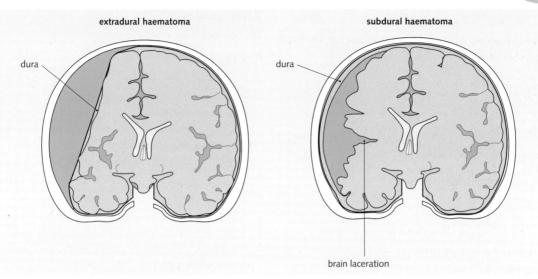

extradural haematoma

dura

subdural haematoma

dura

brain laceration

Fig. 36.6 Location of extradural and subdural haematomas.

- Contralateral hemiparesis.
- Signs of increased intracranial pressure.

Management

An urgent CT scan and evacuation of clot via a burr hole are necessary.

Acute subdural haematoma

Background

Acute subdural haematoma (Fig. 36.6) is due to the rupture of the veins bridging the space between the arachnoid mater and the dura mater.

Clinical presentation

There may not be an associated skull fracture, but there is often underlying brain injury.

Management

Emergency evacuation is required, but there is a high mortality rate.

Chronic subdural haematoma

Background

A trivial injury in the elderly may go unnoticed, but it may tear a vein between the arachnoid and dura mater.

Clinical presentation

A haematoma slowly enlarges by absorption of cerebrospinal fluid. There is a slow neurological deterioration with drowsiness, headache and hemiplegia.

Management

Treatment is by evacuation.

Subdural haemorrhages are more common in patients taking warfarin, *elderly, alcoholics .*

Intracerebral haematoma

The neurological signs of intracerebral haematoma depend on the area of brain affected. It is diagnosed by CT scan and management is conservative.

Diffuse brain injury

Diffuse brain injury is more common than a localized haematoma after a vehicle accident. Rapid head motion with acceleration and deceleration forces causes coup and contrecoup injuries.

This causes diffuse axonal injury, cerebral oedema and diffuse microscopic damage throughout the brain.

The patient is unconscious and full supportive treatment is given while awaiting improvement.

If the patient has a brainstem injury he or she is comatose and may have a decerebrate or decorticate posture. There is associated autonomic dysfunction, with a high fever, hypertension and sweating.

If the patient is unconscious, there is a 5–10% chance that he or she has a cervical spine injury.

LIMB INJURIES

Clinical presentation

Limb injuries are very common. The bones may be fractured and joints dislocated. The injury may be compound, which increases the risk of infection. There may be associated neurological or vascular injury (Fig. 36.7).

Management

Assessment includes examination to check the pulses and detect any neurological or functional deficit and any soft tissue injuries.

Any dislocation is reduced, fractures are immobilized and soft tissue injuries are debrided. If there is a vascular injury, it is important to get proximal and distal control of the bleeding vessel. If the injury is significant then surgical exploration and repair may be necessary.

Fig. 36.7 Signs of vascular injury

haemorrhage
expanding haematoma
abnormal or absent pulses
impaired distal circulation
decreased sensation
increasing pain

Suspect smoke inhalation or thermal injury to the airway if there is:

- Altered consciousness.
- Direct burns to the face.
- Hoarseness/stridor.
- Soot in the nostrils or sputum.
- Drooling of saliva.

BURNS

Management

The assessment of any patient who has burns includes a full history and examination, looking for signs of smoke inhalation or thermal injury, which may cause oedema of the airway and may necessitate intubation. Blood gases should be measured.

The area affected is assessed using the 'rule of nines' (Fig. 36.8) and the thickness of the burns is assessed as:

- First degree or superficial—may be due to a scald and characterized by erythema, blisters and sensitivity to pinprick. This heals with normal skin within 14 days.
- Second degree or partial thickness—caused by scalds, contact or flame burns of thick skin.
- The lesions are pink with white areas that have dull pinprick sensation. These heal within 3–4 weeks, but with poor-quality skin and hypertrophic scars.
- Third degree or full thickness—caused by chemicals, flames, contact burns or scalds. These burns appear dark and leathery and are painless. They can only heal by epithelialization from the edges, and so form contracted scars.

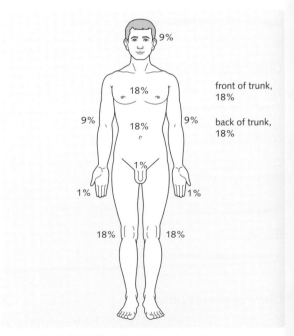

Fig. 36.8 'Rule of nines' for estimating area burned.

The raw surface of a burn loses a large quantity of fluid in the first 24–48 hours, so adequate resuscitation is vital for burns of more than 15% of body surface area (BSA).

The fluid requirement with colloid solution is calculated as:

Volume of fluid required (mL/unit time) = [total percentage of burn × weight (kg)] / 2

for the first four 4-hour periods, and then 6-hourly.

Patients who have burns are closely monitored for pulse, blood pressure and urine output.

Simple wound dressings are sulphadiazine creams or povidone-iodine solution to prevent infection.

Full-thickness burns need early skin grafting.

If the burns are extensive, the patient is catabolic and requires nutritional support and strong analgesia.

The prognosis depends on the extent of the burns, the age of the patient and other medical conditions. There is a 50% mortality rate for patients who have burns covering more than 50% BSA, and those who survive are faced with disabilities and multiple further operations.

Further reading

American Association for the Surgery of Trauma (AAST) http://www.aast.org

American College of Surgeons 1997 *Advanced Trauma and Life Support Program: Abdominal Trauma Course Manual*, 5th edn. American College of Surgeons, Chicago

Anderson ID (ed.) 1999 *Care of the Critically Ill Surgical Patient*. Arnold, London

Driscoll P, Gwinnutt C, LeDuc Jimmerson C, Goodall O 1994 *Trauma Resuscitation: The Team Approach*. Macmillan, London

Harbecht BG 2005 Is anything new in adult blunt splenic trauma? *Am J Surg* 190: 273–278

Hettdziewulski P, Papini R, Dziewulski P, Barret JP 2005 *ABC of Burns*. BMJ Publications, London

NICE Guidelines. *Head Injury*. http://www.nice.orguk

Richardson JD 2005 Changes in the management of injuries to the liver and spleen. *J Am Coll Surg* 200: 648–669

Segelov PM 1990 *Complications of Fractures and Dislocations*. Chapman and Hall, London

Settle JAD 1996 *Principles and Practice of Burns Management*. Churchill Livingstone, Edinburgh

Skinner D, Driscoll P 2006 *ABC of Major Trauma*. BMJ Publishing Group, London

Learning objectives

You should be able to:

- Understand how postoperative complications are classified.
- Know how to investigate a patient with postoperative pyrexia.
- Define oliguria and its significance in the postoperative surgical patient.
- Understand the difference between maintenance fluid management and fluid resuscitation.
- Define hypovolaemic shock.
- Know the symptoms and signs of a pulmonary embolus.
- Understand when wound dehiscence classically occurs.
- Know the important steps in the treatment of septic shock.
- Know the risk factors for the development of DVT and the measures taken to prevent it.
- Understand the modes available for analgesia administration and the use of the analgesic ladder.

For a successful surgical outcome, there are important issues to be addressed in the preoperative, intraoperative and postoperative stages.

The preoperative period is a time of preparation for the upcoming surgery. It often begins with the patient attending a pre-admission clinic and meeting with specialist nursing staff and the anesthetist. Depending on the type of surgery to be undertaken, the patient is given information regarding:

- Temporary cessation of certain drugs, e.g. aspirin or warfarin in advance of the surgery.
- Necessary bowel preparation (before colorectal surgery).
- Methicillin-resistant *Staphylococcus aureus* (MRSA) status of the patient by taking swabs from nose, throat and groin.

It is an opportunity for baseline investigations to be carried out, e.g. blood tests including blood group (group and save), electrocardiogram, chest X-ray. Specialist investigations may also be carried out at this stage (e.g. vocal cord testing to exclude preoperative laryngeal nerve palsy in patients undergoing thyroid or parathyroid surgery). Written consent for the surgery may be taken at this time if not previously done in the outpatient clinic. The patient is again given the opportunity to ask questions about the surgery and the immediate postoperative period. If the patient does not attend a pre-admission clinic all the above is carried out on the ward on the day of the admission.

The postoperative period is very important for monitoring the patient to prevent immediate and long-term complications (Fig. 37.1). After the operation, patients spend some time in the recovery bay, where they are monitored until they are ready to return to the ward or high-dependency unit. Some patients who are seriously ill are transferred directly to the intensive care unit.

All of the patient's vital functions are monitored—airway, heart rate, blood pressure, conscious level, temperature (Fig. 37.2), respiratory rate and depth, oxygen saturation and urine output—and the wound is assessed.

Complications are usually classified as:

- Immediate—within the first 24 hours.
- Early—occurring in the first 2–3 weeks postoperatively.
- Late—occurring at any subsequent period after discharge from hospital.
- General—affecting any of the body systems.
- Local—specific to the operation.

Fig. 37.1 Clinical features and management of postoperative complications

Complication	Time postoperatively	Cause	Signs and symptoms	Management
respiratory depression	<24 h	airway obstruction, GA or excess analgesia	↓RR, ↓ conscious level, cyanosis	clear airway, reverse GA or effect of analgesia
hypovolaemia	<24 h	haemorrhage, inadequate fluid replacement, sepsis	↓BP, ↑HR, ↓ urine output	intravenous fluids—blood or colloids; antibiotics for sepsis
atelectasis	24–48 h	poor analgesia, smoking, previous chest problems	↑temp., ↑RR, ↓O$_2$, ↓AE bases of lungs	analgesia, physiotherapy, nebulizers
respiratory infection	>48 h	poor analgesia, smoking, previous chest problems	↑temp., ↑RR, ↓O$_2$, ↓AE and crepitations; sputum production	analgesia, physiotherapy, nebulizers and antibiotics
deep vein thrombosis (DVT)	5–10 days	operations causing immobility (e.g. pelvic, orthopaedic), oral contraceptive use, malignancy	↑temp., leg swollen, tender calf	Doppler ultrasound or venogram; anticoagulation
pulmonary embolus (PE)	5–10 days	DVT, immobility, no signs of DVT in 50% of cases	present as pleuritic chest pains, multiple small PEs, or massive PE with collapse or death	ECG, V/Q scan, anticoagulation
wound infection	5 days	haematoma, contamination at operation, corticosteroid use, diabetes mellitus, malignancy, jaundice, long-duration operation	↑temp. with red, tender and swollen wound	antibiotics
urinary tract	5 days	immobility, catheterization	↑temp., confusion in elderly, dysuria	antibiotics ± drainage infection
wound dehiscence	5–10 days	poor operative technique, infection, haematoma, corticosteroid use	red serous discharge from wound, protruding intestine	resuscitation, return to theatre to repair wound
paralytic ileus	>4–5 days	normal response, but if occurs after >4–5 days there may be intra-abdominal pathology or ↓K+	NG aspirate, abdominal distension	resuscitation, NG aspiration, correct electrolytes
acute gastric dilatation	2–5 days	vomiting, ↓BP, ↑HR associated with paralytic ileus		NG aspiration
anastomotic dehiscence	5–10 days	poor operative technique, infection, diabetes mellitus, vascular insufficiency	↓BP, ↑temp., ↑HR, peritonitis	resuscitation, laparotomy, antibiotics, lavage, defunction bowel
secondary haemorrhage	7–10 days	infection of suture line	↓BP, ↑HR, bleeding	resuscitation to stop haemorrhage
pseudomembranous colitis		following prolonged antibiotic use, due to Clostridium difficile toxin	diarrhoea, dehydration, abdominal pain	resuscitation, oral vancomycin

AE, air entry; BP, blood pressure; ECG, electrocardiogram; GA, general anaesthetic; HR, heart rate; K$^+$, potassium ions; O$_2$, Oxygen; NG, nasogastric; temp., temperature; RR, respiratory rate; V/Q scan, ventilation/perfusion scan.

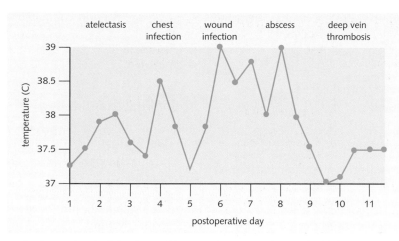

Fig. 37.2 Postoperative temperature chart showing possible causes of a postoperative pyrexia with the average time of onset in days.

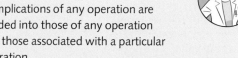

Complications of any operation are divided into those of any operation and those associated with a particular operation.

Certain symptoms and signs commonly present in the postoperative period and when identified and dealt with promptly and correctly prevent deterioration and complications.

POSTOPERATIVE PYREXIA

Many patients become pyrexial in the postoperative period and it is important that the clinician establishes the cause for this and institutes the correct treatment. The likely cause of the pyrexia is dependent not only on the type of operation the patient has had, but also on the time after operation.

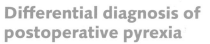

Core temperature is approximately 1û°C higher than axillary temperature.

A low-level pyrexia is common in the hours following surgery. This reflects the trauma of surgery, anaesthetic and the effects of blood transfusion.

Differential diagnosis of postoperative pyrexia

The differential diagnosis of postoperative pyrexia is given in Fig. 37.3.

History to focus on the differential diagnosis of postoperative pyrexia

Operation

It is important to know what operation has been performed. Some infections are more common following large bowel procedures than small bowel or gastric operations.

Fig. 37.3 Differential diagnosis of postoperative pyrexia

Time post-op	Pathology
first 24 hours	trauma response and pre-existing sepsis
24–72 hours	pulmonary atelectasis and chest infection
3–7 days	chest infection, wound infection, pelvic collection or abscess, urinary tract infection, anastomotic dehiscence and wound dehiscence
7–10 days	deep vein thrombosis, pulmonary embolus

223

The site of operation is also important in deciding the likely source of any sepsis, for example:

- Urinary tract infection is likely following a cystoscopy.
- Cholangitis is a risk in a patient who has obstructive jaundice.

Associated symptoms

In order to elicit the patient's symptoms, it is necessary to ask direct questions about the following:

- Shortness of breath, productive cough, pleuritic chest pain—chest infection.
- Pain in wound, discharge—wound infection.
- Abdominal pain (worse on movement or breathing) and distension—intra-abdominal collection.
- Frequency, dysuria, haematuria, offensive urine—urinary tract infection.
- Calf pain, swelling of leg—deep vein thrombosis (DVT).

Examination of patients who have postoperative pyrexia

Each system should be thoroughly examined and temperature, pulse, blood pressure and urine output should be noted.

> Features of septicaemia are rigors, high temperature, tachycardia, hypotension and warm peripheries.

Respiratory system

On examination, the respiratory rate, oxygen saturation and use of accessory muscles should be noted. The chest is examined systematically for signs of atelectasis, infection or effusion.

Wound

The wound should be inspected for signs of infection, including:

- Erythema—cellulitis.
- Swelling.

- Higher temperature compared with surrounding skin.
- Fluctuance.
- Discharge.

Abdominal examination

Following abdominal operations signs of deep infection include:

- Swinging pyrexia (Fig. 37.2)—suggesting abscess formation.
- Tenderness away from the scar.
- Peritonism—indicating local inflammation.
- Palpable swelling—due to a large collection, or more frequently an inflammatory mass.
- Abdominal distension and absent bowel sounds—prolonged ileus.
- Abdominal rigidity suggestive of generalized peritonitis may be due to anastomotic dehiscence.

Rectal examination should be performed. A pelvic abscess may be palpable as a boggy swelling through the rectal wall.

Legs

A DVT should be suspected if the following are present:

- Unilateral swelling of the leg.
- Increased temperature of the swollen leg compared with the other.
- Firm tender calf.

Clinical examination is, however, unreliable and further investigation should be performed (see below).

Investigation of patients who have postoperative pyrexia

An algorithm for the investigation and diagnosis of postoperative pyrexia is given in Fig. 37.4.

Blood tests

Full blood count

This may show a high white cell count, suggesting an infective cause. However, trauma of any kind (e.g. accident or surgical insult) can lead to a raised white cell count. Overwhelming sepsis may cause a low white cell count.

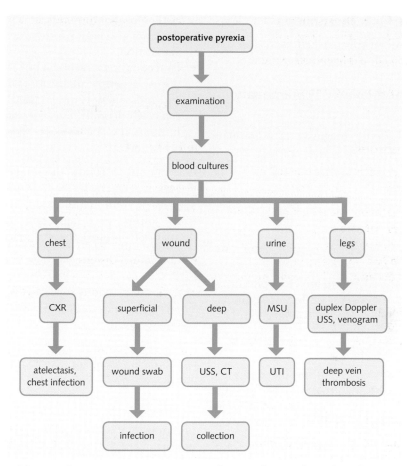

Fig. 37.4 Investigation and diagnosis of postoperative pyrexia. (CT, computed tomography; CXR, chest radiography; MSU, midstream urine; USS, ultrasound scan; UTI, urinary tract infection.)

Blood cultures

These should be requested for any pyrexial patient. The results will not be available until 48 hours later, but these can guide clinicians on the choice of antibiotics as well as give clues to the likely source of sepsis.

All culture specimens should be taken before starting antibiotics.

Chest radiography

This may show signs of:

- Collapse.
- Consolidation.
- Pleural effusion.
- Large pulmonary emboli—may show up as more lucent areas of lung (usually wedge shaped).

Electrocardiography

This is usually normal (except perhaps for a tachycardia) if there are small pulmonary emboli. If there is a large pulmonary embolus, the electrocardiogram may show the following classic features:

- Tall peaked P wave in lead II—due to right atrial dilatation.
- Right axis deviation—due to right ventricular dilatation and hypertrophy.
- S1, Q3, T3 pattern—a deep S wave in lead I and Q wave and inverted T wave in lead III associated with right ventricular strain.

Arterial blood gases

In a severe chest infection, there may be a low pO_2 and high pCO_2. Pulmonary embolism usually results in a normal pO_2 and a low pCO_2 due to hyperventilation.

225

Ventilation/perfusion scanning

This is used to reveal mismatched perfusion and ventilation defects to identify pulmonary emboli.

Computed tomography (CT) pulmonary angiography

This is also used for the diagnosis of pulmonary embolus.

Midstream urine

Urine should be sent for microscopy and culture to elucidate any infection.

Ultrasonography

An ultrasound scan is useful to look for collections, either superficial or deep. Collections can be visualized and drained under ultrasound control.

Computed tomography

Small interloop abscesses within the abdomen are often not visible on ultrasound because the gas- and fluid-filled bowel loops obscure the view. CT is useful for visualizing these collections and particularly those in the retroperitoneal area of the abdominal cavity.

POSTOPERATIVE PAIN

It is very important to make sure that patients are free from pain postoperatively so that they can avoid some of the complications associated with immobility, such as:

- Respiratory infection.
- DVT.
- Pressure sores.
- Urinary retention.

Patients who have been warned and prepared preoperatively for the postoperative period have reduced postoperative anxiety and analgesic needs. The strength of the analgesia and its mode of administration depend on the type of operation:

- Major abdominal or thoracic operations require opiates, which can be given continuously intravenously or using a patient-controlled analgesia (PCA) system. Alternative routes are epidural or intramuscular injections, but the latter give poor control due to erratic absorption.
- Pain of minor surgery can be controlled by the use of simple analgesics or non-steroidal anti-inflammatory drugs (NSAIDs), which can be given orally or rectally. Nerve blocks or infiltration of the wound with local anaesthetic are beneficial.

It is helpful to follow the analgesic ladder when prescribing. Changing from simple to opioid-based analgesics, combination regimens, and converting from short- to long-acting preparations can dramatically improve the analgesic effects.

Good postoperative analgesia:
- Improves respiratory function.
- Reduces cardiac demands.
- Reduces the risk of DVT (patients mobilize earlier).

Increasing postoperative pain or pain that is unremitting despite escalation of analgesia should raise concern. In the case of increasing abdominal pain, peritonitis should be excluded. This could be due to postoperative bleeding; another example is biliary peritonitis from a bile leak after a cholecystectomy. Severe calf pain after vascular surgery such as a femorodistal bypass may be indicative of compartment syndrome. Some vascular surgeons perform routine fasciotomies for this reason.

POSTOPERATIVE OLIGURIA

Oliguria or reduced urine output is defined as a urine output of less than 0.5 mL/kg/hour. It is a problem junior doctors are commonly asked to address in the postoperative patient. It may be a sign of acute renal failure or shock and the causes of these conditions must be excluded. Other causes must be excluded, such as a blocked catheter. It is more commonly a sign of inadequate fluid replacement following surgery and may be corrected by starting or speeding up intravenous fluid resusciatation. A fluid challenge can be useful in confirming the response of the patient and carefully monitoring for the development of pulmonary oedema before starting fluid replacement therapy. During a fluid challenge, a bolus of fluid is given rapidly over a short period of time (e.g. 200 mL over 15–30 minutes).

Postoperative fluid requirements depend on the type of operation performed and whether it is a maintenance or a replacement fluid regimen.

Normal homoeostasis is maintained with 2–3 litres/24 hours of crystalloid fluid, depending on the age and weight of the patient and insensible losses.

Adequate fluid replacement is monitored by checking:

- Heart rate.
- Blood pressure.
- Urine output (which should be at least 0.5 mL/kg/hour).

If the patient is very unwell and has cardiovascular impairment it may be helpful to insert a central venous pressure (CVP) line to monitor fluid replacement.

Maintenance requirements for 24 hours is 1 litre of normal saline and 2 litres of 5% dextrose solution.

Potassium supplements are not necessary for 48 hours because antidiuretic hormone is secreted initially and there is retention of sodium and potassium. Subsequently at least 60 mmol of potassium chloride every 24 hours are necessary if the patient is on a minimal oral intake. If there are excess losses as a result of vomiting, fistula or diarrhoea, the requirements are increased.

If there has been blood loss, it should be replaced. If the patient is actively bleeding, colloid solutions can be used until blood is available. This stays in the circulation and draws extracellular fluid into the circulation by osmotic pressure so it is better than a crystalloid solution for maintaining blood pressure.

Colloid fluids are more effective than crystalloid fluids in maintaining blood pressure.

The blood pressure may be normal in the presence of significant loss of circulating volume.

SHOCK

Background

Shock is defined as an inability to maintain adequate tissue perfusion and oxygenation. It may be:

- Hypovolaemic—inadequate circulatory volume due to haemorrhage or plasma losses or extracellular fluid depletion.
- Cardiogenic—the heart is unable to maintain cardiac output because of infarction or arrhythmia.
- Septicaemic—the presence of bacterial endotoxins causes peripheral vasodilatation and capillary permeability so the circulatory capacity is increased, but fluid leaks from the circulation.
- Anaphylactic—reaction to an antigen and as a result vasoactive substances cause vasodilatation and capillary permeability.

Clinical presentation

Clinical features of shock are:

- Weak, rapid pulse.
- Hypotension.
- Hypoxia.
- Confusion.
- Decreased urine output.

In the initial stages of septic shock, the peripheries may be warm and the patient may have a bounding pulse resulting from a hyperdynamic circulation.

All the above individually are common reasons for a junior doctor to be called to review a postoperative patient. Early identification of the features of shock ensures rapid treatment and therefore prevention of further deterioration or complications.

Whatever the original cause, the patient needs intensive monitoring and treatment to improve tissue perfusion and oxygenation to prevent further complications.

The main treatments are:

- Oxygenation.
- Fluid replacement.
- Treatment of sepsis or other cause.
- Control of arrhythmias.
- Use of inotropes to improve cardiac and renal function.

Complications of shock

Shock may precipitate acute respiratory distress syndrome (ARDS), acute renal failure, disseminated intravascular coagulation (DIC), acute hepatic failure and stress ulceration. Patients may then develop systemic inflammatory response syndrome (SIRS), which may progress to multiorgan failure (MOF).

Each organ that is failing carries a mortality rate of 30%.

Acute respiratory distress syndrome

This is often precipitated by trauma, chest injury, sepsis and pancreatitis. As part of sepsis, toxins damage the endothelium of the lung capillaries—the lungs become oedematous and fibrin and microaggregates collect in the interstitial spaces, so gas transfer is affected and the oxygen saturation decreases. A chest radiograph shows diffuse pulmonary infiltrates. Treatment is ventilation and supportive measures.

Acute renal failure

This is usually secondary to hypovolaemia or sepsis, which cause acute tubular necrosis (ATN). The urine output is less than 20 mL/hour and the urea and potassium then start to increase.

The patient is dialysed until the kidney recovers, which should take 1–3 weeks if the acute renal failure is due to ATN. This is evident by a diuretic phase and the production of unconcentrated urine.

Disseminated intravascular coagulation

In sepsis, the clotting factors are activated, so widespread intravascular clotting occurs and then spontaneous haemorrhage. The diagnosis is confirmed by the presence of high levels of fibrin degradation products (FDPs).

Treatment of disseminated intravascular coagulation is with intravenous heparin to prevent clotting, and normal clotting factors are given.

ANTICOAGULATION

Surgical operations predispose to DVT because, postoperatively, the clotting factors and the number and stickiness of the platelets increase. During the operation, the limbs are immobilized and the muscle pump does not function, so there is stasis in the veins.

Risk factors for the development of DVT are:

- Age—over 40 years old.
- Oral contraceptive use.
- Obesity.
- Diabetes mellitus.
- Polycythaemia.
- Varicose veins.

An increased risk for developing DVT is associated with:

- Operations for malignancy.
- Pelvic operations.
- Orthopaedic operations on the lower limbs.

Prevention of DVT is by use of thromboembolic compression stockings, administration of subcutaneous low molecular weight heparin and use of pneumatic calf compression intraoperatively.

Patients may also be on anticoagulants preoperatively. Warfarin has a long half-life and takes several days to be cleared from the body and several days to reach a therapeutic level once restarted. A patient on warfarin for a metallic heart valve, for example, who is having an elective hernia repair will have had to stop taking warfarin a few days days prior to the operation to avoid intraoperative bleeding. However, the patient will require earlier admission for daily international normalized ratio (INR) blood levels. Once the INR drops to below what is acceptable for metalic heart valve prophylaxis the patient will require an intravenous heparin infusion. Heparin has a short half-life. The infusion is stopped a few hours before going to theatre and restarted a few hours after. Warfarin can be restarted once the patient is over the immediate postoperative period. Warfarin may take several days before an adequate INR level is achieved. The patient is started on their preoperative dose of warfarin. Further dosing will depend on the INR levels, and only when the appropriate INR level is reached is the heparin infusion discontinued. Reaching the target INR will take longer without the loading doses but it is a safer way, especially in the elderly and in patients on medication that affects the INR. The same warfarin loading regimen and heparin cover is applied in treatment of a DVT, with the heparin being low molecular weight heparin given as a subcutaneous injection rather than a continuous infusion. Patients who are on warfarin for AF or recurrent DVTs should stop warfarin, but do not need intravenous heparin perioperatively. They are prescribed subcutaneous low molecular weight heparin, as for prophylaxis.

EVIDENCE-BASED ANTIBIOTIC THERAPY

Prophylactic antibiotics

Prophylactic antibiotics are used to prevent infection from contamination of a wound. They should not be given to prevent other postoperative infections (e.g. chest infection). The risk of infection depends on the operation performed.

Wounds are defined as:

- Clean—the mucosal surfaces are not breached and there is no local infection.
- Potentially contaminated—the mucosal surfaces are breached and exposed (e.g. elective gastrointestinal operation).
- Contaminated—there is established local infection or tissue soiling (e.g. peritonitis).

The choice of antibiotic depends on the likely pathogens that occur at various sites. Antibiotics should be given intravenously at induction of anaesthesia to facilitate high concentrations in the operation site at the time when contamination occurs. A number of well-controlled trials have advised single-dose prophylaxis over multiple doses. However, if an operation is prolonged then an additional dose is advised to maintain a sufficiently high concentration. Patients requiring prophylactic antibiotics are those who have:

- Potentially contaminated operations or instrumentation of an infected site (e.g. endoscopic retrograde cholangiopancreatography for bile duct stones).

- Damaged or prosthetic heart valves or who have a prosthesis (e.g. hip prosthesis).

Prophylactic antibiotics should be given if any prosthesis is present or is to be inserted. hip, valve.

Antibiotic selection

Most hospitals have antibiotic protocols in place to guide the surgeon. When choosing an antibiotic, consider the most likely organisms to be encountered and local resistance patterns.

Postoperative antibiotics

As with prophylactic antibiotics, postoperative antibiotics should be aimed against the most likely causative organism (empirical treatment) or based on microbiology results (e.g. blood cultures). In general, surgeons treat with antibiotics longer than is necessary, as there is difficulty in distinguishing between contamination, infection and inflammation. An expert forum has recently addressed this issue and has produced guidelines, which are summarized in Fig. 37.5.

Antibiotics, and particularly intravenous antibiotics, account for a sizeable proportion of a hospital's pharmacy budget. Excessive antibiotic use results in superinfections and antibiotic resistance (e.g. MRSA).

Fig. 37.5 Guidelines for the duration of antibiotic therapy following surgery

contamination	prophylactic antibiotics only
removable infection	prophylactic antibiotics + 24 h of intravenous antibiotics
mild infection	prophylactic antibiotics + 48 h of intravenous antibiotics
moderate infection	prophylactic antibiotics + up to <5 days of intravenous antibiotics
severe infection	prophylactic antibiotics + ≥5 days of intravenous antibiotics

Excessive antibiotic use is unnecessary, expensive, and results in superinfections and antibiotic resistance.

Following surgery, a patient should be carefully monitored for signs of ongoing infection, including:

- Pyrexia.
- Tachycardia.
- Rising white cell count/C-reactive protein (WCC/CRP).

If ongoing infection is suspected blood cultures should be taken and intravenous broad-spectrum antibiotics given.

Other important factors to consider before prescribing antibiotics are:

- Age—some antibiotics are contraindicated in children.
- Renal and hepatic function—many antibiotics are metabolized or excreted by the liver and kidneys.
- Pregnancy—most antibiotics are contraindicated in pregnancy.
- Prosthetic material—infections related to prosthetic material rarely respond to antibiotics.
- Allergies.

POSTOPERATIVE NUTRITION

Many patients undergoing gastrointestinal operations are malnourished preoperatively and have an increased risk of postoperative morbidity and death because of:

- Decreased resistance to infection.
- Impaired wound healing.

A history of recent weight loss is suggestive of malnutrition. Malnutrition can be assessed by body mass index [BMI = weight (kg)/height^2 (m^2)]; other anthropometric measures include mid-arm muscle circumference and triceps skin-fold thickness. Preoperative feeding may be of benefit to selected patients.

If patients are malnourished or experience complications of the operation so they cannot resume eating within a few days they should be fed. It is better to feed enterally because the integrity of the gut mucosal barrier and secretion of gut hormones and enzymes are maintained. The feed is given via a fine-bore nasogastric tube or gastrostomy or jejunostomy tube. If gastrointestinal function is satisfactory the feed can be a complete polymeric feed but, if the digestive enzymes are inadequate, an elemental feed is given.

Enteral nutrition is cheaper and safer than parenteral nutrition.

Total parenteral nutrition (TPN) should be given via a CVP line to some patients who have a short gut, pancreatitis or a high-output fistula. Possible complications are:

- Vascular damage.
- Haemopericardium.
- Haemopneumothorax.
- Thrombosis.
- Line sepsis.

The nutritional effects need to be closely monitored.

Prolonged TPN feeding can affect the liver, bones and immune system.

POSTOPERATIVE DRAINS

It is very common for a patient to return to the ward following surgery attached to a variety of lines, drains and tubes. These are invariably a cause of anxiety for the patient and require careful monitoring by the staff. The first step in their management is being clear about what they are and what their output should be if any. Reading the operative note is crucial. It helps distinguish intra-abdominal drains from feeding tubes and tells where each tube is lying and therefore what its function should be. Their output should be carefully documented daily. The volume and nature of the effluent is important. For example, small amounts of haemoserous effluent coming from a drain placed in the gallbladder bed after a laparoscopic cholecystectomy is normal. The same amount of bile-stained fluid from the same drain is indicative of a bile leak and will need further investigation and treatment. The volume of all fluids lost daily should be considered when calculating the fluid balance.

Further reading

Bagshaw SM, Bellomo R 2007 Acute renal failure-critical illness and intensive care. *Surgery* **25**: 391–398

Chan O (ed.) 2007 *ABC of Emergency Radiology*. BMJ Publications, London

Coakes J, Schuster-Bruce MJL 2007 Gastrointestinal dysfunction-critical illness and intensive care. *Surgery* **25**: 388–390

Colquhoun MC, Handley AJ, Evans TR (eds) 2003 *ABC of Resuscitation*. BMJ Publications, London

Hari MS, Mackenzie IMJ 2007 Respiratory failure – critical illness and intensive care. *Surgery* **25**: 380–387

NICE Guidelines. 2003 *Preoperative Tests*. http://www.nice.org uk.

NICE Guidelines. 2007 *Recognition of Response to Acute Illness in Adults in Hospital*. http://www.nice.org uk.

NICE Guidelines. 2007 *Venous Thromboembolism (Surgical)*. http://www.nice.org uk.

Paterson-Brown S 1997 *Emergency Surgery and Critical Care*. WB Saunders, London

Ridley S 2005 The recognition and early management of critical illness. *Ann Roy Coll Surg Engl* **87**: 315–322.

Robarts WM, Parkin JV, Hobsley M 1979 A simple clinical approach to quantifying losses from the extracellular and plasma compartments. *Ann Roy Coll Surg Engl* **61**: 142–145

Skinner D, Driscoll P 2006 *ABC of Major Trauma*. BMJ Publications, London

Truswell AS 2003 *ABC of Nutrition*. BMJ Publications, London

Weed HG 2003 Antimicrobial prophylaxis in the surgical patient. *Med Clin North Am* **87**: 59-75

Principles of cancer management

Learning objectives

You should be able to:

- Describe the general features of advanced malignancy.
- List the necessary factors for an effective screening programme.
- Understand the histological occurrence that takes place before a cancer can spread.
- Understand why cancers are staged.
- Name three complications of radiotherapy.
- Understand the aims of palliative care.

Cancer accounts for 1 in 4 deaths in the UK. It is the uncontrolled proliferation of abnormal cells. Tumour cells dedifferentiate so they become less like the parent cells and their growth is no longer inhibited by contact with neighbouring cells, but they have the capacity to invade and destroy adjacent normal structures—the lymphatic and venous channels.

Tumour size depends on the cell cycle time, growth fraction and the number of cells lost from the tumour surface. For a tumour to be palpable, there are at least 109 cells, and in most cases more.

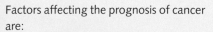

Factors affecting the prognosis of cancer are:

- Histological type.
- Size of tumour.
- Stage at presentation.
- Age of patient.
- Treatment available.

A simple classification of tumours is benign or malignant, primary or secondary.

Background

Most cancers are idiopathic, but there are some direct causal relationships:

- Smoking and lung cancer.
- Chemical exposure in the dye industry and bladder cancer.
- Ultraviolet radiation and skin cancer.
- Genetic abnormality resulting in familial polyposis coli and colon cancer.

Clinical presentation

There are several presentations of malignant disease:

- Specific symptom related to a localized cancer (e.g. breast cancer, skin cancer).
- Symptoms caused by the primary cancer (e.g. haemoptysis and lung cancer or rectal bleeding and rectal cancer).
- Systemic symptoms caused by the cancer (e.g. anaemia due to gastric cancer).
- Systemic symptoms related to ectopic hormone production (e.g. ectopic adrenocorticotrophic hormone production).
- Symptoms of metastatic disease (e.g. jaundice from liver secondaries or bone pain from bone metastases).

General features of advanced malignancy include malaise and weight loss, but it is hoped that most patients present before these systemic signs develop, when the cancer is more likely to be treatable and curable.

Other syndromes related to malignancy are:

- Ectopic antidiuretic hormone secretion causing hyponatraemia.
- Neurological syndromes.
- Skin lesions such as dermatomyositis and acanthosis nigricans.

233

SCREENING FOR CANCER

...is the process of investigating an asymptomatic population that is at risk of a disease. The aim is to reduce the mortality rate from the disease. For screening to be effective, the disease must have:

- A high population incidence.
- A detectable presymptomatic stage.

The test needs to be acceptable, cheap, reproducible, sensitive and specific to the disease. Once detected, there should be treatment available. For screening to be cost-effective, there should be high compliance by the population at risk.

In the UK, there are national screening programmes for breast cancer, cervical cancer, and bowel cancer. Recommended regimens for screening are:

- Breast cancer—50–70-year-old women—3-yearly bilateral mammograms.
- Cervical cancer—20–64-year-old women—5-yearly cervical smears.
- Bowel cancer—60–69-year-old men and women—2-yearly fecal occult blood testing with colonoscopy follow-up if abnormal.

Screening for early gastric cancer by barium meal and gastroscopy is carried out in Japan.

Spread of cancer

Invasive cancer means that the basement membrane has been breached and that the tumour is capable of spreading into the adjacent tissues, especially the lymphatics and venous channels, so the cells can be transported to other fertile sites to form a secondary metastasis. The cells adhere to the vascular endothelium and the basement membrane is digested by the release of enzymes such as collagenase, which facilitates invasion of the tissue parenchyma. Fig. 38.1 shows the routes of cancer spread

Epithelial cancers spread via the lymphatics and bloodstream, sarcomas spread via the bloodstream.

Complications of malignancy may be local, metastatic or systemic (including paraneoplastic syndromes).

STAGING OF CANCER

The extent and degree of malignancy of a tumour are defined clinically and pathologically. This helps to plan treatment and gives an indication of the prognosis.

Pathological staging is based on the TNM classification (i.e. the extent of the tumour, nodes and metastases).

Further tests such as blood tests for tumour markers and imaging by chest radiograph, computed tomography (CT) scan and bone scan may be required to assess the patient.

Histological grading refers to:

- Degree of differentiation of the tumour.
- Degree of nuclear polymorphism.
- Mitotic rate.

Treatment depends on the stage of the disease.

There is often a multidisciplinary approach, which uses a combination of surgery, chemotherapy, radiotherapy or hormonal treatment. Different forms of treatment may be appropriate at different time periods of the disease (e.g. mastectomy for breast cancer and radiotherapy 10 years later for a bone secondary).

Grading quantifies the aggressiveness of a cancer. Staging quantifies the extent of a cancer. Staging is of greater clinical value.

OPERATIONS FOR MALIGNANT DISEASE

Operations may be required at different times in the disease process. The main types of operation are:

- Diagnostic biopsies—for example, lymph node biopsy to diagnose lymphoma.
- Primary excision—excision of the primary lesion with a margin of normal tissue in the longitudinal and lateral directions. This is usually combined with excision of the blood supply and the associated lymphatic drainage and nodes.

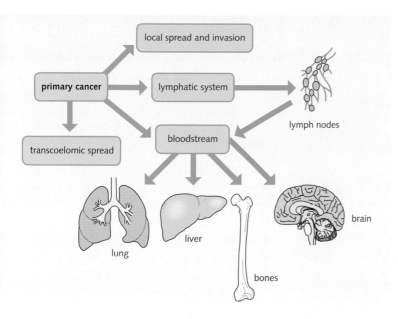

Fig. 38.1 Routes of cancer spread.

- Palliative surgery—it may not be possible to excise the primary tumour because of its invasion into vital structures, but surgery may be performed to relieve symptoms (e.g. gastroenterostomy for antral gastric cancer or defunctioning colostomy for inoperable rectal cancer). Surgical excision may be appropriate even if metastases are present (e.g. mastectomy for a fungating breast cancer).
- Reconstructive surgery—after radical resection of some tumours, the defect may need a reconstructive operation (e.g. pectoralis major flap after a head and neck operation, or a transverse rectus abdominis myocutaneous flap for breast reconstruction).

General surgery has now become subspecialized in an attempt to improve the outcomes of patients with cancer.

RADIOTHERAPY FOR MALIGNANT DISEASE

Tissues vary in their sensitivity to radiotherapy; for example, squamous cell carcinomas are more sensitive than adenocarcinomas. There are several indications for the use of radiotherapy:

- Primary treatment—for some skin cancers, carcinoma of the larynx or squamous cell carcinoma of the oesophagus.
- Preoperative—to reduce the tumour mass.
- Postoperative adjuvant treatment after excision of primary tumour—to decrease the chance of local recurrence.
- Palliative—for bone metastases, superior vena caval obstruction or spinal cord compression.
- Systemic treatment—whole body irradiation of leukaemic patients having a bone marrow transplant.

Mechanism of action of radiotherapy

External beam radiotherapy from a linear accelerator produces high-energy X-rays that interact with the molecules of the body tissues leading to ionization and the release of high-energy electrons, which cause secondary damage to adjacent molecules, including DNA, via oxygen-dependent reactions. Large tumours are therefore more difficult to treat because hypoxic areas are more resistant to radiotherapy.

Some of the DNA damage cannot be repaired, resulting in chromosomal abnormalities that prevent normal mitosis of cells, so they die when they try to divide. Tumour cells are no more sensitive than normal cells to DNA damage, but are less able to repair it.

The dose is fractionated to allow normal cells time to recover. Before radiotherapy is carried out there is careful planning of the fields so that the maximum dose is given to the smallest volume of tissue.

The aim of radiotherapy is to deliver a measured dose of radiation to a tumour with minimal damage to the surrounding normal tissues.

Complications of radiotherapy

These are usually due to the effect of radiotherapy on normal tissues. The sensitivity to damage and its expression depends on the differing proliferation characteristics of each tissue. Early effects on different tissues include the following:

- Skin—desquamation.
- Mucosa of upper gastrointestinal tract—mucositis, oesophagitis.
- Intestine—vomiting, diarrhoea, ulceration, bleeding.
- Bladder—cystitis.

Tissues affected by late effects of radiotherapy include:

- Gonads—infertility.
- Thyroid gland—hypothyroidism.
- Bowel—strictures due to impaired vascularity and fibrosis.
- Heart—ischaemic heart disease.
- Lymphatics—lymphoedema.

Recently, brachytherapy has been introduced.

This involves the placement of a radioactive source (seeds, needles, wire implants) into a body cavity or tissue to deliver radiation over short distances.

CHEMOTHERAPY FOR MALIGNANT DISEASE

The aim of chemotherapy is to selectively destroy malignant cells while sparing the normal cells, but the drugs interfere with the cell division of both normal and abnormal cells. The rate of proliferation of tumour cells varies in the tumour's lifetime:

- In the early stages of tumour growth, the growth fraction is high.
- As the tumour enlarges, the growth fraction is low as the growth rate slows.

Chemotherapy is therefore less effective for larger tumours. The chemotherapy kills a constant fraction of the cells, not a constant number.

There are four groups of chemotherapeutic agents:

- Alkylating agents.
- Antimetabolites.
- Vinca alkaloids.
- Antimitotic antibiotics.

There are many different drugs and treatment schedules for different tumour types and the side-effect profiles are variable.

Most cytotoxic chemotherapies are administered intravenously as a bolus or short infusion.

Role of chemotherapy

The role of chemotherapy differs from case to case and may be:

- Curative—it is the main form of treatment for lymphomas and leukaemias.
- Adjuvant—as an extra treatment for micrometastases after the main tumour has been surgically excised (e.g. breast cancer).
- Neoadjuvant or preoperative—to reduce the tumour mass before operation.
- Palliative—to delay progression and control symptoms of metastatic disease.

Complications of chemotherapy

The main complications of chemotherapy are:

- Metallic taste for 2–3 days.
- Bone marrow toxicity—causing anaemia, thrombocytopenia, decreased white cell count and increased risk of infection.
- Mucositis.
- Nausea and vomiting—because of the effect on the chemoreceptor trigger zone. The introduction of the 5-HT$_3$ antagonist ondansetron in combination with dexamethasone has dramatically improved the quality of life of patients undergoing chemotherapy.
- Diarrhoea—because of the effects on the rapidly dividing cells of the gastrointestinal tract.
- Alopecia—occurs after 18–21 days with some drugs. Alopecia is reduced by the use of 'cold caps' (i.e. gel-filled hats that are chilled in the freezer) which reduce blood-flow to the scalp.

HORMONAL THERAPY FOR MALIGNANT DISEASE

Some tumours are hormone sensitive and therefore drugs that alter the hormone balance are effective as primary treatment or adjuvant treatment (e.g. the ovaries can be suppressed by luteinizing hormone-releasing hormone (LHRH) agonists—to treat breast cancer).

PALLIATIVE CARE

Many patients who have cancer reach a stage where cure is not possible and the aim of treatment is relief of symptoms to improve the quality of remaining life so that it is as comfortable and as meaningful as possible. The approach focuses on the whole patient and his or her family, who are all coping with a mixture of emotions—anxiety, denial, anger, despair, depression and fear.

Palliative care is a multidisciplinary team approach to provide psychological support and symptomatic control for the patient. Patients' main fears are uncontrollable pain and death. It is very important that communication is good and honest and that there are realistic targets and expectations at this difficult time.

Further reading

Austoker J 1994 Screening for cervical cancer. *BMJ* **309**: 1241–1248

Austoker J 1994 Screening for ovarian, prostatic and testicular cancers. *BMJ* **309**: 315–320

Beahrs OH 1991 Staging of cancer. *CA Cancer J Clin* **41**: 121–125

Casciato DA, Lowitz BB 2000 *Manual of Clinical Oncology*, 4th edn. Little Brown, Boston

Elmore JG, Armstrong K, Lehman CD, Fletcher SW 2005 Screening for breast cancer. *JAMA* **293**: 1245–1256

Fallon M (ed) 2006 *ABC of Palliative Care*. BMJ Publications, London

Horwich A 1995 *Oncology: A Multidisciplinary Textbook*. Chapman & Hall, London

Jatoi I, Anderson H 2005 Cancer screening. *Curr Probl Surg* **42**: 620–682

Langenhoff BS, Krabbe PFM, Wobbes T, Ruers TJM 2001 Quality of life as an outcome measure in surgical oncology. *Br J Surg* **88**: 643–652

McArdle CS 1990 *Surgical Oncology: Current Concepts and Practice*. Butterworths, London

NICE Guidelines 2005 *Referral for Suspected Cancer*. http://www.nice.org.uk

Priestman TJ 1989 *Cancer Chemotherapy: An Introduction*, 3rd edn. Springer, Berlin

Ruoslahti E 1996 How cancer spreads. *Sci Am* **275**: 72–77

Weinberg RA 1996 How cancer arises. *Sci Am* **275**: 62–70

HISTORY, EXAMINATION AND COMMON INVESTIGATIONS

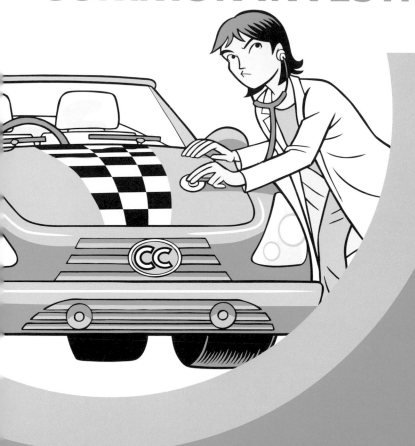

Clerking a surgical patient

Learning objectives

You should be able to:

- Document in a systematic fashion the history taken for any given presenting complaint.
- List the important information that should be included, even if negative, in the systems review.
- Appreciate the importance of accurate and legible documentation of patient details, date, time, place of consultation, responsible consultant, name and contact details of clerking doctor.

Taking an accurate and detailed history from a patient is a critical stage in making the diagnosis and provides vital information. It is important to listen and observe, let the patient tell the story in his or her own words, then use questions to clarify points. It involves acquiring information about the present problems and supplementing this with background information about related symptoms, general health, and past medical history.

Many patients who are referred to surgeons do not need to have an operation, but require the diagnostic skills of surgeons. A surgical operation may not be the first mode of treatment but, if it is contemplated, it is important that the surgeon is aware of the patient's general health and past history, which may influence:

- The type of operation that can be performed.
- The type of anaesthesia.
- The risks associated with the operation.

When clerking a surgical patient, always remember to:

- Introduce yourself to the patient.
- Be polite and try to establish a rapport with the patient to help them feel at ease.
- Maintain eye contact.
- Give the patient time to express his or her thoughts.

Always remember to observe:

- The general surroundings of the patient.
- The general demeanour of the patient—anxious, in pain, comfortable, well, unwell.

Remember that the clerking of a patient is a record of your encounter with the patient and, when you are qualified, it is an important hospital document so it must be accurate, legible and signed.

HISTORY

This should include the following information:

- Patient details—patient's name, age, address, marital status, occupation.
- Date, time and place of consultation (e.g. accident and emergency department, outpatient clinic).

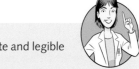

A clerking should be accurate and legible and contain:

- Patient's name and details at the top of every page.
- Date and time.
- The name of the consultant responsible.
- Your name clearly written and signed.
- Your bleep/contact number.

Presenting complaint

This is a brief statement of the reason for consulting the doctor.

History of presenting complaint

After the patient has given a brief summary of the problem, it is important to obtain a more detailed history of the symptoms in a chronological order.

For all the symptoms mentioned, further details are required regarding:

- Duration.
- Progression.
- Frequency.
- Severity.
- Exacerbating and relieving factors.
- Any associated symptoms.

With clinical experience, vital clues from the history allow pattern recognition, so the doctor can then ask more specific questions to aid the diagnostic process.

It is always important to define what the patient means by terms such as diarrhoea, constipation or indigestion because each patient has a different experience.

Past medical history

All previous admissions to hospital, operations, any problems with anaesthesia (e.g. difficult intubation) and any unpleasant experiences (e.g. postoperative vomiting or awareness during a procedure) are documented because this will affect the patient's reaction to future operations. The patient is asked specifically about whether he or she has or has had any of the following conditions:

- Tuberculosis.
- Rheumatic fever.
- Valvular heart disease.
- Myocardial infarction.
- Cerebrovascular accident.
- Diabetes mellitus.
- Jaundice.
- Epilepsy.

Systematic enquiry

Although the patient may present with a very specific problem (e.g. a hernia), it is important to assess all systems because general health and past medical history will influence the need for an operation and the type of operation that is considered appropriate (Fig. 39.1).

Drug history

Ask about current medication and any recent changes of medication. Many patients cannot remember the names and dosages of their medication, so obtain accurate information from general practitioner records, repeat prescriptions or labels on bottles.

Obtain information about allergic reactions and define what the patient means by an allergy—the usual symptoms are rash, oedema and difficulty breathing, but many people mention nausea and diarrhoea or 'thrush' as allergic reactions. Specific drugs that should be noted before an operation include:

- Diuretics—these reduce the potassium level and this may lead to cardiac instability.
- Insulin and diabetic medication.
- Aspirin and anticoagulants—risk of bleeding.
- Asthma medication—inhalers may need to be changed to nebulizers pre- and postoperatively.
- Cardiac medication and antihypertensives—should be continued.
- Anticonvulsants—should be continued.
- Corticosteroids—long-term use results in adrenal suppression and therefore corticosteroid supplements are required to cope with the stress of surgery.

Family history

Questions are asked about any illnesses that appear to occur in the family and the cause of death of first-degree relatives. If a patient presents with a change of bowel habit and has a family history of colon cancer, this obviously causes the patient anxiety and should also concern the doctor.

There may be a family history of anaesthetic problems (e.g. familial deficiency of pseudocholinesterase in which patients cannot metabolize short-acting muscle relaxants given during anaesthesia).

Social history

When a patient is seen in hospital, it is important to remember that this is an abnormal environment where the patient feels vulnerable, so obtain some more information on the patient's normal environment, including:

- Occupation.
- Social circumstances—home, relatives, other people who are affected by the patient's illness.

Fig. 39.1 Systematic enquiry

System	Features to ask about
general	night sweats, pyrexia, jaundice, anorexia, fatigue, weight changes
cardiovascular system	chest pain, angina, exercise tolerance palpitations ankle swelling shortness of breath on exertion or lying flat, paroxysmal nocturnal dyspnoea intermittent claudication
respiratory system	cough, sputum production, haemoptysis wheezing or asthma—frequency of attacks—severity of symptoms shortness of breath, exercise tolerance
gastrointestinal system	indigestion, gastro-oesophageal reflux, dysphagia abdominal pain, vomiting, nausea bowel habit—frequency, change, difficulty rectal bleeding appetite, weight loss
genitourinary system (male)	frequency, nocturia dysuria, haematuria hesitancy, urinary stream, dribbling impotence, libido
genitourinary system (female)	menarche, menopause, pregnancies, contraception menstrual history—length of cycle, date of last menstrual period vaginal discharge dyspareunia
central nervous system	headaches, fits, faints paraesthesia, weakness dizziness, vertigo
musculoskeletal system	muscle aches, pains arthritis, poor mobility, neck stiffness

- If elderly or dependent, are social services involved?
- Financial problems that may be exacerbated by the illness.
- Smoking—average consumption and duration.
- Alcohol—average number of units per week.
- Drug abuse.
- Recent foreign travel.

illnesses. Operative risks are increased in these patients, especially if they have cardiovascular or respiratory disease. Preoperatively, it is therefore important to:

- Accurately diagnose and assess medical conditions.
- Optimize medical conditions before surgery.
- Consider potential drug interactions.

INFLUENCE OF CO-EXISTING DISEASE IN OPERATIVE INTERVENTION

Approximately 50% of patients who have an operation, particularly elderly patients and those undergoing an emergency operation, have concurrent medical

IMPORTANT MEDICAL CONDITIONS

Cardiovascular conditions

The key cardiovascular conditions to consider, together with the major practical points to remember for operative intervention, are:

- Ischaemic heart disease—important to maintain adequate coronary artery perfusion.
- Myocardial infarction—use of a general anaesthetic within 6 months of a myocardial infarction increases the risk of a further myocardial infarction.
- Valvular heart disease—antibiotic prophylaxis is needed to prevent endocarditis.
- Mitral stenosis and atrial fibrillation—anticoagulation may be necessary.
- Severe aortic stenosis—important to maintain adequate blood pressure and coronary artery perfusion.
- Arrhythmias—stabilize preoperatively and maintain medication perioperatively.
- Hypertension—often associated with ischaemic heart disease—if diastolic blood pressure is higher than 110 mmHg it should be stabilized before surgery if possible.
- Congestive cardiac failure—if not controlled preoperatively there is a risk of further deterioration during anaesthesia.
- Pacemaker—take precautions with diathermy during surgery.

If a patient has suffered a myocardial infarction within 3 months, their risk of a further myocardial infarction under anaesthetic is 25%.

Respiratory conditions

The key conditions to consider for the respiratory system, together with the major practical points to remember for operative intervention, are:

- Asthma—optimize the condition preoperatively.
- Chronic obstructive airways disease—if there is chronic sputum production, the patient has an increased risk of respiratory infection because general anaesthesia increases the viscosity of secretions and reduces the action of the cilia. Postoperative pain may inhibit respiratory effort.
- Smoking—increased risk (sixfold) of postoperative problems. It causes mucous hypersecretion, impaired tracheobronchial clearance mechanisms, small airway narrowing and decreased immune function. It also increases carbon monoxide concentration in the blood and decreases oxygen-carrying capacity.

The carbon monoxide has a negative cardiac inotropic effect and this is a risk if the patient has ischaemic heart disease. Stopping smoking 12–24 hours preoperatively has a beneficial effect on the cardiovascular system, but patients need to stop smoking 6 weeks preoperatively to gain any beneficial effect on respiratory function.

Gastrointestinal conditions

The key conditions to consider for the gastrointestinal system, together with the major practical points to remember for operative intervention, are:

- Acid reflux, hiatus hernia, oesophagitis—with these conditions there is a risk of reflux at induction of anaesthesia and a risk of aspiration of gastric contents into lungs. The anaesthetist will prescribe antacids and histamine H_2-receptor antagonists and apply gentle pressure to the cricoid cartilage to prevent stomach contents passing into the lungs at induction before intubation.
- Obesity—this is associated with increased morbidity and mortality rates because of the risk of cardiovascular and respiratory problems, difficult venous access and increased risk of thromboembolic events postoperatively, and because the operation may be technically more difficult.

Endocrine conditions

The key conditions to consider for the endocrine system, together with the major practical points to remember for operative intervention, are as follows.

Diabetes mellitus

Operations result in impaired glucose tolerance with metabolic disturbances. Diabetics are more prone to cardiovascular problems and problems associated with autonomic neuropathy, and have an increased risk of infection.

To avoid prolonged periods of hypoglycaemia, a diabetic patient should be placed at the start of an operating list.

Thyroid disorders

Local problems of a mass in the neck may result in difficult intubation. If the patient is euthyroid preoperatively and has no specific problem normal medication should be maintained.

Adrenal disorders

The problems associated with these disorders are as follows:

- Excess glucocorticoid results in problems due to increased glucose levels, increased blood pressure and electrolyte disturbances.
- Excess mineralocorticoid results in decreased potassium levels, increased sodium levels and hypertension.
- Insufficient mineralocorticoid results in decreased sodium levels and increased potassium levels, and the patient needs intravenous hydrocortisone and close monitoring of cardiovascular status.
- Excess catecholamine causes hypertension and cardiac arrhythmias.

Blood disorders

Disorders to consider together with the major practical points to remember for operative intervention are:

- Anaemia—if chronic and haemoglobin is less than $10\,g/dL$ the patient needs transfusion (at least 48 hours preoperatively if it is to be effective).
- Haemoglobinopathy—if the patient is homozygous for sickle cell anaemia, there is a risk of sickle cell crisis if hypoxia occurs during operation, so the patient is kept hydrated, warm and oxygenated.
- Haemophilia—need to give appropriate clotting factors preoperatively.

Chronic renal failure

Correct electrolytes preoperatively by dialysis. Patients have an increased risk of cardiovascular problems, anaemia, electrolyte disturbances, blood coagulation problems and infection.

Hepatocellular disorders

These include:

- Portal hypertension, ascites, jaundice, abnormal clotting—associated with a perioperative mortality rate of more than 50%.
- Obstructive jaundice—associated with a risk of postoperative renal failure due to endotoxins from gut flora.

Alcohol and drug abuse

Particular aspects to consider include the following:

- Chronic abuse of alcohol and narcotic drugs induces hepatic enzymes so a larger dosage of anaesthetic drugs may be required to be effective.
- Problems of withdrawal due to hospital admission and operation.
- Increased risk of associated human immunodeficiency virus or hepatitis B infection, so take precautions.

Neurological disorders

Disorders to consider, together with the major practical points to remember for operative intervention, are:

- Epilepsy—maintain normal medication.
- Cerebrovascular accident—increased risk of progression or further cerebrovascular accident.

Rheumatoid arthritis

The anaesthetist is concerned with neck movements because of the risk of difficult intubation or subluxation if neck with an unstable atlantoaxial joint is hyperextended—so need cervical spine radiography.

COMMON PRESENTING SYMPTOMS

This section concentrates on common presenting symptoms and some specific details that should be obtained in the history.

'No man's opinions are better than his information' (Paul Getty 1960).

Dysphagia (difficulty in swallowing)

Specific features that should be elicited include:

- Duration of symptoms—acute (i.e. bolus obstruction) or progressive over a few months (implies malignancy).

- Severity of symptoms—is it dry food, semisolids, fluids or even saliva that the patient cannot swallow?
- Where does the blockage seem to be?
- A history of gastro-oesophageal reflex or hiatus hernia—may suggest a benign peptic stricture.
- Association with chest infections—for example aspiration pneumonia.
- Sensation of 'double swallowing'—symptom of pharyngeal pouch.

Vomiting

Vomiting is an active process and involves violent contraction of the abdominal musculature forcibly expelling the gastric contents in a retrograde fashion. It is usually associated with gastrointestinal pathology, but it may be neurogenic, as Ménière's disease, or associated with medication. Features of vomiting are shown in Chapter 3 (Fig. 3.1).

Abdominal pain

If the patient complains of abdominal pain, a detailed history should be obtained regarding onset, site of pain, radiation, character, severity, duration, frequency, aggravating and relieving factors and any associated symptoms (Fig. 39.2). Ask the patient to describe the pain in his or her own words, and they will often use descriptions such as gripping, burning, throbbing or stabbing pain:

- Colicky pain—suggests obstruction of a hollow viscus. It is gripping in nature and fluctuates from peaks of intensity to complete relief. It is always severe and makes the patient restless.

- Somatic pain—severe localized pain due to inflammation of the parietal peritoneum from localized or generalized peritonitis. It is aggravated by movement so the patient lies still.
- Burning pain—signifies mucosal injury or inflammation such as oesophagitis.

The site of the abdominal pain is related to the embryological development of the gut:

- Epigastric pain—foregut (oesophagus, stomach, duodenum).
- Central and periumbilical pain—midgut (duodenum, small intestine, right colon).
- Suprapubic pain—hindgut (mid-transverse colon, left colon, rectum).

The site of abdominal pain is related to the embryological development of the gut.

The nature and sites of different types of abdominal pain are summarized in Fig. 39.2, together with their possible diagnoses.

Change of bowel habit and rectal bleeding

If a patient complains of a change of bowel habit, it is important to define the previous bowel habit (i.e. frequency and consistency of motion and colour).

Fig. 39.2 Nature, site and possible diagnosis of abdominal pain

Nature	Site	Possible diagnosis
burning pain relieved by food	epigastrium	peptic ulceration
burning pain—worse on lying or bending	retrosternal	gastro–oesophageal reflux
severe constant pain relieved by leaning forward	epigastrium	pancreatic disease
increasing intensity	right hypochondrium, scapula	gallbladder disorder
sudden onset, severe, constant	generalized	peritonitis—perforated viscus
intermittent colicky	central and lower abdomen	bowel obstruction
severe colicky pain	loin, groin, scrotum	ureteric colic

Everyone has their own idea of what is 'normal'. Constipation may mean infrequent bowel action or difficulty in evacuation or hard stool. Diarrhoea may mean increased frequency and number of bowel actions or change of consistency.

Associated symptoms are:

- Passage of blood or mucus.
- Tenesmus (i.e. a sensation of incomplete evacuation of the rectum).

If there is rectal bleeding, it is important to know its relationship to defecation (i.e. is the blood mixed with feces, or separate and occurring after defecation). If it is:

- Bright red and fresh, it is probably arising from the anal canal or low rectum.
- Dark red and mixed with the stool, it is coming from the upper rectum or sigmoid colon.

Jaundice

If the presenting complaint is jaundice then associated features are colour of urine and feces and any history of pruritus. Associated symptoms are anorexia, nausea, abdominal pain, weight loss and pyrexia.

Clues to the aetiology may come from a history of gallstones, drug history, a history of foreign travel and contact with infectious illnesses such as hepatitis.

Lump

If the patient complains of a lump then clarify the duration of the history:

- When did the lump appear?
- Is there any change in size or consistency?
- Is there any pain or tenderness or inflammation?
- Are there any associated symptoms, such as bleeding or discharge?

If a hernia is suspected:

- Does the lump disappear spontaneously?
- Are there any precipitating factors, such as chronic cough, constipation, urinary difficulties or history of heavy lifting?
- Has there been any episode of colicky abdominal pain, vomiting and tenderness of the lump that may suggest obstruction?

Breast problems

Breast complaints are usually of a breast lump, breast pain or nipple discharge.

Features of a breast lump are:

- Its relationship to the menstrual cycle—has it changed in size with the cycle?
- Is there any associated discomfort?

Benign lumps often show cyclical variation.

If there is a discharge, its colour and whether it is from a single duct or many ducts are relevant.

If the complaint is of breast pain then its intensity and relationship to the menstrual cycle need to be clarified.

A history of breast problems is not complete unless there is a record of the menstrual history, including:

- Age of menarche.
- Number of pregnancies.
- Age at first pregnancy.
- Use of oral contraceptive or hormone replacement therapy.
- Any family history of breast cancer.

Thyroid disorders

Does the patient have any symptoms of hypo- or hyperthyroidism, such as:

- Weight gain, lethargy, constipation, cold intolerance, dry hair—hypothyroidism.
- Weight loss, anxiety, tremor, palpitations, heat intolerance, diarrhoea—hyperthyroidism.

Are there any symptoms due to compression (e.g. dysphagia, dyspnoea, hoarse voice).

Peripheral vascular disease

If the patient complains of a cramp-like pain in the calf while walking that is relieved by rest, it suggests intermittent claudication (Latin claudicare—to limp). The claudication distance reflects the severity of the symptoms. The pain is due to ischaemia and the accumulation of metabolites such as lactic acid during exertion.

Rest pain is constant severe pain in the legs that is worse at night and often made easier by sleeping in a chair. This implies critical ischaemia and may be exacerbated by infection or ulceration. Associated problems are diabetes mellitus, ischaemic heart disease and cerebrovascular disease. There is usually a history of smoking.

Urinary symptoms

The main symptoms are:

- Dysuria (i.e. painful micturition).
- Frequency—how often the patient micturates.
- Nocturia—micturition at night.
- Urgency—poor control.
- Hesitancy with poor stream and terminal dribbling—suggest outflow obstruction.
- Haematuria—blood in the urine needs to be defined as macroscopic or microscopic.

Questions need to be asked about whether the blood is fresh or altered and whether it occurs:

- At the start of micturition—suggesting that it comes from the urethra.
- Throughout micturition—therefore possibly from the kidney or bladder.
- At the end of micturition—comes from the prostatic bed.

Examination of a surgical patient

Learning objectives

You should be able to understand the principles of :

- General abdominal examination.
- Breast examination.
- Ulcer examination.
- Peripheral vasculature examination.
- Groin and scrotum examination.
- Neck and thyroid examination.
- Trauma patient examination.

Examination of any patient should be conducted in a systematic manner to ensure that nothing is missed. The extent of the 'surgical' examination does vary according to the situation—it is brief in the outpatient clinic for removal of a skin lesion, and more comprehensive if the patient is an emergency admission and has acute abdominal pain.

Examination often focuses on a specific anatomical region but, if operative intervention is contemplated, the cardiovascular, respiratory and central nervous systems should be fully assessed preoperatively.

Before touching the patient, gain an overall assessment of the patient—is the patient anxious, relaxed, in pain, well or unwell?

Remember to ask the patient if they have pain. Hurting the patient is unforgivable.

EXAMINATION OF SPECIFIC SURGICAL CONDITIONS

Examination of an ulcer

An ulcer is defined as an area of discontinuity of the surface epithelium and can occur internally or externally. The basic structure and characteristic shapes of ulcers are shown in Chapter 18, Fig. 18.2.

Certain characteristics of the ulcer provide clues regarding the nature of the ulcer. Any description of the ulcer should include:

- Anatomical site.
- Floor.
- Base and edges.
- Size.
- Shape.
- Surrounding skin.
- Regional lymph nodes.

Examination of a lump or swelling

A lump may be visible on inspection, but may not be evident until palpation. The important features of a lump are:

- Anatomical site and anatomical plane (e.g. intracutaneous, subcutaneous, intramuscular).
- Size—measurements rather than comparison with objects!
- Shape, colour, temperature.
- Tenderness—if there is inflammation.
- Mobility of mass in relationship to skin and deep structures.
- Consistency—soft, hard, firm, rubbery.
- Transillumination—in darkened surroundings, a light is shone through a swelling to see whether it transmits the light and therefore contains fluid.

- Fluctuation—another test for fluid, which is tested in two planes at right-angles.
- Pulsations and thrills—real or transmitted.

An intramuscular mass is less obvious if the muscles are contracted.

GENERAL EXAMINATION OF THE PATIENT

The following should be assessed in the general examination of the patient:

- Height and weight.
- Pulse, blood pressure, temperature.
- State of hydration—skin turgor and elasticity, sunken eyes.
- Anaemia, jaundice, cyanosis.

Common clinical signs and aetiologies

Examination of the hands (Fig. 40.1) and skin (Fig. 40.2) can reveal signs that aid in the diagnosis.

EXAMINATION OF THE BREAST

This requires removal of the clothes to the waist, a warm environment and the presence of a chaperone. Many women will be embarrassed by the examination, so be as sensitive as possible. Examination of the breast also includes examination of regional lymph nodes—axilla and supraclavicular fossa.

Inspection of the breast

Initial inspection is performed with the patient sitting up with hands by the side (Fig. 40.3A). Features to look for are:

- Any asymmetry.
- Distortion.
- Nipple abnormality.

Fig. 40.1 Hand signs and their significance.

Examination of the hands	
Sign	**Diagnostic inference**
clubbing	inflammatory bowel disease, chronic lung disease, congenital heart disease
leukonychia (white patches on nails)	may be normal, liver disease
koilonychia (brittle or spoon-shaped nails)	iron deficiency anaemia
pallor of nail and palmar creases	anaemia
Dupuytren's contracture (thickening and shortening of palmar fascia causing a flexion deformity)	liver disease, epilepsy, idiopathic, familial
palmar erythema	liver disease
nicotine stains	chronic smoker
splinter haemorrhages	vasculitis, infective endocarditis
tremor and sweaty palms	thyrotoxicosis, anxiety
flap	carbon dioxide retention, hepatic encephalopathy
joint deformities	rheumatoid arthritis
Heberden's nodes of terminal interphalangeal joints	osteoarthritis

Fig. 40.2 Skin signs and their significance.

Examination of the skin	
Sign	**Diagnostic inference**
petechiae (red or blue lesions in skin deep to the epidermis)	suggests capillary fragility
spider naevi (central arterial dot from which several dilated vessels radiate)	liver disease
telangiectasia (dilatation of superficial veins)	hereditary, alcoholism, radiotherapy
cutaneous striae	previous pregnancy, weight loss, Cushing's syndrome
purpura, ecchymoses	bleeding abnormality
erythema ab igne	chronic pain
xanthelasma, arcus senilis	hyperlipidaemia
collateral veins	obstruction of normal circulation

- Redness.
- Inflammation.
- Peau d'orange skin.

The patient then lifts her arms above her head, which accentuates any distortion or skin dimpling and allows inspection of the inframammary fold (Fig. 40.3B).

The nipple and areola are inspected for ulceration or inversion, which may be long-standing or of recent onset. Accessory nipples are very common and can occur anywhere from axilla to groin.

Palpation of the breast

The patient then lies flat or semirecumbent with her arms elevated above the head. The 'normal' breast is palpated first. If the patient is premenopausal the best time for examination is 7–10 days after a period when benign nodularity decreases. Palpation is with the flat of the fingers and is performed in a systematic fashion to incorporate all quadrants of the breast, including areola and axillary tail (Fig. 40.4). If any nipple discharge occurs, its colour and whether it originates from a single duct or multiple ducts is noted.

If a breast lump is identified, note its characteristics of:

- Size.
- Shape.
- Position.
- Borders.
- Consistency.
- Skin tethering.

Muscle fixation is tested by asking the patient to contract the pectoralis major muscle and then testing mobility.

Palpation of the axilla

The axilla is palpated when the patient is sitting upright or in a semirecumbent position. The patient's left arm is supported by the examiner's left arm so the muscles are relaxed. The examiner palpates the left axilla with his right hand, and vice versa. Palpation starts at the apex of the axilla, followed by the medial (chest) wall, anterior wall, (pectoral muscles) and posterior wall (subscapularis muscle). Any nodes identified are described by:

- Number.
- Consistency.
- Mobility.

EXAMINATION OF THE NECK

Inspection of neck and thyroid

The neck is inspected from the front to look for any obvious masses such as an enlarged thyroid, lymph nodes or salivary glands.

Dilated superficial veins may imply right ventricular failure or superior vena cava obstruction.

If the swelling is a thyroid gland, it will move on swallowing because it is invested by the pretracheal fascia, which is attached to the hyoid bone.

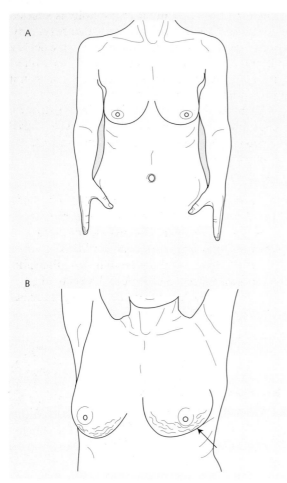

Fig. 40.3 Patient positions for breast examination.
(A) Initial inspection is carried out with the patient sitting up with her hands by her side. (B) The patient is then asked to lift up her arms. This may reveal asymmetry (arrow) due to underlying disease as shown here.

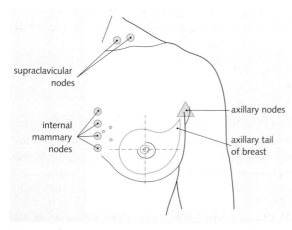

supraclavicular nodes

internal mammary nodes

axillary nodes

axillary tail of breast

Fig. 40.4 Lymphatic drainage of the breast.

The thyroid is bilobed, with the isthmus lying over the second and third tracheal rings. The gland may be uniformly or partially enlarged.

Palpation of neck and thyroid

The thyroid gland is palpated by the examiner standing behind the patient. Palpation may demonstrate a diffusely enlarged gland or a solitary nodule. The consistency of the thyroid is either smooth, multinodular or hard and fixed. The swelling may extend to the superior mediastinum if its inferior margin is impalpable. The trachea may be deviated by a unilateral swelling.

A midline swelling that moves when the tongue is protruded is a thyroglossal cyst.

Auscultation of a thyroid goitre may demonstrate a bruit if it is a hypervascular thyrotoxic goitre. There may be stridor if there is involvement of the recurrent laryngeal nerve or compression of trachea by a large goitre.

Examination of the thyroid is not complete without looking for signs of hypothyroidism or thyrotoxicosis and the eye changes of exophthalmos, lid lag and ophthalmoplegia.

If palpation of the neck reveals enlarged lymph nodes their position and characteristics should be described and all anatomical areas that drain to those nodes should be examined to identify the primary lesion.

When examining a patient's thyroid, a glass of water is necessary to enable the patient to swallow.

EXAMINATION OF THE ABDOMEN

The regions of the abdomen are shown in Fig. 40.5. In a warm environment, the patient lies supine with one pillow. The abdomen is exposed from the xiphisternum to the pubic area.

Inspection of the abdomen

The inspection consists of noting:

- Abdominal wall movement on respiration.
- Scars, striae, ostomies.
- Distension and contour of abdomen.
- Peristalsis and pulsation.

The extent of abdominal wall rigidity is affected by the state of the individual's musculature (elderly, frail patients may have minimal muscle tone despite peritonitis, but younger people have 'board-like' rigidity). Patients taking corticosteroids may not exhibit the classic signs of peritonism.

If there is diffuse peritonism, deep palpation should not be carried out. If there is localized tenderness, the rest of the abdomen should be examined more deeply.

Specific clinical signs include:

- Tenderness over McBurney's point (one-third of the distance between the anterior superior iliac crest and the umbilicus)—suggests localized peritonism associated with appendicitis.
- Murphy's sign—localized tenderness in the right hypochondrium, accentuated while palpating the area during deep inspiration—a sign of acute cholecystitis.

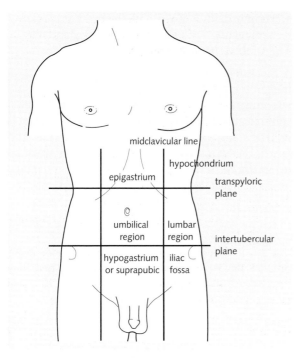

Fig. 40.5 Anatomical regions of the abdomen.

midclavicular line
hypochondrium
epigastrium
transpyloric plane
umbilical region
lumbar region
intertubercular plane
hypogastrium or suprapubic
iliac fossa

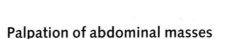

During palpation of the abdomen, watch the patient's facial expression.
Never forget to examine hernial orifices if the patient has an acute abdomen.

- Dilated veins and bruising.
- Erythema ab igne.

Palpation of the abdomen

The examiner should have warm hands! He or she kneels by the bed or raises the bed so that the arm is parallel to the abdomen. Palpation is carried out with the flat of the fingers. Initially, it is light, then deeper, and then the organs and masses are palpated.

Acute abdomen

In the acute situation, the patient will be apprehensive. Palpation starts in an area that is not painful so that there is no voluntary muscle spasm to confuse the picture.

If there is any peritonitis, the peritoneum is inflamed and the overlying muscles become tense due to stimulation of the somatic nerves supplying the abdominal parietes. The pain is made worse by movement or pressure and the act of coughing, or simple percussion over the affected area may produce marked pain—this is diagnostic of peritonitis.

Palpation of abdominal masses

Liver and gallbladder

The lower edge of the liver may be palpable normally. Palpation of the liver starts from the right iliac fossa and proceeds towards the right hypochondrium. The patient breathes in and out as the examiner's hand moves. If a liver edge is found then its characteristics are noted. It may be:

- Smooth.
- Craggy.
- Tender.
- Enlarged (note the degree of enlargement).

A normal gallbladder is not palpable but, if it is distended, it may be a round, smooth swelling palpable at the liver edge in the midclavicular line.

Spleen

The spleen lies beneath the left ninth, tenth and eleventh ribs on the abdomen's posterolateral wall.

It has to be enlarged by 1.5–2 times the normal size before it is palpable. It enlarges medially and inferiorly, so it projects below the costal margin towards the right iliac fossa. There is a notch on its medial aspect. Palpation therefore starts from right iliac fossa and moves towards the left hypochondrium.

Kidneys

Normal kidneys are not palpable, but an enlarged kidney may be palpable as a mass in the loin, which moves on respiration and is ballotable when examined bimanually (i.e. one hand anteriorly and one posteriorly).

The characteristics and anatomical position of any abdominal mass will give vital clues to its aetiology (see Chapter 5, Fig. 5.1).

Percussion of the abdomen

This is useful if the abdomen is distended. A resonant note suggests gaseous distension of a viscus. If the note is resonant centrally and becomes dull in the flanks, there may be fluid present. This can be confirmed by examining the patient when he or she is lying on one side and the dullness then shifts. A fluid thrill may also be present if there is ascites.

Auscultation of the abdomen

The stethoscope is used to listen for bowel sounds, which may be:

- Absent despite listening for 2 minutes—suggests an adynamic ileus.
- Hyperactive—implies increased peristaltic activity.
- High-pitched and tinkling—occur when fluid is moving around in a distended obstructed loop of intestine.

A succussion splash occurs when the stomach is obstructed and full of fluid and it is heard when the patient is moved from side to side.

Bruits may be heard over narrowed arteries.

Rectal examination

Examination of the abdomen is not complete without a rectal examination. Women who have acute abdominal pain should also have a vaginal examination. The rectum is examined with the patient in the left lateral position with knees flexed. The perianal region is inspected for:

- Signs of inflammation.
- Fistula.

- Fissures.
- Skin tags.
- Prolapsed haemorrhoids.

A lubricated finger is then gently inserted but, in the presence of acute problems, this may be too uncomfortable. If possible, the tone of the anal sphincter is assessed. Each wall of the rectum is palpated for local tenderness, inflammation and mucosal lesions, and the size and consistency of the prostate is noted. In the acute situation deep tenderness may be associated with:

- Acute appendicitis.
- Salpingitis.
- Prostatitis.

A ballooned rectum may be found in a patient who has pseudo-obstruction.

EXAMINATION OF A HERNIA

If a groin hernia is suspected, the patient should be examined standing up because it may reduce when the patient lies down. Observe the position of the swelling—if it descends towards the scrotum this is likely to be an indirect inguinal hernia. Palpation over the swelling as the patient coughs produces a cough impulse.

A reducible indirect inguinal hernia can be controlled by pressure over the deep ring (halfway between the anterior superior iliac spine and the pubic tubercle).

The patient then lies down. If the swelling disappears immediately, it is a direct inguinal hernia. If the swelling has to be reduced, but is controlled by pressure over the deep inguinal ring (halfway between the pubic symphysis and the anterior superior iliac spine), it is an indirect inguinal hernia.

A femoral hernia is most commonly seen in women and is found below the inguinal ligament; the neck is below and lateral to the pubic tubercle.

If a hernia is inflamed, tender and irreducible then it is probably acutely obstructed and the contents are at risk of strangulation.

Other hernias may be visible when the patient is standing, but not when the patient is lying. They may be visible by asking the patient to cough or lift their legs or head off the bed by contracting the rectus abdominis muscles.

EXAMINATION OF A SCROTAL SWELLING

A varicocoele is best palpated with the patient standing.

Patients can be examined lying or standing. If there is a scrotal swelling, the first step is to see whether it is possible to get above the swelling; if it is not, the swelling is an inguinoscrotal hernia.

If the swelling is a scrotal swelling:

- Is it uni- or bilateral and does the swelling transilluminate?
- Can the testis be felt separately and does it feel normal in size, shape and lie?
- Are there any signs of inflammation?

Descriptions of scrotal swelling and their diagnoses are given in Fig. 40.6.

EXAMINATION OF PERIPHERAL VASCULATURE

Inspection of peripheral vasculature

General inspection of the limbs may show the effects of ischaemia, such as pallor, hair loss, inflammation and gangrene. If the patient is hanging the leg over the edge of the bed then it may imply rest pain.

Remember when examining a limb to expose the other limb first.

Palpation of peripheral vasculature

Gentle palpation will reveal temperature differences and gentle pressure on the nailbeds will indicate the speed of capillary return. All the peripheral pulses are palpated and the character of the pulsation is noted. The limb is examined for areas of paraesthesia.

Auscultation may demonstrate bruits over narrowed vessels.

A diagram of anatomical positions of peripheral pulses is shown in Fig. 40.7.

Buerger's test

The patient lies down and both legs are lifted, keeping the knees straight. The legs are supported by the examiner while the patient flexes and extends the ankles and toes to the point of fatigue. If the blood supply is defective, the sole of the foot becomes pale and the veins are guttered. The feet are lowered and the patient adopts a sitting position. In 2–3 minutes, a cyanotic hue spreads over the affected foot. This sequence signifies that a major limb artery is occluded.

To palpate the popliteal pulse, ask the patient to bend his knee, place both of your thumbs on the tibial tuberosity and palpate with all eight fingers.

Scrotal swellings	
Description	**Diagnosis**
painless swelling of testis	testicular tumour
horizontal lie of testis, painful	testicular torsion
cystic swelling separate from testis	epididymal cyst
transilluminable swelling of scrotum, testis impalpable	hydrocoele
tender epididymis	epididymitis
distended veins—'bag of worms'	varicocoele

Fig. 40.6 Scrotal swellings and their significance.

Fig. 40.7 Anatomical positions of peripheral pulses.

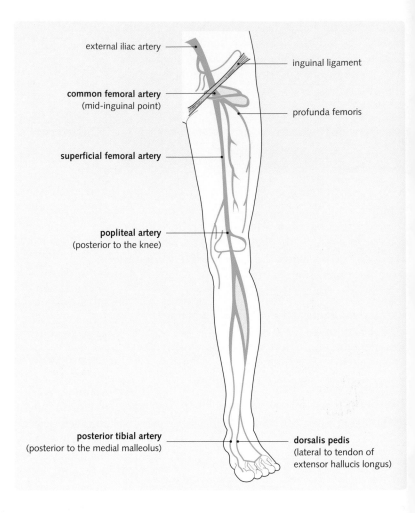

external iliac artery

inguinal ligament

common femoral artery
(mid-inguinal point)

profunda femoris

superficial femoral artery

popliteal artery
(posterior to the knee)

posterior tibial artery
(posterior to the medial malleolus)

dorsalis pedis
(lateral to tendon of
extensor hallucis longus)

EXAMINATION OF VARICOSE VEINS

Fig. 40.8 shows a diagram of normal venous drainage of the leg.

Inspection of varicose veins

With the patient standing and in good light, the legs are inspected from the front and behind to assess the anatomical distribution of the varicosities affecting the long and short saphenous veins and their effects on the tissues, such as hyperpigmentation, varicose excema, venous flares, oedema, lipodermatosclerosis and ulceration. The groin is inspected to look for a saphena varix.

Palpation of varicose veins

Sometimes the veins are not obvious on inspection, but are palpable.

Tests that can be carried out when palpating veins include:

- Cough impulse.
- Trendelenburg's test.
- Percussion.

With the cough impulse test, fingers are placed over the long saphenous vein just below the saphenous opening, the patient coughs and there is a palpable fluid thrill if the saphenofemoral junction is incompetent.

In the percussion test, the examiner's left fingers are placed below the saphenous opening and the

The saphenofemoral junction is found 4 cm below and lateral to the pubic tubercle.

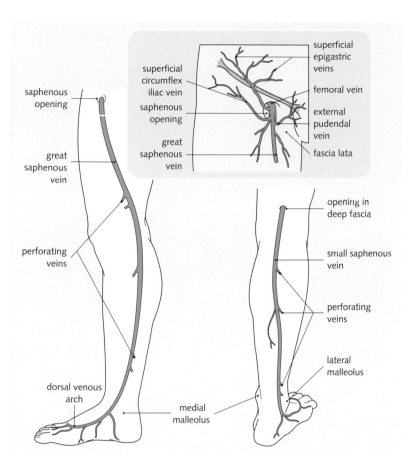

Fig. 40.8 Normal venous drainage of the leg.

other hand taps the varicosities. If the valves are incompetent then the impulse will be transmitted up the vein to the saphenous opening.

During Trendelenburg's test, the patient lies on the couch and the leg is elevated to drain the blood from the veins. Fingers are placed firmly over the saphenous opening or a tourniquet is placed around the leg. Maintaining the pressure the limb is lowered and the patient stands. If the varicose veins have been controlled then the main incompetence is at the saphenofemoral junction. If there is partial filling of the lower varicose veins, it implies that some of the lower perforating veins are also incompetent.

EXAMINATION OF A PATIENT WHO HAS MULTIPLE INJURIES

Trauma is the leading cause of death in the first four decades of life. The quality of the initial assessment has a significant influence on the final outcome.

Principles of trauma management have now been well defined to improve standards of care.

Patient management consists of:

- Primary survey.
- Resuscitation.
- Secondary survey.

Assessment of a multiple injured patient should be performed by a trauma team consisting of:
- Four doctors.
- Five nurses.
- One radiographer.

The aim is to detect the life-threatening injuries first and to prevent further damage to vital organs from hypoxia and hypovolaemia (Fig. 40.9).

Fig. 40.9 Areas to be examined carefully in patients who have suffered multiple trauma. (JVP, jugular venous pressure.)

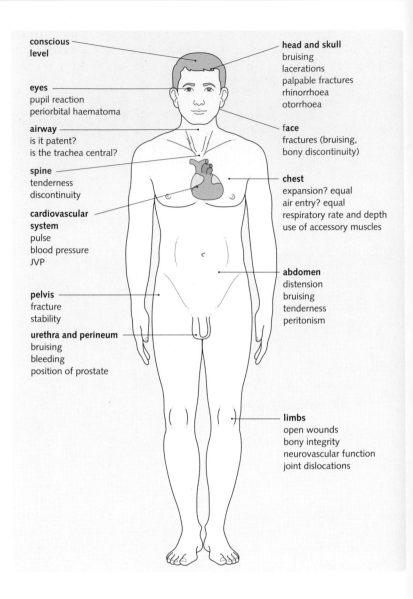

conscious level

eyes
pupil reaction
periorbital haematoma

airway
is it patent?
is the trachea central?

spine
tenderness
discontinuity

cardiovascular system
pulse
blood pressure
JVP

pelvis
fracture
stability

urethra and perineum
bruising
bleeding
position of prostate

head and skull
bruising
lacerations
palpable fractures
rhinorrhoea
otorrhoea

face
fractures (bruising, bony discontinuity)

chest
expansion? equal
air entry? equal
respiratory rate and depth
use of accessory muscles

abdomen
distension
bruising
tenderness
peritonism

limbs
open wounds
bony integrity
neurovascular function
joint dislocations

Fig. 40.10 Glasgow coma scale

Eye opening		Voice response		Best motor response
				obeys commands
		alert and orientated	5	localizes pain
spontaneous	4	confused	4	flexes to pain
to voice	3	inappropriate	3	abnormal flexion to pain
to pain	2	incomprehensible	2	extends to pain
no eye opening	1	no voice response	1	no response to pain

The secondary survey then looks for the non-life-threatening injuries that may have significant long-term effects if not treated properly.

Any unconscious patient should be assessed carefully, with particular attention to maintaining a patent airway, blood pressure, pulse and adequate respiration. The conscious level is assessed using the Glasgow Coma Scale (Fig. 40.10) by monitoring three features that change with the conscious level:

- Stimulus needed to cause eye opening.
- Verbal response.
- Best motor response.

The Glasgow Coma Scale is a reproducible scale, so any change in level can be detected and communicated easily. A fully conscious person has a score of 15, while the deepest level of coma scores 3. A score of 8 or less indicates coma.

Learning objectives

You should be able to:

• Identify some of the commonly used abbreviations in medical notes.
• Become familiar with a common layout for the initial clerking of a surgical patient.

SAMPLE CLERKING

A sample surgical clerking is shown in Fig. 41.1. Abbreviations used in this sample medical clerking are:

GP	General Practitioner
PC	Presenting Complaint
HPC	History of Presenting Complaint
PMH	Past Medical History
SH	Social History
JVP	Jugular Venous Pressure
I	First heart sound
II	Second heart sound
I–II+O	Murmurs
PR	Rectal examination
RUQ	Right Upper Quadrant
oHx	No History
DM	Diabetes Mellitus
IHD	Ischaemic Heart Disease
CVA	Cerebrovascular Accident
EP	Epilepsy
NKA	No Known Allergies
Fam H	Family History
T	Temperature
oJ/A/Cy/Cl/O/L	No Jaundice, Anemia, Cyanosis, Clubbing, Oedema, Lymphadenopathy
HR	Heart Rate
HS	Heart Sounds
RR	Respiratory Rate
A/E	Air Entry
B/L	Bilateral
oL	No Palpable Liver
oS	No Palpable Spleen
oK	No Palpable Kidney
oH	No Palpable Hernia
+Ve	Positive
oMasses	No palpable Masses
BS	Bowel Sounds
N	Normal
oBlood	No Blood
NS	Nervous System
GCS	Glasgow Coma Scale
PERLA	Pupils Equal, Reacting to Light and Accommodating
ΔΔx	Differential diagnosis
CVS	Cardiovascular System
RS	Respiratory System
Abds	Abdominal Systems
NBM	Nil By Mouth
IVI	Intravenous Infusion
FBC	Full Blood Count
U&E	Urea and Electrolytes
LFT	Liver Function Text
CXR	Chest X-ray
AXR	Abdominal X-ray
ECG	Electrocardiogram
DH	Drug History
o.d.	once daily

Hospital No: X349182
SMITH, Freda
29/4/40
20/06/05 19:30   ♀ 65 yr old retired secretary   Referred by GP – seen in GOPD

PC   Acute onset of
           (R) UQ, duration 5 hrs

> 1. Presenting complaint should be brief, but it is necessary to include duration of symptoms.

HPC   Pain constant and severe
           Radiates to back
           Vomited (x3) - bile stained
           Episodes of colicky (R) UQ pain $^6/_{12}$
           Intolerance of fatty food
           o Hx of jaundice
           o change of bowel habit

> 2. Mention the relevant negatives.

PMH   Hypertension DX 1995
           Appendicectomy aged 10 years
           Hysterectomy aged 45 years
           °DM/IHD/CVA/Ep/Renal

> 3. A useful way of recording important negatives on one line.

DH   Lisinopril 10mg od

> 4. Always record the dose and frequency of any drugs.

Allergies NKA   Non smoker

           Alcohol - occasional < 20 units/week

Fam H   Mother underwent cholecystectomy   SH   Lives with husband
           aged 45 years   Retired factory worker
                                                          No social package

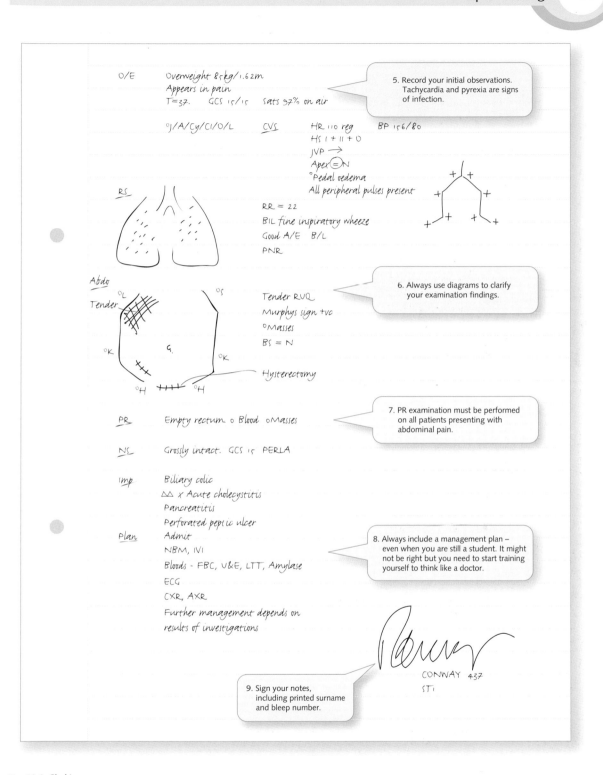

O/E   Overweight 85kg/1.62m
       Appears in pain
       T=37.   GCS 15/15   Sats 97% on air

> 5. Record your initial observations. Tachycardia and pyrexia are signs of infection.

°J/A/Cy/Cl/O/L   CVS   HR 110 reg   BP 156/80
                         HS I + II + 0
                         JVP →
                         Apex = N
                         °Pedal oedema
                         All peripheral pulses present

RS   RR = 22
                         BIL fine inspiratory wheeze
                         Good A/E B/L
                         PNR

Abdo   Tender RUQ
Tender   °L   °S   Murphys sign +ve
                         °Masses
                         BS = N
       °K   G.   °K
                         Hysterectomy
       °H   °H

> 6. Always use diagrams to clarify your examination findings.

PR   Empty rectum. 0 Blood 0Masses

> 7. PR examination must be performed on all patients presenting with abdominal pain.

NS   Grossly intact. GCS 15 PERLA

Imp   Biliary colic
       ΔΔ x Acute cholecystitis
       Pancreatitis
       Perforated peptic ulcer
Plan   Admit
       NBM, IVI
       Bloods - FBC, U&E, LTT, Amylase
       ECG
       CXR, AXR
       Further management depends on
       results of investigations

> 8. Always include a management plan – even when you are still a student. It might not be right but you need to start training yourself to think like a doctor.

CONWAY 437
STi

> 9. Sign your notes, including printed surname and bleep number.

Fig. 41.1 Clerking.

Investigation of a surgical patient

After clerking the patient, a list of differential diagnoses is formulated. This will aid the selective planning of further investigations. When planning further investigations, it is important to remember:

- If the patient is an acute admission, there is a limit to the investigations that can be requested in the middle of the night.
- Do not order a long list of investigations hoping that one will provide the answer.
- Students should try and see as many investigations being carried out as possible so that they are aware of the nature of the tests and what the patients have to experience.
- Some tests are very straightforward, but others require specialists to perform them.

Before ordering an investigation, ask yourself 'What is the question I want answered?'.

ASSESSMENT BEFORE GENERAL ANAESTHESIA

Young fit patients may require no investigations before a minor elective operation, but any patient who has a history of respiratory or cardiovascular problems needs to be assessed by:

- Electrocardiography (ECG)—to detect arrhythmias, ischaemic changes, previous myocardial infarction and evidence of hypertrophy. This is not required if the patient is under 40 years of age, asymptomatic, and has no risk factors.
- Chest radiography—the incidence of abnormalities is 10% in patients over 40 years and 25% in patients over 60 years of age. A chest radiograph is not required if the patient is asymptomatic, has no risk factors and is under 50 years of age. A chest radiograph can show signs of chronic lung disease, cardiomegaly and cardiac failure.

Whenever possible, preoperative assessment should be performed prior to admission.

Specialized tests of respiratory and cardiovascular function

These are:

- Echocardiography—to assess valvular heart disease and ventricular function.
- Exercise ECG—to diagnose angina and assess severity.
- 24-hour ECG—if the patient has a history of intermittent arrhythmias.

- Peak expiratory flow rate—to assess asthma.
- Lung function tests—to measure forced expiratory volume in 1 second and forced vital capacity to assess lung function in patients who have chronic lung disease.
- Blood gas analysis—an arterial blood sample is analysed for oxygen and carbon dioxide levels. If these are abnormal, they may indicate the possibility of postoperative chest problems.

Blood tests

Full blood count

Measurements include:

- Haemoglobin level—decreased in anaemia, increased in polycythaemia and dehydration.
- Mean corpuscular haemoglobin and mean corpuscular volume—decreased in iron deficiency anaemia.
- Mean corpuscular haemoglobin—increased in vitamin B_{12} or folate deficiency, or alcoholism.
- White cell count—increased if there is infection. Neutrophilia results from bacterial infection, lymphocytosis from viral infection, and eosinophilia from allergy. White cell count is decreased in overwhelming infection.
- Platelets—increased if there has been recent haemorrhage, after splenectomy, or in myeloproliferative disorders. Platelets are decreased if there is hypersplenism and in some autoimmune conditions (e.g. idiopathic thrombocytopenic purpura).

> Puzzling blood results need to be discussed with the haematologist or biochemist.

Urea and electrolytes

It is important to know the patient's preoperative renal function, especially if the patient is to have an emergency or major operation. Increased urea and creatinine may be due to dehydration or renal impairment. It is also important to know the potassium level, because if it is less than 3 mmol/litre the patient has an increased risk of developing cardiac arrhythmias.

Glucose

A random sample may reveal undiagnosed diabetes mellitus, particularly in the elderly. If the patient is known to be diabetic then the glucose needs to be stabilized preoperatively.

Blood transfusion

Many elective operations do not require a blood transfusion, but the patient's blood is grouped and the serum saved in case it is needed. Blood donations are now separated into a large number of different components so they can be used specifically. Whole blood is only given for acute haemorrhage. Other components of blood are used as follows:

- Packed cells—given for symptomatic anaemia or urgent operation. Platelet concentrates have to be ABO/Rhesus compatible and are given if the platelet count is less than 40×10^9/litre.
- Clotting factors—can be infused as fresh frozen plasma and are used if there is bleeding, massive transfusion or disseminated intravascular coagulation (DIC).
- Specific clotting factors—these are cryoprecipitate (factor VIII, von Willebrand's factor, fibrinogen) and factor VIII and factor IX concentrates.

Adverse effects of transfusion are:

- Pyogenic febrile reaction.
- Hypersensitivity reaction to platelet and leukocyte antigens—causes a mild pyrexia.
- Anaphylactoid reaction—may cause hypotension and bronchospasm.
- Acute haemolytic reaction—due to ABO incompatibility. The clinical features are pain at the infusion site, chest pain, fever, rigors, hypotension, flushing, DIC and renal failure. Treatment is to stop the transfusion and treat the symptoms; the patient may need dialysis.
- Metabolic haemostatic complications of a massive rapid transfusion—hypothermia, acidosis and lack of clotting factors.
- Transmission of infectious diseases such as hepatitis C—occurs in less than 0.1% of transfusions. Blood donations in the UK are screened for hepatitis B and human immunodeficiency virus (HIV) infection.

No medical or surgical condition justifies a transfusion of less than 2 units.

Specialist blood tests

You should be aware of the following specialist blood tests:

- Clotting screen—this includes the platelet count, prothrombin time and thromboplastin time. This is performed if the patient is anticoagulated or jaundiced, or has a hepatic disorder or history of excessive bleeding.
- Sickle cell test—should be performed on all patients who come from the Middle East, Indian subcontinent, Africa or Mediterranean areas.
- Liver function tests—these include bilirubin, hepatic transaminases, albumin, alkaline phosphatase and γ-glutamyl transferase. Increased bilirubin and very high transaminases suggest hepatitis, but increased bilirubin and alkaline phosphatase suggest biliary obstruction or hepatic metastases.
- Hepatitis screen—if jaundiced or past history of hepatitis, because the patient may be an asymptomatic carrier.
- Amylase—measured in all cases of acute abdominal pain, because if it is higher than 1000 IU/litre it is diagnostic of acute pancreatitis, but it can also be elevated in renal impairment or if the patient has a perforated viscus or ischaemic bowel.
- Erythrocyte sedimentation rate and C-reactive protein (an acute-phase protein)—elevated in inflammatory conditions, infection and tissue injury.

Tumour markers

These are substances present in the body in a concentration that is related to the presence of a tumour, but they may not be tumour specific (Fig. 42.1). They can be used to monitor response to treatment and early diagnosis of recurrence.

Microbiological tests

If any infection is suspected, specimens should be taken before starting antibiotics so that they can be examined microscopically and cultured to detect the organisms and their sensitivities (MCS).

- Pus swabs—can be taken from a wound, ulcer or abscess.
- Midstream urine (MSU)—if urinary tract infection suspected. A pure culture of more than 10^5 organisms/mL is diagnostic.
- Blood cultures—these should be taken (using a sterile technique) from any patient who has a rigor or temperature of 39°C, which are signs of bacteraemia.

Classification of preoperative state

The criteria defined by the American Society of Anesthesiologists for classification of the preoperative state are given in Fig. 42.2.

INVESTIGATION OF THE GASTROINTESTINAL TRACT

Plain radiography

In the acute situation, an erect chest radiograph and an abdominal radiograph are helpful. A chest

Marker	Tumour
human chorionic gonadotrophin (HCG), α-fetoprotein (AFP)	testicular tumours
carcinoembryonic antigen (CEA)	colon cancer
CA125	ovarian cancer
prostatic-specific antigen (PSA)	prostatic cancer
AFP	hepatocellular carcinoma
CA19–9	pancreatic cancer

Fig. 42.1 Tumour markers

Fig. 42.2 Classification of preoperative state—American Society of Anesthesiologists' criteria

Class	Definition
1	healthy patient
2	mild systemic disease; no functional limitations
3	severe systemic disease with functional limitation
4	severe systemic disease that is a constant threat to life
5	moribund patient not expected to survive 24 h with or without operation

radiograph will demonstrate gas under the diaphragm (Fig. 42.3). Its presence indicates a perforated viscus, but its absence does not exclude the diagnosis.

An abdominal radiograph can demonstrate several structures:

- Small bowel dilatation (Fig. 42.4)—central loops of bowel with complete lines due to the plicae circulares. It is abnormal if the small bowel is dilated.
- Colonic dilatation—this is recognized by the peripheral position of the colon and incomplete lines across the bowel due to the haustra. It can be normal.
- Gas in the biliary tree—may be due to a fistula from the gallbladder to the duodenum, which may present as a gallstone ileus.
- Loss of psoas shadow—due to retroperitoneal pathology.

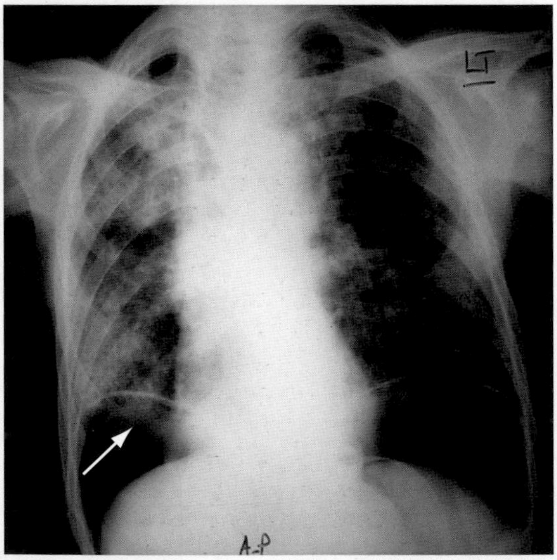

- Calcification—a feature of 90% of renal tract calculi and 10% of gallstones.
- Vascular calcification—of an aneurysm and atheromatous vessels.

A lateral decubitus abdominal radiograph can be performed if the patient is suspected to have an intra-abdominal perforation and is unable to sit upright.

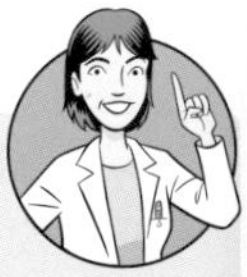

When looking at an abdominal radiograph it is helpful to start by identifying the rectum and working out the course of the bowel proximally. Remember the sigmoid colon can be a long loop that may extend medially all the way to the centre of the X-ray if on a long mesentery. Similarly, the transverse colon loop may flop all the way into the pelvis and the lower aspect of the X-ray if again on a long mesentery.

Fig. 42.3 Erect chest radiograph showing free gas under the diaphragm (arrow) and a chest infection.

Contrast studies

These can provide an assessment of diseases of hollow organs. Double contrast means that barium is given initially and then the viscus is distended with air, which this demonstrates mucosal detail. These investigations include:

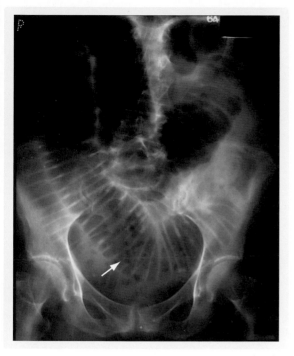

Fig. 42.4 Abdominal radiograph demonstrating small bowel dilatation (arrow).

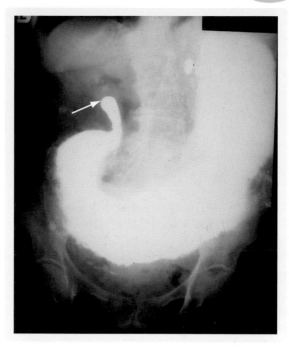

Fig. 42.5 Barium meal. This barium meal shows gross gastric distension due to pyloric obstruction (arrow).

- Barium swallow—initial investigation for dysphagia because it can assess the position and length of a stricture or define the anatomy of a hiatus hernia. It is also a dynamic test for observing oesophageal motility.
- Barium meal—useful for assessing the stomach and duodenum if endoscopy is impossible (Fig. 42.5).
- Barium meal and follow-through—a nasogastric tube is passed into the stomach and barium is passed down it and then it moves into the small intestine. Radiographs are taken over a period of a few hours to monitor the progress of the barium. It is useful for assessing small bowel diseases such as Crohn's disease.
- Barium enema—a single contrast study can be performed on unprepared bowel if colonic obstruction is suspected. A double contrast study can be used to assess mucosal problems after the use of aperients to clear the colon.

The rectum is poorly visualized by barium enema and therefore a rigid sigmoidoscopy should also be performed.

Ultrasonography

This is a diagnostic technique that uses high-frequency sound waves to generate an image. The interfaces of different body tissues reflect the sound waves as echoes, which are converted into electrical impulses and then into images. It is very useful for examination of the biliary and urogenital systems, because the contrast between fluid-filled organs, normal tissues and calculi can lead to variations in echogenicity.

Ultrasonography is a painless investigation, but is operator dependent.

Practical aspects of note when using ultrasound for investigating different parts of the body include the following:

- Abdominal ultrasound—patients are starved for a few hours before the test to reduce bowel gas. The procedure is useful for assessing the liver, gallbladder, biliary tree, pancreas, aneurysms, inflammatory masses and kidneys.
- Pelvic ultrasound—the patient's bladder should be full because this provides a better contrast background than air-filled bowel. This is useful for assessing gynaecological pathology and pregnancy.
- Intraluminal ultrasound—ultrasound probes can be passed down the oesophagus to assess the extent

of oesophageal tumours and through the anal canal to assess rectal tumours or the anal sphincters.

- Intraoperative ultrasound—at laparotomy, probes can be used to identify intrahepatic and small pancreatic tumours such as insulinomas.
- Interventional ultrasound—biopsies and cytopathology can be taken from intra-abdominal masses using ultrasound guidance. Fluid collections can be aspirated and hydronephrotic kidneys can be drained.
- Contrast ultrasound—ultrasound-specific contrast agents have led to improved image resolution in renal and peripheral vascular disease, malignancy and gynaecology.

Computed tomography

Computed tomography (CT) is a technique that produces cross-sectional images of the body. The CT scanner takes many digital images in different directions and these are fed into a computer, which constructs the cross-sectional image. The system is very sensitive, so differences in tissue density can be recognized and a detailed two-dimensional image is formed. The recent introduction of spiral CT has allowed accurate reconstruction of images in different planes or three dimensions. A CT scan showing a renal carcinoma is shown in Fig. 42.6.

Ionizing radiation is the main disadvantage of CT.

Magnetic resonance imaging

Magnetic resonance imaging (MRI) is a newer diagnostic tool based on the fact that an externally applied magnetic field causes protons in tissues to align in the direction of the magnetic field. By applying a second smaller magnetic field, in the form of a radiofrequency pulse, perpendicular to the main magnetic field the alignment of the protons is changed. When the radiofrequency pulse is stopped the protons return to equilibrium, and in so doing produce another radiofrequency signal. This is the MR signal, which is amplified and transformed by the computer into an image.

Magnetic resonance imaging is particularly useful for imaging the central nervous system, but it also produces very high-quality images of the rest of the body. The differences between vessels, tumour, inflammatory

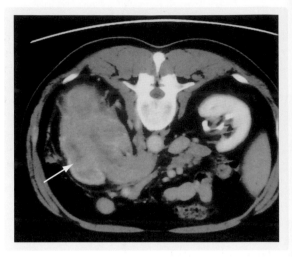

Fig. 42.6 Computed tomography scan showing renal carcinoma (arrow).

lesions and surgical scars is more easily demonstrated with MRI scans than with CT scans. The presence of any metal, however, produces a marked artefact.

Radionuclide imaging

Radionuclide imaging techniques use radioisotopes to depict function rather than anatomy. The principle is that an inhaled, injected or ingested pharmaceutical compound labelled with a suitable radionuclide is concentrated in the organ under review and the emitted radiation is detected by a gamma camera. Using the appropriate isotopes, the technique can be used to look at the brain, bones, thyroid, kidney, bowel and liver.

Radiolabelled red cells can be used to investigate bleeding from the gastrointestinal tract. If a Meckel's diverticulum is suspected, technetium pertechnetate can be used to look for ectopic gastric mucosa. Technetium iminodiacetic acid derivatives (HIDA) can be used to investigate hepatobiliary function. These derivatives are taken up by the hepatocytes and excreted in the bile, with accumulation in the gallbladder and small intestine. This technique can be used to investigate cholecystitis and cholestasis, detect bile leakage, and for assessment after hepatic transplantation.

Isotope-labelled white cell scans are able to detect localized areas of inflammation in the abdomen and other parts of the body.

Endoscopic techniques

The development of fibre-optic endoscopes and video viewing has revolutionized the diagnosis and management of gastrointestinal pathology. Diagnostic biopsies, excision of polyps, injection of sclerosants, insertion of stents and removal of stones can be carried out via the endoscope. Most of the examinations are performed under sedation, although most people can tolerate a diagnostic gastroscopy after local anaesthesia to the pharynx only. The examinations include:

- Oesophagogastroduodenoscopy (OGD)— examines the oesophagus, stomach and first two parts of the duodenum.
- Endoscopic retrograde cholangiopancreatography (ERCP)—a side-viewing scope that views the duodenum and allows contrast to be injected into the biliary tree, extraction of gallstones, biopsies of pancreatic lesions and insertion of stents.
- Sigmoidoscopy—a rigid scope used in the outpatient clinic to examine the rectum and distal sigmoid colon. A flexible scope will reach the splenic flexure of the colon.
- Proctoscope—a small rigid instrument to examine the anal canal.
- Colonoscopy—a flexible instrument that can examine the colon from the rectum to the caecum. Biopsies can be taken and polyps snared and retrieved.

Intraoesophageal pH monitoring and manometry

Probes are passed via the nose into the oesophagus to monitor the pH and measure the sphincter pressures. Similar probes can be used in the anal canal to measure sphincter pressures.

Percutaneous transhepatic cholangiography

In a case of obstructive jaundice with a dilated biliary tree, it may not be possible to gain access with ERCP, but contrast can be injected via a tube that has been passed through the skin into a dilated bile duct to outline the biliary tree and, if necessary, a stent can be passed via the same route to bypass the obstruction.

INVESTIGATION OF BREAST PROBLEMS

Several investigations are used to investigate breast pathology:

- Mammograms (Fig. 42.7)—these are low-dose radiographs used to image the breast. They are not used routinely for women under 35 years of age because of their lack of sensitivity in dense glandular breasts. The technique can demonstrate mass lesions, spiculated lesions and microcalcification, which can be benign or malignant.
- Ultrasound—this is useful (particularly in young women) for distinguishing between solid and cystic lesions. It can be used to perform image-guided biopsies of impalpable lesions.
- Fine-needle aspiration cytology (FNAC)—a 21-gauge needle can be used to aspirate cysts or obtain cells from solid lesions. Cytopathologists can distinguish between benign and malignant cells.

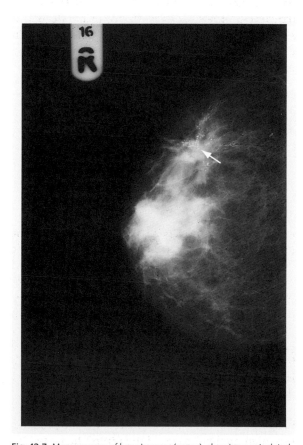

Fig. 42.7 Mammogram of breast cancer (arrow), showing a spiculated lesion with malignant microcalcification.

- Tru-cut biopsy—after local anaesthetic a core biopsy can be taken to obtain a precise pathological diagnosis.
- MRI—This is being used in some centres for additional assessment of invasive lobular cancers, to aid detection of recurrent disease, to aid diagnosis of problems associated with breast implants and is a potential screening method for women at high risk of developing breast cancer due to genetic abnormalities.

Fine-needle aspiration cytology (FNAC) should be performed on all thyroid nodules.

A mammogram may show another impalpable abnormality in the same or the contralateral breast.

INVESTIGATION OF THYROID DISEASE

The following investigations can be used to test for thyroid disease:

- Thyroid function tests—thyroxine (T_4), tri-iodothyronine (T_3) and thyroid-stimulating hormone (TSH). An elevated T_4 suggests thyrotoxicosis. A low T_3 and a high TSH indicate hypothyroidism.
- Thyroid antibodies—these give an indication of autoimmune disease. Antithyroglobulin and antimitochondrial antibodies are elevated in Hashimoto's disease. Long-acting thyroid stimulating antibody (LATS) is diagnostic of Graves' disease.
- Ultrasound scan—provides a simple outline of the shape of the thyroid gland and can distinguish whether a lump is solid or cystic.
- Thoracic inlet view or a chest radiograph—will demonstrate tracheal displacement if compressed by a retrosternal goitre.
- Radioisotope scan—technetium pertechnetate can be used to assess thyroid function. Generalized high activity suggests Graves' disease. A highly active nodule suggests a toxic nodule, and a cold nodule may indicate a tumour.
- FNAC—this is used to assess thyroid nodules.
- CT—this is used to assess the degree of retrosternal extension in retrosternal goitres.

VASCULAR INVESTIGATIONS

Vascular investigation techniques include:

- Doppler ultrasound.
- Duplex scanner.
- Ankle/brachial pressure index.
- Arteriography.
- Digital subtraction arteriography (DSA).
- Magnetic resonance angiography is increasingly used as it avoids the risk of embolization.

With Doppler ultrasound, probes can be used to detect arterial and venous blood flow. The Doppler effect is a change in frequency of a sound due to the relative movement of the source of the sound and the observer. The duplex scanner method is a pulsed Doppler combined with real-time ultrasound screening, and a computer-generated picture can be used to assess flow and anatomy in the peripheral vessels, especially the carotid artery.

To measure the ankle/brachial pressure index, a Doppler probe can be used to locate the posterior tibial arterial signal. A proximally placed sphygmomanometer cuff is inflated to find the pressure at which the signal disappears and reappears on deflation. The mean of the pressures can be compared with the pressure in the arm (i.e. systemic pressure):

Ankle/brachial pressure index (ABI) = ankle pressure/brachial pressure (%)

The ankle/brachial pressure index gives an indication of the severity of any reduction in flow and can be used as a non-invasive monitoring tool.

The ankle/brachial pressure index tends to be spuriously high in diabetic patients.

The retrograde (Seldinger) transfemoral arteriogram is the standard imaging technique for defining the precise abnormalities of the peripheral vascular system. The catheter is passed into the unaffected side and passed up the iliac vessels and down the affected side. Contrast medium is injected to outline the vascular system and define the level and extent of any narrowing and any collateral circulation. This can be combined with angioplasty (i.e. balloon dilatation of the vessel if there is a short segment of atherosclerosis). The risks associated with these procedures are:

- Haematoma formation.
- Initiation of intimal dissection.
- Dislodgement of thrombus.
- False aneurysm formation at the site of catheter insertion.

Digital subtraction arteriography is a new technique that is superseding the need for translumbar aortograms or arteriograms via the brachial route if both femoral vessels are included. The dye is injected into a peripheral vein and the pictures obtained are almost as good as those of conventional arteriograms, but dilutional problems result in inferior pictures of the distal vascular tree. DSA 'subtracts' the bony image and enhances the arteriographic profile.

UROLOGICAL INVESTIGATIONS

The tests to be considered in urological investigations include:

- Blood tests.
- Midstream urine.
- Imaging.

Blood tests

Measurement of blood urea and creatinine levels indicate renal function, and a creatinine clearance provides an estimation of the glomerular filtration rate.

Calcium, uric acid and phosphates are measured if there is stone disease.

Prostatic-specific antigen is a tumour marker for prostatic cancer.

Midstream urine

A ward dipstick can demonstrate the presence of glucose, ketones, blood, bilirubin and protein and pH.

A urine dipstick test positive for blood should be confirmed by microscopic examination of the urine.

Microscopic examination will reveal the presence of red cells, white blood cells, casts, crystals and organisms.

A culture showing more than 10^5 bacteria/mL of a pure growth is diagnostic of a urinary tract infection.

More than three red blood cells per high-power field is abnormal and more than five white cells per high-power field suggests pyuria; if this is sterile, it may be due to tuberculosis.

Urine cytology can detect transitional cell carcinoma cells.

Imaging of renal tract

The different methods of imaging for the renal tract are:

- Abdominal radiograph, kidneys, ureters and bladder (KUB view)—this may show renal calculi, renal size or abnormal calcification (e.g. phleboliths, calcified gallstones, calcified vessels).
- Ultrasound—this is a non-invasive test that can be used to delineate the kidneys, show any evidence of obstruction (i.e. hydronephrosis) or the presence of solid or cystic lesions, measure postmicturition residual volume and assess prostate size. It can also be used to guide percutaneous renal biopsies or nephrostomy tubes. Transrectal ultrasound can be used to assess the prostate and prostatic biopsies can be obtained transrectally.
- Intravenous urography (IVU)—contrast medium (iodine based) is injected intravenously and is rapidly excreted by the kidneys if they are functioning normally. The investigation delineates the kidney and the pelvicalyceal system and it can show abnormal anatomy, such as a duplex system, obstruction to flow due to a calculus, or a filling defect in the renal calyx, ureter or bladder.
- Aortography—the renal arteries may be defined by aortography. Stenosis of the renal artery or abnormal tumour circulation can be demonstrated. In selected cases renal artery arteriography can be combined with transluminal angioplasty for renal artery stenosis.
- CT scan—used to assess the local spread of renal tumours.

- Radionuclide scan—this can be used to demonstrate anatomical differences between the kidneys and provide dynamic imaging of the renal tract, particularly in the presence of urinary tract obstruction. Technetium-labelled diethylene triamine penta-acetic acid (DPTA) can provide information on renal perfusion, function and the presence of obstruction. Technetium-labelled dimercaptosuccinic acid (DMSA) is taken up by the tubules and can be used to demonstrate the cortex and assess renal size and function.

Cystoscopy

The usual method for investigating the bladder is cystoscopy—rigid or flexible. It can usually be performed under local anaesthetic and sedation in the outpatient clinic. It allows direct visualization of the bladder and ureteric openings. Biopsies can be taken to assess suspicious lesions of the bladder mucosa.

Bladder neoplasms and the prostate can be resected via the cystoscope—transurethral resection of the prostate (TURP) and transurethral resection of the tumour (TURT).

Ureteric calculi can be removed via ureteroscopes and dormia baskets passed via the cystoscope into the ureters.

A urethroscope is used to visualize the urethra.

Urodynamics

This is dynamic assessment of the storage and voiding function of the urinary tract.

Flow rate

Urine flow rate is measured to assess the rate and pattern of voiding.

Cystometry

This involves measurement of intravesical pressures during filling and voiding and is useful for differentiating between urge and stress incontinence.

Videocystometry

This involves filling the bladder with contrast medium during cystometry, so that bladder activity can be observed on a fluoroscope during the filling and voiding phases.

Further reading

Roberts GM, Hughes JP, Hourihan MD 1998 *Clinical Radiology for Medical Students*, 3rd edn. Butterworth–Heinemann, Oxford

Royal College of Radiologists referal guidelines 2007 *Making the Best Use of Clinical Radiology Services*, 6th edition. http://www/rcr/ac/uk

Introduction to the operating theatre

Learning objectives

You should be able to:

- Understand the general layout of an operating theatre department.
- List important considerations when creating a theatre list.
- Know the basics about what to wear and how to scrub in theatre.

The operating theatre can be an intimidating environment when encountered for the first time. It can also be dangerous both for the patient and staff when things go wrong. A basic understanding will hopefully make the first visit to the operating theatre the memorable experience it ought to be.

LAYOUT

All operating theatre departments have a common layout, which includes:

- Reception—theatre lists are submitted here after they have been discussed with the theatre sister in charge. The patient log is also recorded here.
- Holding bay—the patient enters this bay on arrival. Consent and personal details are checked here.
- Operating theatres—each consists of the main operating room, the anaesthetic room, the scrub room, the sluice, the prep room. One usually enters the main operating room through the scrub room.
- Recovery bay—the patient is monitored here in the immediate postoperative period. Vital signs, neurology, and drain output are closely recorded.

THE THEATRE LIST

The list of patients and their intended operations is submitted to the theatre department the day before the relevant operating session. The list must be in clear legible handwriting or ideally should be typed. Important details to include are:

- Patient details, including the admission ward.
- Operation site and side, with no abbreviations.
- Additional intended procedures and any additional instruments required (e.g. sigmoidoscope)
- The position the patient is required to be in for the operation (e.g. lithotomy)
- High-risk patients should be clearly identified.

In prioritizing patients for an elective operating list, it is important to be aware that:

- Carriers of resistant bacterial strains (e.g. MRSA) go at the end of the list as the operating theatre needs to be decontaminated after the procedure.
- Diabetic patients and children are given priority.
- Clean procedures (e.g. breast surgery) are prioritized before dirty procedures (e.g. incision and drainage of abscess).

THEATRE APPAREL

Before entering the operating theatre, outside clothes must be removed and scrubs worn. In addition, a hat, theatre shoes and mask are also required. Senior theatre sisters and students will wear a different colour hat so as to be distinguished from the rest of the staff. Depending on the operation, further protective wear may be required. Masks with a protective visor are advised for those scrubbed not wearing protective glasses, particularly in vascular operations. If a laser is used in the operation then all staff may need to use specially designed protective glasses. For orthopaedic surgery involving metal prostheses, specially designed masks and gowns are used (Charnley exhaust gown) and the surgery is carried out within an area of laminar air flow in the main operating room to reduce the risk of infection. If lavage (washout) is planned or a large volume of fluid is anticipated (e.g. in a laprotomy for small bowel obstruction or perforation), a plastic apron worn over the scrubs but beneath the sterile gown helps protect from getting wet.

SCRUBBING

Before starting, the gown and gloves should be opened if not done so already by theatre staff. Jewellery should be removed (simple wedding bands are permitted but they should be loose enough to allow soap to wash underneath). Scrubbing should include the hands and arms all the way to the elbows and rinsing of the soap should be in the direction of hand to elbow. Brushes should be used only to clean fingernails, which should be kept trimmed. Any abrasions or lacerations of the hands should be covered with a waterproof dressing prior to scrubbing. The most common scrubbing protocol lasts 10 minutes and suggests the use of either chlorhexidine or povidone-iodine soap.

- 1-minute fingernail scrub.
- 3-minute wash going all the way to the elbow.
- 3-minute wash going to mid forearm.
- 3-minute wash concentrating on the hands and wrists.

The base of the thumb, the medial aspect of the hand, the wrist, and the centre of the palm are often not satisfactorily clean after scrubbing when inspected under ultraviolet light, and therefore special attention should be paid to these areas.

When drying, the direction should be again from fingertips to elbow, disposing of the towel after the elbow has been reached. Donning the gown should be carried out with care not to touch anyone or anything not sterile. A theatre staff member will tie the back of the gown. A closed technique of donning gloves should be followed (i.e. this should be done with hands covered by the ends of the gown sleeves). There are often posters displaying the steps of this technique in theatres but, more commonly, the beginner is taken through this process by the scrub sister. Double gloving offers added protection. In orthopaedic procedures, green gloves are worn underneath regular gloves, providing a clearer indication if the top glove rips. Once fully gowned and gloved, keep hands close to the chest and keep out of the way of non-scrubbed theatre staff so as not to become de-sterilized as they move around doing their various jobs in preparing the patient and the theatre equipment.

GENERAL TIPS

- Introduce yourself to theatre sister in charge and to the operating surgeon before the operation begins.
- Take the opportunity to observe and discuss the anaesthetic management of the patient both pre- and postoperatively with the anaesthetic team in theatre.
- Surfaces covered by green or blue drapes are sterile. Do not touch unless scrubbed.
- Keep noise to a minimum during the surgery. Although most surgeons and theatre sisters maintain a fairly informal atmosphere in the operating room, it is good practice to request permission from the scub nurse before speaking to the operating surgeon during an operation.
- A member of the surgical team should always stay with the patient at all times and accompany the patient to the recovery bay.
- Operations require stamina as one is often standing for a long period of time. Make sure you are adequately prepared for this, particularly if you are going to be scrubbed.
- Do ask questions and ask to scrub. After all, it is the best way to learn!

Index

Note: Page numbers in **bold** refer to figures and tables.